GUIDELINES FOR THE USE OF PSYCHOTROPIC DRUGS

A Clinical Handbook

GUIDELINES FOR THE USE OF PSYCHOTROPIC DRUGS

A Clinical Handbook

Edited by

HARVEY C. STANCER, Ph.D., M.D., F.R.C.P.(C)
Clarke Institute of Psychiatry
University of Toronto

PAUL E. GARFINKEL, M.S., M.D., F.R.C.P.(C)
Toronto General Hospital
University of Toronto

VIVIAN M. RAKOFF, M.A., M.B., F.R.C.P.(C)
Clarke Institute of Psychiatry
University of Toronto

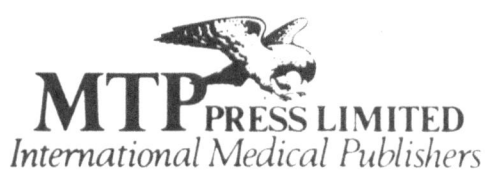
MTP PRESS LIMITED
International Medical Publishers

Published in the UK and Europe by
MTP Press Limited
Falcon House
Lancaster, England

Published in the US by
SPECTRUM PUBLICATIONS, INC.
175-20 Wexford Terrace
Jamaica, NY 11432

ISBN 978-94-011-7620-0   ISBN 978-94-011-7618-7 (eBook)
DOI 10.1007/978-94-011-7618-7

This volume is dedicated to
Magda, Dorothy, and Gina

Contributors

William H. Anderson, M.D. • Assistant Clinical Professor of Psychiatry, Harvard Medical School; Acute Psychiatry Service, Massachusetts General Hospital, Boston, Massachusetts

Jack D. Barchas, M.D. • Nancy Pritzker Laboratory of Behavioral Neurochemistry and Stanford Mental Health Clinical Research Center, Department of Psychiatry and Behavioral Sciences, Stanford University School of Medicine, Stanford, California

Philip A. Berger, M.D. • Department of Psychiatry and Behavioral Sciences, Stanford University School of Medicine, Stanford, California

Janel S. Carino, M.D. • Research Psychiatrist, Dept. of Psychopharmacology, New York State Psychiatric Institute, New York, New York

Daniel E. Casey, M.D. • Clinical Investigator, Medical Research, Psychiatry and Neurology Services, Veterans Administration Medical Center, Portland, Oregon; Associate Professor, Department of Psychiatry, School of Medicine, Oregon Health Sciences University, Portland Oregon

Guy Chouinard, M.D. • Clinical Psychopharmacology Unit, Allan Memorial Institute, Royal Victoria Hospital, Montreal; Department of Psychiatry, McGill University, Montreal; Research Department, Hospital Louis-H. Lafontaine, Montreal, Quebec, Canada

Bruce M. Cohen, M.D., Ph.D. • Assistant Professor of Psychiatry, Harvard Medical School, Cambridge, Massachusetts; Associate Director, Mental Health Clinical Research Center, McLean Hospital; Chief, Clinical Biochemistry Laboratory, Mailman Research Center, McLean Hospital, Belmont, Massachusetts

Robert M. Cohen, M.D., Ph.D. ● Staff Psychiatrist, Clinical Neuropharmacology Branch, National Institute of Mental Health, Bethesda, Maryland

Stephen H. Curry, Ph.D. ● Professor and Director, Division of Clinical Pharmaco-kinetics, J. Hillis Miller Health Center, University of Florida, Gainesville, Florida

John M. Davis, M.D. ● Director of Research, Illinois State Psychiatric Institute, Chicago, Illinois

Lynn E. DeLisi, M.D. ● Staff Psychiatrist, National Institute of Mental Health, Bethesda, Maryland

Lee E. Emory, M.D. ● Psychiatrist, Titus Harris Clinic, Galveston, Texas

Barry D. Garfinkel, M.D. ● Associate Professor, Director, Division of Child and Adolescent Psychiatry, University of Minnesota Medical School

Jes Gerlach, M.D. ● Department AEH, Sct Hans Hospital, Roskilde, Denmark

Alexander H. Glassman, M.D. ● Chief, Clinical Psychopharmacology, New York State Psychiatric Institute, New York, N.Y.; Professor of Psychiatry, College of Physicians and Surgeons, Columbia University, New York, New York

Paul Grof, M.D. ● Director, Affective Disorders Program, Hamilton Psychiatric Hospital, Hamilton, Ontario, Canada; Professor, Department of Psychiatry, McMaster University, Hamilton, Ontario, Canada

John Gunn, M.D., Ph.D. ● Professor of Forensic Psychiatry, University of London; Institute of Psychiatry, London, United Kingdom

Lawrence B. Guttmacher, M.D. ● Medical Staff Fellow, Clinical Neuropharma-cology Branch, National Institute of Mental Health, Bethesda, Maryland

Leo G. Hollister, M.D. ● Professor of Medicine, Psychiatry and Pharmacology, Stanford University School of Medicine, and Veterans Administration Medical Center, Palo Alto, California

Stephen J. Hucker, M.D. ● Chief of Forensic Service, Clarke Institute of Psy-chiatry, Assistant Professor of Psychiatry, University of Toronto, Ontario, Canada

Robert Kellner, M.D., Ph.D. • Professor of Psychiatry and Director of Research, Department of Psychiatry, University of New Mexico School of Medicine, Albuquerque, New Mexico

Thomas A. Kent, M.D. • Department of Pharmacology, University of Kansas Medical Center, Kansas City, Kansas

Roy King, Ph.D., M.D. • Department of Psychiatry and Behavioral Sciences, Stanford University School of Medicine, Stanford, California

Malcolm Lader, M.D. • Professor of Clinical Psychopharmacology, Institute of Psychiatry, University of London, London, England

Robert Linden, M.D. • McLean Hospital, Belmont, Massachusetts

Markku Linnoila, M.D., Ph.D. • Staff Psychiatrist, Clinical Psychobiology Branch, National Institute of Mental Health, Bethesda, Maryland

Walter, J. Meyer, III, M.D. • Departments of Pediatrics and Psychiatry and Behavioral Sciences, The University of Texas Medical Branch, Galveston, Texas

Dennis L. Murphy, M.D. • Chief, Clinical Neuropharmacology Branch, National Institute of Mental Health, Bethesda, Maryland

Karl O'Sullivan, M.D. • Assistant Professor, McMaster University, Hamilton, Ontario, Canada; Program Director, Haldimand Brant Ward, Hamilton Psychiatric Hospital, Hamilton, Ontario, Canada

W. Z. Potter, M.D., Ph.D. • Acting Chief, Clinical Psychobiology Branch, National Institute of Mental Health, Bethesda, Maryland

Sheldon H. Preskorn, M.D. • Associate Professor of Psychiatry and Pharmacology, Department of Psychiatry and Director, Psychopharmacology Laboratory, The University of Kansas, College of Health Sciences and Hospital, Kansas City, Kansas

Allen Raskin, Ph.D. • Chief, Anxiety Disorders Section, Pharmacologic and Somatic Treatments Research Branch, National Institute of Mental Health, Rockville, Maryland

Alan L. Rubin, M.D. • San Francisco, California

Joan Rubinstein, M.D. • Illinois State Psychiatric Institute, Chicago, Illinois

Mary V. Seeman, M.D. • Professor, Department of Psychiatry, University of Toronto; Clarke Institute of Psychiatry, Toronto, Ontario, Canada

Edward M. Sellers, M.D., Ph.D. • Director, Clinical Institute, Addiction Research Foundation, Toronto, Ontario, Canada; Professor, Departments of Pharmacology and Medicine, University of Toronto, Ontario, Canada

Susanne Steinberg, M.D. • Clinical Psychopharmacology Unit, Allan Memorial Institute, Royal Victoria Hospital, Montreal; Department of Psychiatry, McGill University, Montreal, Quebec, Canada

Siu W. Tang, M.D. • Director, Clinical Psychopharmacology and Psychopharmacology, Clarke Institute of Psychiatry, Toronto; Assistant Professor, Departments of Psychiatry and Pharmacology, University of Toronto, Toronto, Ontario, Canada

Joe P. Tupin, M.D. • Professor and Chairman, Department of Psychiatry, University of California, Davis School of Medicine, Sacramento, California

Gavin Tennant, M.D. • Medical Director, St. Andrew's Hospital, Northampton, England, United Kingdom

Per Vestergaard, M.D. • Senior Registrar, The Psychopharmacology Research Unit, Aarhus University Institute of Psychiatry; The Psychiatric Hospital, Risskov, Denmark

George Voineskos, M.D. • Professor, Department of Psychiatry, University of Toronto; Chief, Primary Care Service, Clarke Institute of Psychiatry, Toronto, Ontario, Canada

Jerry J. Warsh, M.D., Ph.D. • Associate Professor, Departments of Pharmacology and Psychiatry, University of Toronto; Head, Section of Biochemical Psychiatry, Clarke Institute of Psychiatry, Toronto, Ontario, Canada

Paul A. Walker, Ph.D. • Psychologist, San Francisco, California

Daniel R. Weinberger, M.D. • Chief, Section on Clinical Neuropsychiatry and Neurobehavior, National Institute of Mental Health, Saint Elizabeth's Hospital, Washington, D.C.

Richard Jed Wyatt, M.D. • Chief, Adult Psychiatry Branch, Intramural Research Program, National Institute of Mental Health, St. Elizabeth's Hospital, Washington, D.C.

Preface

... to the Clinician

Although huge quantities of drugs are dispensed daily by psychiatrists, there appears to be insufficient concern about the short and long term effects of these exogenous agents on the recipients — our patients. Many clinicians have been trained at a time when knowledge of clinical psychopharmacology was superficial at best, and recent trainees do not necessarily have access to newer, constantly changing, relevant information. The busy clinician is frequently dependent upon the limited knowledge dispensed by the drug company representatives and naturally shys away from many of the more esoteric contributions appearing in the literature. Because of the foregoing issues, the Executive of the Clarke Institute of Psychiatry of the University of Toronto, with the financial support of the Ministry of Health of the Government of Ontario, organized an international symposium on May 14-17, 1982, to bring together some of the acknowledged experts in clinical psychopharmacology. This book is, in part, a reflection of that symposium.

The editors are aware that a contributed volume, however tightly edited, is not necessarily a textbook. Notwithstanding this, it was thought to be important to assemble expert opinion on current important issues, of immediate concern to the practicing clinician. With this in mind, the chapters have been organized around five themes. Schizophrenia, Affective disorders, and Anxiety, are clearly important since they are the major targets of drug use in psychiatry. The recent development of Emergency Psychiatry, and the medical and legal issues concerning the use of high dose potent drugs, necessitated a section on this topic. A section on Forensic Psychiatry was included to alert the reader to the use of drugs in certain personality disorders.

To make this book useful to the clinician, each section has been organized to deal first with the most practical issues and then to examine more theoretical issues. Thus, the editors have attempted to distill the most relevant new information at the beginning of each section, under the heading "Hints for the Clinician." For those more interested in the underlying evidence, a summary and critique of the entire section has been written by the Chairmen who presided over the proceedings of the original conference. The chapters that follow constitute the information we believe is at the cutting edge of clinical psychopharmacology. For completeness, the interested reader will find one or two chapters at the end of each section devoted to theoretical considerations including an assessment of future directions.

Obviously, any book may fall short of projected goals. The editors regret that there could not be an opportunity to include other experts in this clinical psychopharmacology update. Nevertheless, we hope that this book provides an opportunity for practicing clinicians to gain knowledge about the newest information which could be useful to them in their clinical practice.

June 1983   Harvey C. Stancer
                                                          Paul E. Garfinkel
                                                          Vivian M. Rakoff

ACKNOWLEDGEMENT

The editors are grateful to Fred Bradley who so diligently helped in the organization of the symposium that served as the impetus for this book and to Isabel Kelly for her technical assistance.

Contents

SECTION I.   AFFECTIVE DISORDERS

Contents

SECTION III.   ANXIETY

SECTION IV. EMERGENCY PSYCHIATRY

SECTION V. FORENSIC PSYCHIATRY

Contents

Affective Disorders

Hints for Clinicians

GENERAL CONSIDERATIONS

The further away the physician gets from the typical "vegetative syndrome," the less predictable the drug's response. Minimizing unwanted effects is one of the most important considerations in selection of an antidepressant.

ORTHOSTATIC HYPOTENSION

The most common important unwanted effect of tricyclic antidepressants is orthostatic hypotension. There is obviously a difference in the autonomic sensitivity in depressed patients. This hypotensive effect can lead to serious trauma in patients and more consideration should be given to this effect in the treatment of patients. Moreover, the orthostatic hypotension is not dose related. Thus, one cannot reduce the drug to diminish orthostatic hypotension. When it occurs, one should change to a new tricyclic antidepressant. Interestingly, there is not a greater incidence of orthostatic hypotension in healthy old people, but it is increased if they are on sodium or fluid restricted diets of diuretics. Nortriptyline is said to have caused less orthostatic hypotension than some other tricyclics. It is not true that tricyclics adversely affect left ventricular function.

CARDIOVASCULAR EFFECTS

In healthy humans with normal cardiovascular function, there are likely to be few problems with tricyclic medication; in the aging population, the most important consideration is not the age, but the illnesses concomitant with aging. Tricyclics all affect conduction but heartblock does not occur in the normal heart as a result of tricyclic medication. With regard to arrhythmias, these usually occur only in overdose, not in therapeutic doses.

It is important to note that adaptation takes place during the administration of tricyclic medication. If patients do not have heart rate effects early, then it is unlikely that they will have a problem. Conduction changes are such that the PR interval and the QRS interval will increase modestly. These, however, have no clinical significance. Newer evidence suggests that some of the previous concerns regarding anticholinergic effects on the heart may not have been correct, for example, the belief that doxepin is a safer drug than nortriptyline because of the effects on the heart may not be correct.

The reputation for cardiotoxicity associated with tricyclic medication has stemmed primarily from the cardiac effects these drugs have in overdose. However, these effects do not occur with therapeutic doses in the healthy heart. The clinician should be attentive to the possibility of the development of 2:1 heartblock, if patients with bundle branch block are placed on tricyclics. Therefore, the patients with bundle branch block should probably only be placed on these drugs with extreme caution. As hypertension occurs fairly frequently in the aged population, it is important to note that antidepressant drugs can diminish the efficacy of antihypertensive compounds. Thus, clonidine and guanethidine have a reduced effect if given concomitantly with most antidepressant medication. Furthermore, diuretics can cause relative volume-depletion and increase the likelihood of orthostatic hypotension developing with tricyclic drug treatment.

COMBINED MAOI AND TRICYCLIC

With regard to the combined treatment of MAO inhibitors with tricyclic antidepressants, previous studies were marred by low or, probably, subtherapeutic doses. There is some evidence that the atypical depressives said to respond to MAO inhibitors are in fact those with significant anxiety. While it has been accepted for some years that MAO inhibitors combined with tricyclic antidepressants might be more effective than either one alone, there have been very few controlled studies supporting the efficacy of combined use. It is also likely that the dangerousness of combined use has been exaggerated, but this question too has not been well investigated. However, there is experimental support for the use of tryptophan combined with an MAO inhibitor; the two together are more effective than either one alone. It now seems clear that the hypertensive crisis or "cheese reaction" is a peripheral sympathetic nervous system syndrome which responds to adrenergic blocking agents such as phentolamine. It is interesting that some prominent side effects such as orthostatic hypotension during monoamine oxidase inhibitor use do not develop before the two or three weeks commonly associated with the time expected for efficacy.

BLOOD LEVELS

While it may be useful to monitor blood levels of tricyclic antidepressants, present knowledge regarding the pharmacokinetics of these drugs make it difficult to judge their clinical significance. The monitoring of blood tricyclic levels at present is most useful in treatment-resistant cases or where toxicity occurs at low doses. While the therapeutic blood levels may be known for a few tricyclics, at the present time it is probably safer to consider that drug levels are being assessed experimentally. Other important indications for assessing blood levels are situations in which patients are on other nonpsychiatric medications, or in high risk populations, so as to monitor the effects of a given dose. The monitoring of plasma concentration of MAO inhibitors is even less useful than that for tricyclics. This is understandable; the effects of the MAO inhibitors are on the MAO enzyme. It may be preferable to measure the enzyme effect rather than the level of the MAO inhibitor itself. The previous view that phenelzine efficacy is related to whether an individual is a slow or fast acetylator has been shown not to be true. However, it has been found that higher phenelzine doses than previously used, that is in the order of 60-90 mg a day yield greater than 80-85% enzyme inhibition and greater efficacy.

OVERDOSE

In considering toxicity or overdose, it is important to remember that absorption continues long after the drug has been swallowed. The clinician can be misled by plasma levels as the level has not reached the study state. Moreover, the high risk of serious toxicity is the result of the low therapeutic index (median toxic concentration divided by median effective concentration) of the tricyclics. This is further aggravated in cases of increased age or pre-existing cardiac problems or interaction with other drugs of similar toxicity. Overdose usually affects the brain and cardiovascular system. Because of effects on the brain, respiration is reduced. This eventually leads to grand mal seizures. The more serious cardiovascular effects lead to impairment in intracardiac conduction and bundle branch block and arrhythmias result; plasma concentrations of greater than 1000 nanograms per ml are associated with such overdoses. In such high ranges, there is a local anesthetic effect and thus cardiotoxic effects. Cleansing the blood by filtering through charcoal and resins are often used in treatment for overdose. Hypotensive shock is treated by fluid replacement. Forced diuresis, peritoneal dialysis and hemodialysis are ineffective ways of speeding drug elimination. Alkalanization appears to be an effective and safe means to reverse toxicity once absorption has occurred. Such alkalanization can be accomplished by either hyperventilation and/or the administration of sodium bicarbonate. It is interesting that the single most correctible cause of fatality, in one series studied, was insufficient attention to the maintenance of adequate respiration by mechanical support systems. When recurrent TCA-induced seizures occur, treatment with intravenous diazepam or phenytoin is preferable to either physostigmine because of the increased risk of further seizures, or barbiturates, because of the increased risk of further respiratory depression.

LITHIUM CARBONATE

Lithium carbonate has been shown repeatedly to be the best prophylactic treatment for recurrent manic depressive psychosis and frequently for recurrent unipolar depressions. A recent study has shown that antidepressants such as amitriptyline are also useful as a prophylactic treatment for recurrent unipolar depressions. Carbamazepine is a useful prophylactic treatment for lithium nonresponders; the most efficacious use of carbamazepine reported thus far is for the rapid cycling group who suffer from at least four episodes per year.

A practical rule of thumb for the use or prophylactic lithium is that it should be instituted after the second episode in bipolar patients and after the third episode in unipolar patients. It is presently considered (on the basis of controlled studies) that a lower limit of dose of 0.5 mmol is prophylactically effective. This differs from earlier recommendations of average serum lithium concentrations between 0.6 and 1.2 mmols per litre. Obviously, some patients may not show satisfactory prophylactic response with the lower level and for such patients higher average serum lithium concentrations may be necessary. Lithium intoxication may develop relatively early in treatment, in particular within the first six months. These intoxications are frequently iatrogenic in origin and can be avoided. Conjunctive treatment with tricyclic antidepressants which may be helpful, may also increase the number of patients who complain of tremor. It may also increase the risk of mood instability, since antidepressant drugs can antagonize the stabilizing effect of lithium. On the other hand, lithium when added to tricyclics has been shown to convert some nonresponders into responders.

With regard to physiology, long-term lithium treatment leads to a urinary concentrating defect in many patients. This may manifest as clinically significant polyuria in 10 to 20% of chronically treated patients, and infrequently as a vasopressin-resistant diabetes insipidus-like syndrome. Polyuria and polydipsia are known to be reversible with discontinuation of the medication; whether this is also true for the urinary concentration defect is not known. The impairment of renal concentrating ability is correlated to both the duration of lithium treatment and the serum lithium concentration. Renal functional changes which may develop during long-term lithium treatment do not present a contraindication for the continuation of treatment. However, these changes underline the need for careful selection of patients for lithium so that only the patients who really need the treatment and are likely to benefit from it receive lithium treatment for extended periods. The renal changes also make it imperative to monitor lithium treatment carefully.

Lithium affects thyroid function in almost everyone. However in subjects with adequate thyroid reserve, who can compensate for the effects of lithium, effects are transient and without clinical relevance. Slightly decreased T4 and elevated TSH levels are found in about one third of the patients on long-term lithium maintenance. In most cases the interference of lithium with thyroid function remains sub-clinical. Significant hypothyroidism requiring thyroid supplements has been observed in 15 to 25% of lithium treated patients. Thyroid requirements are said to change over time and patients who require a thyroid supplement at one point in time may not require it later.

Dramatic weight gain is observed only during the first year, and takes place mainly in obesity-prone lithium responders. The increase in bodyweight is a real increase in tissue mass and is considered to be independent of fluid retention. Most explanations for the weight gain refer to the insulin-like effect of lithium on body metabolism, gluconeogenesis and increase in glycogen storage. Weight gain on lithium can be both effectively treated and prevented by substantially reducing carbohydrates or caloric intake. In suitable patients a carefully scheduled intermittent treatment with a period of four to six weeks off lithium usually produces dramatic weight reduction in lithium-induced obesity.

There is no good evidence that ordinary lithium treatment adversely affects memory or other neuropsychological functions in patients with primary affective disorder. During the initial stage of lithium treatment, hand tremor is quite frequent and may be observed in half of all patients. In long-term treatment the most common problem, with respect to the gastrointestinal system, is an increased tendency for loose stool. Benign reversable EKG changes are quite common among patients on long-term lithium. They manifest mainly as T wave flattening or inversion. Leucocytosis is relatively common and may to some degree occur in the majority of patients on lithium therapy. Psoriasis is frequently exacerbated by long term lithium treatment and is a relative contraindication to such long-term treatment.

Studies on teratogenic effects have not documented an overall increase in malformations; however, the prevalence of cardiovascular malformations was greater than expected and one cannot exclude the possibility of teratogenic potential of lithium for the developing heart.

Finally, as the cell membrane transport of lithium changes with age, and older patients tend to achieve intracellular concentration with the same blood lithium levels, it is advisable to treat older patients with a lower dosage to produce a lower plasma lithium level.

1

Summary of the Guidelines
for Use of Antidepressants and Lithium

JERRY J. WARSH

The rational use of drugs in the treatment of any disease process requires comprehensive knowledge of the phenomenology and natural history of the disorder as well as an understanding of the pharmacokinetics (disposition, turnover, and metabolism of the drug in body compartments), pharmacodynamics (interaction of the drug with its specific site of action) and toxic effects of the agent. Knowledge of the exact etiopathology of the disorder is extremely helpful but is not an absolute requirement affecting rational drug use. The antidepressant medications currently available for the treatment of affective disorders have been in use for slightly more than two decades, having been discovered serendipitously in the mid 1950s. Until recently the clinical usage of these agents has, for the most part, evolved empirically. In the last five years this situation has begun to change as techniques have been developed permitting the measurement of these agents in plasma, and the description of the pharmacokinetics, pharmacodynamics, and mechanisms of toxicity of these agents.

In this section on antidepressant agents the authors focus their presentations on the use of antidepressants and lithium in relation to the above requirements for the rational use of drugs. The therapeutic efficacy of these agents is not a major part of the focus of this section as this has already been clearly established and thoroughly reviewed (Kupfer and Detre 1978; Klein et al., 1980). Nor is anything other than brief consideration given to the biochemical and neuropharmacological actions of these drugs except where this bears directly upon the knowledge of the clinical use of these agents. The purpose of this volume is to define the current guidelines for the optimal use of these agents and

7

to identify areas of lack of knowledge which, through further research, would improve their clinical use. It is within the context of these constraints that the authors have surveyed the use of currently available antidepressant medications.

TRICYCLIC ANTIDEPRESSANTS

Turning first to the tricyclic antidepressant (TCA) drugs, these agents are characterized by relatively low therapeutic indices and broad spectra of pharmacological activity including adrenergic, anticholinergic, serotonergic, and histaminergic effects, as well as membrane stabilizing actions at higher tissue concentrations (see Potter; also Preskorn and Kent, both in this volume). These characteristics taken together with the now well established phenomenon of marked interindividual differences in rate of metabolism and clearance of TCAs (Potter et al., 1981) and the new awareness of the effects of physiological and pathological changes in aging on drug response, set the framework for understanding their therapeutic actions, side effects and toxicity in clinical use. This same framework forms the foundation for guidelines in the use of these agents and point of embarkation for new research to enhance our knowledge of the action and use of these drugs.

Dr. Potter outlines the theoretical and practical concerns which arise out of the pharmacokinetic variance among TCAs. It is well established that marked interindividual differences in TCA metabolism can lead to a wide range of plasma concentrations for a fixed oral dose (as much as 40-fold). This could account in part for the development of side effects, toxicity, and poor response to medications (Preskorn and Kent, this volume) particularly when such variations in metabolism and clearance are considered along with the multiplicity of actions of these drugs and changes in clearance with aging and disease (Glassman and Carrino, this volume; Potter et al., 1981). Recognition of this pharmacokinetic variance stimulated critical examination of the utility of plasma TCA drug level monitoring to predict optimal blood levels either for therapeutic response or the lower concentration limits signalling the potential to develop side effects and toxicity. To date, however, only in the instance of nortriptyline has a true therapeutic range (window) been identified, while for imipramine a lower therapeutic limit has been defined (Potter, this volume; Potter et al., 1981; Risch et al., 1981). Specific ranges of therapeutic plasma levels have not been conclusively demonstrated for other TCAs and considerable investigation is required to resolve this issue.

Several possible factors may contribute to the confusion regarding plasma TCA levels and response. First, heterogeneity of depressive disorders and differences in severity of depression may create confusion in establishing relationships between plasma levels and response. For example, several studies suggest the existence of subgroups of depressive illness in which there are different underlying putative neurotransmitter disturbances. This may account for the fact that certain cases may be more responsive to certain antidepressants rather than others, with greater selectivity towards one rather than another brain neurotransmitter system (Maas, 1975). In this case relationships between plasma level and response could be observed only by first identifying the appropriate subgroup of patients and then employing a drug with the required selectivity. To accomplish this requires the development of biological markers of sufficient selectivity and sensitivity to identify such subgroups and a much better understanding of the clinical pharmacodynamics and selectivity of antidepressant action.

Clinical subtype and severity of depression may need to be considered also when evaluating therapeutic plasma drug levels if linear correlations between plasma level and response only hold for certain subtypes of depressive disorder or range of severity of illness, (e.g., Glassman et al., 1977). The relationship of pharmacologically active metabolites or combinations of parent compound and metabolite to response are additional issues that need to be resolved to establish the utility of determining plasma TCA levels in order to optimize therapeutic efficacy. For example, the hydroxylate metabolites of TCAs also have biological activity and may contribute to response or side effects. If active metabolites act synergistically with the parent drug then complex relationships may be expected between the sum of the plasma concentrations of parent and active TCA metabolites, and response. These issues remain to be explored and resolved. Finally, aging with its attendant changes in drug metabolism and pharmacodynamic response may also affect the relationships between plasma drug level and response: the altered sensitivities of aging patients to parent drugs and metabolites may result in response and/or side effects at lower plasma levels. The pharmacological basis for this is considered by Dr. Glassman (this volume) and will be touched on later in this summary.

Although many issues remain to be resolved before the ultimate utility of plasma drug level monitoring is established, there are several relatively clear-cut indications for determination of plasma TCA levels. These include: evaluation of compliance, failure to respond, exaggerated response, high risk patients and polypharmacy (Potter, this volume). For drugs such as nortriptyline and imipramine, plasma levels may be used to maximize the likelihood of response. These are the only two drugs for which consistent evidence of a therapeutic window (nortriptyline) or minimal plasma concentrations for response (imipramine) has been reported.

Dr. Preskorn emphasizes the possible value of plasma TCA monitoring to detect and prevent impending toxic effects of TCAs. This group of drugs is highly lipophilic and exhibits a high degree of protein binding; factors leading to marked tissue accumulation in organs such as liver and heart. However,

Dr. Preskorn notes the excellent correlation between plasma and myocardial tissue TCA concentration, for example, which supports the notion that plasma level monitoring can be useful in establishing and preventing certain types of toxicity. A TCA plasma level in excess of 1 μg/ml is invariably associated with significant impairment of intracardiac conduction. However, cardiotoxicity has been shown to occur in some patients at TCA plasma levels well below this concentration. Possible explanations for this are interindividual differences in end-organ response or preexisting disease states which might lower the threshold for significant toxicity. Another important possibility is that formation of active metabolites may contribute to the net toxic effect on an end organ (Jandhyala et al., 1977). Thus, determination of both parent drug and active metabolites may be necessary to identify the minimal cumulative concentrations clearly predictive of toxicity.

Dr. Glassman is concerned that changes in pharmacological action associated with aging could result in prominent and potentially serious side effects at relatively low plasma concentrations, possibly as a result of altered pharmacodynamic activity. For example, he notes that CNS toxicity, signalled by difficulty with balance, may not occur even at plasma concentrations substantially above those considered to be in a therapeutic range. However, impaired speech may relate more directly to plasma levels and is associated with concentrations above the therapeutic range. Anticholinergic side effects of TCAs in younger patients may produce relatively innocuous side effects (constipation) but in the geriatric patient these could lead to serious complications such as paralytic ileus or confusional psychosis.

Plasma level monitoring itself will not be sufficient to identify and prevent all situations of high risk for toxicity. As with therapeutic response, other biological parameters, which reflect impending end-organ toxicity, are probably necessary to complement plasma level information. Only with such an approach will it be possible to define indices predictive of a wide variety of serious complications attributable to TCAs. At present a great deal of work remains to be undertaken in these areas.

Drs. Potter and Preskorn both consider some of the evidence which explains the range and differences in pharmacodynamic activity observed with currently available TCAs. The monomethylated TCA desipramine shows noradrenergic actions at low concentrations, in keeping with the well established high potency of this drug on NE reuptake. Anticholinergic effects and 5-HT reuptake blocking actions occur at higher concentrations. In contrast, a reverse set of dose response relationships is seen for the tertiary TCA amitriptyline; at high drug concentrations the lidocaine-like actions of these drugs become prominent and account for the cardiac toxicity of these agents at plasma concentrations above 1 μg/ml.

Dr. Potter introduces another important variable in relation to the pharmacological activity of TCAs, namely the formation of biologically active hydroxylated metabolites of TCAs. In the past few years procedures have become available to measure these metabolites in plasma. Quite soon after the introduction of these methods it became apparent that these metabolites occur in substantial concentrations during administration of their respective parent TCAs (Ziegler et al., 1976; Devane and Jusko 1981). Concomitant studies of the neuropharmacology of these metabolites demonstrate significant reuptake blockade and potential receptor effects (Bertilsson et al., 1979; Potter et al., 1979; Langer et al., 1980; Smith et al., 1980). Moreover, the formation of such metabolites has been implicated as a possible factor in some forms of toxicity based on animal studies (Jandhyala et al., 1977). At the present time, however, we do not know the ultimate significance of such active metabolites in relation to clinical response or toxicity. It may be that measurement of hydroxylated metabolites as well as the parent TCAs in plasma will provide more accurate indices of response and toxicity. These are new avenues of research to be undertaken.

Dr. Potter also underlines an area of major current interest, namely the study and elucidation of the clinical pharmacodynamics of these agents. Neuropharmacological studies have given us insights into the possible mechanisms of TCAs responsible for therapeutic and side effects based on receptor changes (Charney et al., 1981). However, we still do not know the specific mechanism(s) responsible for therapeutic action or in some cases certain side effects. Development of clinical biochemical indices of pharmacodynamic activity is an area requiring substantial research and should enhance our understanding of the total pharmacological effect of these drugs, as well as provide clinical tests to assess the potential of developing serious side effects.

Aging presents additional risk factors in the use of antidepressants. The underlying basis for increased risk with age includes altered rates of hepatic metabolism, altered receptor sensitivities, increased occurrence of concomitant medical illness and increased use of medications which may interact with TCAs. The latter drug-drug interaction may occur because of interference with drug metabolism, pharmacodynamic responses or potentiating effects such as might occur between TCAs and quinidine, lidocaine, or dilantin with respect to cardiotoxicity (Preskorn and Kent, this volume).

ANTIDEPRESSANTS IN CHILDREN

One of the main problems confronting TCA treatment in children and adolescents has been the diagnostic indications for use. In view of the lack of clear diagnostic criteria of depressive illness in children, the issue of efficacy of

TCAs becomes even more questionable. Dr. Garfinkel summarizes the literature on pharmacological management of affective disorders in children, taking into account methodology and experimental design, measures of degree of behavioral change, duration of treatment, and side effects. Many deficiencies have been noted in the majority of studies undertaken which make definitive statements about efficacy extremely difficult. Despite the limitations of these studies, the reported efficacy of TCAs and MAOIs lies between 57 and 100 percent. This remains to be solidly supported through large scale studies using designs encompassing the cogent criticisms raised by Dr. Garfinkel.

It is noteworthy that the pharmacological issues identified in the use of TCAs in treatment of depressive disorders in adults also apply in children. Thus, as for adults, there appears to be a lower limit of plasma imipramine and desipramine concentrations for therapeutic response (Weller et al., 1982). The occurrence of cardiotoxic side effects such as first degree heart block are associated with dosages exceeding 3.5 mg/kg bodyweight; clearly it is important to establish whether a relationship exists between such side effects and plasma levels of parent drug and/or metabolites. As in the case of adults, pharmacokinetic variance and pharmacodynamic response are issues requiring considerable investigation to identify indices predictive of optimal response and side effects.

The role of tricyclic antidepressants in treatment of enuresis is much more clearly established. The paradoxical finding of high efficacy at low TCA dose may be explained by the possibility that the CNS anticholinergic effect of these drugs, which saturate at relatively low dosage, mediate the therapeutic effect of TCAs in enuresis. This, however, requires further investigation to substantiate. TCAs may have a role in the treatment of school phobias and attentional deficit disorders but their use in the treatment of these disorders requires considerable further investigation.

MONOAMINE OXIDASE INHIBITORS

Dr. Murphy reviews the current status of monoamine oxidase inhibitors (MAOI) in the treatment of affective disorders, giving us new insights into the neuropharmacology and clinical pharmacology of these drugs. This group of agents has only recently received renewed interest, particularly in the treatment of atypical depression and depressive illness accompanied by prominent anxiety. Concerns about the lack of therapeutic efficacy of these agents and the potential for interaction with dietary pressor amines contributed to the relegation of MAOIs to a secondary role in the treatment of depression; these were usually considered only after failure of response to the TCAs. The findings of recent controlled research studies have altered this view. The MAOI phenelzine appears equally effective compared to the TCA amitriptyline in treatment of depressed outpatients and may have more prominent antianxiety effects. There may also be a role for MAOIs in treatment of anxiety-related disorders. In addition, some MAOIs may be equally efficacious in treatment of a variety of subgroups of depressed patients, i.e., endogenous as well as nonendogenous depressions. These findings emanate from studies selectively evaluating one or another MAOI and at present it is difficult to generalize such results across all MAOIs. Clearly further investigation of such interesting observations is warranted.

The utility of monitoring plasma MAOI levels has received little interest in view of the fact that current agents are irreversible inhibitors of MAO. There is no direct relationship between their plasma steady-state concentrations and the net degree of MAO inhibition. Moreover, there may not be any general utility in determining the degree of platelet MAO inhibition as an index of therapeutic response for this relationship appears to be unique to phenelzine.

With respect to the side effects of MAOIs, the major concern regarding the occurrence of hypertensive crises has been put into a clear perspective in regard to its incidence and mechanisms. The relationship between anticholinergic and hypotensive side effects and drug concentrations has not been explored. Nor have the relationships between aging, co-existing medical illness and drug action been examined in a systematic manner. Thus specific guidelines regarding the use of MAOIs in the aged population and in the presence of cardiovascular, hepatic, or CNS disease remain to be clearly defined.

LITHIUM

Progress in establishing the guidelines for lithium therapy and prophylaxis is far advanced over that for other pharmacotherapeutic modalities used in the treatment of affective disorders. This reflects the better understanding of the clinical pharmacology and toxicology of lithium, which in turn was a direct result of the ease of lithium determination and the characteristics of clearance of lithium via a single outflow without metabolic conversion. The guidelines for lithium use have already been the subject of a number of very current reviews and monographs (Johnson, 1980), thus in this section the presentations attempt only to highlight selective concerns in regard to lithium prophylaxis, maintenance, and toxicity.

Dr. Vestergaard emphasizes the central role of lithium in the treatment of bipolar affective disorders as well as the still unresolved question on the value of lithium versus long-term antidepressants for the prophylaxis of unipolar affective disorder. The recent demonstration of the therapeutic efficacy of carbamepazine (Ballenger et al., 1980; Okuma et al., 1981) in the treatment of bipolar illness unresponsive to lithium adds another dimension in the pharmacotherapy of bipolar affective disorder; the role of this agent in prophylaxis and maintenance still needs to be established.

Criteria for selection of patients for lithium prophylaxis and duration of maintenance therapy remain empirically defined based on the frequency and severity of relapse and age of the patient. With the introduction of biological markers of affective disorders such as the dexamethasone suppression and TRH stimulation test (Caroll et al., 1981; Targum et al., 1982) and sleep studies (Kupfer et al., 1978), the possibilities of identifying patients at high risk for relapse and thus in need of prophylaxis are on the horizon.

In reviewing the administration of lithium for maintenance therapy, Dr. Vestergaard emphasizes the use of a lower range of therapeutic plasma levels (0.5-0.8 mmol/L) than previously recommended, except in those few patients who do not show satisfactory prophylactic response. This approach is directed primarily towards reduction of side effects. However, the dependence of this plasma range on the chemical preparation of lithium employed, the dosing interval, and time of sampling after the last dose are important considerations in evaluating any suggested therapeutic range for prophylaxis and should be standardized by clinicians in treatment of their own patients. Controversy still exists with respect to such issues as the frequency of administration and the value of sustained versus fluctuating blood levels of lithium in relation to prevention of side effects. These are in need of further investigation. Dr. Vestergaard succinctly outlines the considerations and questions still to be resolved regarding monitoring of long-term lithium treatment and problems in compliance; these need no further reiteration here.

Drs. Grof and O'Sullivan indicate that the clinically relevant long-term side effect of lithium administration are mainly those related to the CNS, gastointestinal and neuroendocrine systems, and the kidney. The effects of long-term lithium administration on the kidney has received considerable attention recently; the current consensus of studies and reviews on this issue is that long-term lithium administration does not increase the occurrence of structural changes in healthy kidneys. Nevertheless, as renal functional changes may develop during long-term treatment, careful selection of patients is recommended.

The extent of renal function evaluation prior to and during lithium therapy has been the subject of much discussion. Initial patient evaluation should include urinalysis, serum creatinine concentrations and serum electrolytes. The value of creatinine clearance and fluid deprivation tests as a routine has been questioned (Vestergaard et al., 1982), but are clearly warranted if there are any concerns about preexisting renal disease or abnormal findings found by the above routine examinations. Determination of serum creatinine concentrations at least every 2 to 4 months is indicated in uncomplicated cases receiving lithium prophylaxis (Vestergaard et al., 1982; Ramsey and Cox, 1981), or more frequent intervals of at least monthly or less for patients with abnormalities of renal function.

One should underscore the advice given by Dr. Grof regarding lithium-induced hypothyroidism as the thyroid requirements change over time. Thus, while thyroid supplementation may be required at one point in time it may not be needed at another. This observation indicates the need for review of supplementation, particularly as long-term repletion may permanently suppress thyroid hormone production.

Another issue in need of comment pertains to the cardiac effects of lithium. Although the most common lithium induced EKG changes, T wave flattening or inversion, are benign and reversible, significant conduction defects and rhythm disturbances have occurred in some cases, fortunately an infrequent event. These have included sinus node dysfunction or sinoatrial block and multiple premature ventricular contractions suggestive of ventricular irritability. Moreover, it is noteworthy that there appears to be an increased incidence of significant EKG abnormalities at therapeutic lithium concentrations in persons over 60 years of age (Mitchell and Mackenzie, 1982). In view of these observations careful evaluation of cardiac status is an important part of pre-lithium examination with an EKG obtained for all patients >40 years of age and for any individual with a history or physical findings suggestive of cardiac disease. The latter should be repeated annually and more frequently if EKG abnormalities are detected. Monitoring of pulse rate and rhythm should be a routine in follow-up of patients on long-term lithium. A final point worthy of additional emphasis is the reduced lithium plasma level and dosage required in the elderly, a result of higher intracellular concentrations in the aged.

SUMMARY

There have been major advances in the pharmacotherapy of affective illness over the past 25 years. There is now a considerable armamentarium of medications for treatment and prophylaxis of these disorders which continues to grow rapidly. Currently available groups of thymoleptic drugs are inherently quite safe when used with due consideration of their indications, contraindications and pharmacological effects. However, there are a number of aspects of their pharmacology and interaction with aging and disease states which with further elucidation and understanding may enhance the safe use of these agents and improve therapeutic response. Newer antidepressants currently being introduced in Europe have been developed and screened taking into account the pharmacological profile, side effects, and toxicity of forerunner antidepressants such as TCAs (Shopsin et al., 1981). These newer agents hold the hope of still safer drugs for treatment and prophylaxis of affective illness. However, it is likely that continued vigilance for potential significant side effects and toxicity will always be a requirement in the management of patients receiving any of these agents.

REFERENCES

Ballenger, J.C., Post, R.M., and Bunney, W.E. Carbamazepine in manic-depressive illness: A new treatment. *Am. J. Psychiatry* 137:782-790, 1980.

Bertilsson, L., Mellstrom, B., and Sjoqvist, F. Pronounced inhibition of noradrenaline uptake by 10-hyroxymetabolites of nortriptyline. *Life Sci.* 24:1285-1291, 1977.

Caroll, B.J., Feinberg, M., Greden, J.F., Tarika, J., Albala, A.A., Haskett, F., James, N.McI., Kronfol, Z., Lohr, N., Steiner, M., deVigne, J.P., and Young, E. A specific laboratory test for the diagnosis of melancholia. *Arch. Gen. Psychiatry* 38:15-22, 1981.

Charney, D.S., Menkes, D.B., and Heninger, G.R. Receptor sensitivity and the mechanism of action of antidepressant treatment: Implications for the etiology and therapy of depression. *Arch. Gen. Psychiatry* 38:1160-1180, 1981.

Devane, C.L., and Jusko, W.J. Plasma concentration monitoring of hydroxylated metabolites of imipramine and desipramine. *Drug Intelligence Clin. Pharm.* 15:263-266, 1981.

Glassman, A.H., Perel, J.M., Shostak, M., Kantor, S.J., and Fleiss, J.L. Clinical implications of imipramine plasma levels for depressive illness. *Arch. Gen. Psychiatry* 34:197-204, 1977.

Jandhyala, B.S., Steenberg, M.L., Perel, V.M., Manian, A.A., and Burkley, J.P. Effects of several tricyclic antidepressants on the hemodynamics and myocardial contracility of the anaesthetized dog. *Eur. J. Pharmacol.* 42:403-410, 1977.

Johnson, F.N. *Handbook of Lithium Therapy.* University Park Press, Baltimore, 1980.

Klein, D.F., Gittelman, R., Quitkin, F., and Rifkin, A. *Diagnosis and Drug Treatment of Psychiatric Disorders: Adults and Children.* Williams and Wilkins Co., Baltimore, pp. 276-294, 1980.

Kupfer, D.J., Foster, F.G., Coble, P., Mcpartland, R.J., and Ulrick, R.F. The application of EEG sleep for the differential diagnosis of affective disorders. *Am. J. Psychiatry* 135:69-74, 1978.

Kupfer, D.J., and Detre, T.P. Tricyclic and monoamine oxidase inhibitor antidepressants: Clinical use. *Handbook of Psychopharmacology* 14:199-232, 1978.

Langer, S.Z., Raisman, R., and Briley, M.S. Stereoselective inhibition of (^{3}H)-imipramine binding by antidepressant drugs and their derivatives. *Eur. J. Pharmacol.* 64:89-90, 1980.

Mass, J. W. Biogenic amines and depression. Biochemical and pharmacological separation of two types of depression. *Arch. Gen. Psychiatry* 32:1357-1361.

Mitchel, J.E., and Mackenzie, T.B. Cardiac effects of lithium-therapy in man—a review. *J. Clin. Psychiatry* 43:47-51, 1982.

Okuma, T., Inanaga, K., and Otsuki, S. A preliminary double-blind study on the efficacy of carbamazepine in prophylaxis of manic-depressive illness. *Psychopharmacology* 73:95-96, 1981.

Potter, W.J., Calil, H.J., Manian, A.A., Zavadil, A.P., and Goodwin, F.K. Hydroxylated metabolites of tricyclic antidepressants: Preclinical assessment of activity. *Biol. Psychiat.* 14:601-613, 1979.

Potter, W.Z., Bertilsson, L., and Sjoqvist, F. Clinical pharmacokinetics and psychotropic drugs-fundamental and practical aspects. In: *The Handbook of Biological Psychiatry.* Part VI, Practical Applications of Psychotropic Drugs and Other Biological Treatments. H.M. Van Praag, O. Rafaelson, M. Lader, and A. Sachar, eds. Marcel Dekker, New York, 1981, pp. 71-134.

Ramsey, T.L., and Cox, M. Lithium and the kidney: A review. *Am. J. Psychiatry* 139:443-449, 1982.

Risch, S.C., Janowsky, D.S., and Huey, L.Y. Plasma levels of tricyclic antidepressants and clinical efficacy. In: *Antidepressants: Neurochemical, Behavioral, and Clinical Perspectives.* S.J. Enna, J.B. Malick, and E. Richelson, eds. Raven Press, New York, 1981, pp. 183-217.

Shopsin, B., Cassano, G.B., and Conti, L. An overview of new "second generation" antidepressant compounds: research and treatment implications. In: *Antidepressants: Neurochemical, Behavioral, and Clinical Perspectives.* S.J. Enna, J.B. Malick, and E. Richelson, eds. Raven Press, New York, 1981, pp. 219-251.

Smith, R.C., Misra, C.H., and Leelavothi, D.E. Receptor studies of the effects and blood levels of neuroleptic and antidepressant drugs. *Psychopharmacol. Bull.* 16:84-85, 1980.

Targum, S.D., Sullivan, A.C., and Byrnes, S.A. Neuroendocrine interrelationships in major depressive disorder. *Am. J. Psychiatry* 139:282-286, 1982.

Vestergaard, P., Schou, M., and Thomsen, K. Monitoring of patients in prophylactic lithium treatment. *Br. J. Psychiatry* 140:185-187, 1982.

Weller, E.B., Weller, R.A., Preskorn, S.H., and Glotzbach, R. Steady-state plasma imipramine levels in prepubertal depressed children. *Am. J. Psychiatry* 139:506-508, 1982.

2

Use of Antidepressants in the Geriatric Population

ALEXANDER H. GLASSMAN AND JANEL S. CARINO

Depression is one of the most common of human maladies and is particularly prominent in a geriatric population (Klerman, 1976; Pfeiffer and Busse, 1973). The medical management of the depressed geriatric patient may be complicated by his inability to tolerate drug side effects, by other illnesses from which he may be suffering, or by adverse interactions between antidepressant medications and other medications frequently used in his age group. This chapter outlines a rational approach to the use of tricyclic antidepressants in this population.

DIAGNOSIS

For many years depression was considered to be an illness whose etiology and treatment could be totally explainable in psychological terms. With the introduction of antidepressant drugs, biological etiologies and methods of management have been increasingly emphasized. Although the classical arguments attempting to establish whether this is a biological or psychological illness have in no way been resolved, psychiatrists have come to recognize several different types of depression and there has been some evidence for the validity of these distinctions independent of any absolute understanding of etiology. From this the concept of Major Affective Disorder has emerged. This is a syndrome characterized by dysphoria or depression, associated with the "vegetative" symptoms of insomnia, anorexia, weight loss, psychomotor retardation or agitation, and diminished sexual interest.

One of the major reasons for the clinician to recognize this syndrome is the high likelihood that it will respond to tricyclic antidepressants. What is confusing is that patients without these associated "vegetative" signs are not necessarily nonresponsive to these drugs. Many patients who experience depression as a symptom but who do not have the syndrome of major affective disorder will benefit. Sometimes even in settings where life circumstances are such that one might expect to find patients depressed, they will improve with pharmacologic treatment. However, the further away the physician gets from the typical "vegetative" syndrome, the less predictable the drug's response becomes. In spite of our inability to tell who will respond, double-blind controlled studies involving patients whose depressions are nonvegetative show them to have a better response to tricyclics than to placebo medications (Rickels et al., 1974; Rickels et al., 1981; Goldberg et al., 1981).

Whether because in some biological way humans become more vulnerable to depression as they grow older, or merely because aging exposes us to an increasing number of psychological insults, or a combination of the two, both depression as a vegetative syndrome and depression as an isolated symptom become increasingly common in an aging population. However, since serious and life-threatening medical illnesses can masquerade as depression, any depressed patient who seeks treatment for his or her depression should first receive a thorough medical examination. Not only is it important in the elderly to establish that an affective disorder is not the presenting symptom of an underlying medical illness, but it is also crucial to have a complete understanding of the elderly patient's underlying medical condition. That medical condition and the drugs used to treat it are the factors most likely to determine the safety of tricyclic antidepressant use.

CNS Effects

For the sake of convenience, the more frequent side effects of the tricyclic drugs can be broken down into those occurring in the central nervous system (CNS), in the peripheral autonomic nervous system, and in the cardiovascular system. Ranking just below dry mouth and constipation in frequency, and certainly the most common CNS effect of the tricyclics, is sedation. This effect is sometimes beneficial. Many patients find the more sedative tricyclics particularly helpful with sleep. As a matter of fact, tricyclic drugs can, in many patients, be used in lieu of hypnotic compounds. On the other hand, a number of patients find the sedative effects of these drugs so pronounced that it is difficult, if not impossible, to function. This sedative effect is most pronounced with the dimethylated drugs; that is, doxepin, amitriptyline, and to a somewhat lesser extent, imipramine. On the other hand it is seldom seen with monomethylated compounds: desmethylimipramine, nortriptyline, or protriptyline. Regardless of the drug used these sedative effects are most prominent when drug therapy is initiated or when the dose is raised. For most patients these effects will abate over the first three or four days of drug use. In those patients where sedation is excessive it can usually be avoided by switching to nortriptyline or desmethyl-imipramine.

In spite of the fact that most patients are sedated by these drugs, occasional patients will become agitated or overstimulated by the same compounds. Like sedation, this also usually dissipates over the first few days. However, occasionally it is so severe that patients will not continue medication. Other CNS manifestations of these drugs include intention tremor and hyperreflexia. The intention tremor is rarely severe in a patient who has not previously experienced tremor, but a patient who has a mild pre-existing tremor can experience a significant exacerbation on medication. More troublesome with tricyclics in an older population is the propensity of some patients to have serious difficulty with balance when on these drugs. Although unusual, it can be very incapacitating and can be a reason for discontinuing the medication. When such effects do occur, they do not seem to vary much from one standard tricyclic to another. Insufficient information is available on the newer drugs to make an informed statement about them in this regard.

Many of the adverse effects seen with the tricyclics depend more on an individual patient's propensity to develop a particular effect than they do on the dose of the drug. Many patients show no difficulty with balance even at plasma levels four or five times those usually seen from therapeutic doses. Some people even seem immune to the ordinarily common side effects of dry mouth and constipation. One difficulty that seems to be more dependably related to the plasma level of the drug is impaired speech. This type of CNS complication is practically never seen with therapeutic levels and strongly suggests that the patient's plasma concentration of the drug is excessive. Speech problems of this sort can take the form of difficulty in word finding or stuttering, or of increasing verbal pauses. These difficulties will almost always respond to lowering the oral dose of the drug and seldom interfere with treatment.

Anticholinergic Reactions

Undoubtedly the most common adverse effects of the tricyclic drugs are the anticholinergic effects. In a younger population this anticholinergic activity manifests itself as dry mouth, blurred vision, constipation, and, sometimes, delayed urination. In general, although these effects are common, they usually are of little serious significance. However, in an older population these same effects can take on much more ominous significance. Interestingly, the blurred vision common in younger patients is not as noticeable in older patients because it is an effect on accommodation similar to changes that have already occurred as a result of aging. On the other hand, dry mouth, which is a nuisance in younger patients, may become a more serious problem in a patient with dentures. This dryness can, in the dehydrated patient, occasionally provoke an inflammation of the parotid gland. More commonly, the GI effects of tricyclics that produce constipation in the younger patient can produce fecal impaction and paralytic ileus in the geriatric patient. In a similar way urinary hesitancy in the younger patient can readily become urinary retention in the older depressive. This is particularly true for males with prostatic hypertrophy.

There are significant differences among the traditional tricyclic drugs in their propensity to cause anticholinergic effects. Both desmethylimipramine and nortriptyline in therapeutic dosages probably have significantly less anticholinergic effect than doxepin, amitriptyline or imipramine. Some of the newer drugs coming on the market, like trazodone, are also much less likely to produce anticholinergic effects (Newton, 1981).

Although the peripheral anticholinergic effects of the tricyclics can certainly be troublesome, by far the most distressing anticholinergic effect is central. In younger patients, imipramine probably has some modest effect on memory because of its central anticholinergic effect. In the older patient this effect is often much more marked and can result in an acute confusional psychosis. Although not dangerous, these acute confusional states can be frightening to the patient, his family and the physician.

The peripheral anticholinergic effects of the tricyclics can be dramatically reduced through the use of cholinergic agonists such as bethanechol (Urecholine). However, the use of a monomethylated tricyclic or a newer, less anticholinergic antidepressant is generally preferable. The use of multiple drugs is seldom justifiable, particularly in the elderly. In addition, cholinergic agonists are not effective against the central anticholinergic effects of the tricyclics. Here, the only way of avoiding or coping with these effects is to use a less anticholinergic drug (Branconnier and Cole, 1981). Anticholinergic side effects that are only of nuisance significance in younger patients can become serious problems in the elderly; therefore, in general, an antidepressant drug with reduced anticholinergic effects should be selected for use in a geriatric population.

Cardiac Effects

Certainly the most commonly worrisome adverse events associated with the tricyclics are cardiac. In overdose the tricyclics clearly cause serious adverse consequences, and these cardiac effects are the most frequent cause of tricyclic death. Indeed, tricyclics' reputation for difficulty stems primarily from the cardiac effects these drugs have in overdose. At therapeutic levels the cardiac effects of the tricyclics have, until recently, been poorly understood. It is now reasonably clear that these drugs will, in general, lengthen cardiac conduction times. These changes in otherwise healthy hearts are seldom, if ever, of any clinical consequence. However, in patients with pre-existing conduction disease these same effects can be quite serious (Glassman and Bigger, 1981). Obviously the chance that a patient will have pre-existing conduction disease increases with age. The frequency with which pre-existing conduction disease will result in serious complications when exposed to tricyclics is not clear. The situation is probably similar to that seen with quinidine, a drug which shares many characteristics with the tricyclics. Although the specific risk is not clear, patients with bundle branch blocks should be placed on these drugs with extreme caution and not without clearcut indications. If patients with bundle branch blocks are placed on tricyclics, the clinician should be attentive to the possibility of the development of 2:1 heart block. Since imipramine, like quinidine, acts to suppress ectopic pacemakers, patients whose pacemakers are below the SA node are at risk for idioventricular rhythms or asystole if given imipramine. The relationship between tricyclic use and sinus node disease itself is not clearly understood, but given the experience with quinidine, which may exacerbate sinus node disease, it is likely that caution should be used in treating patients with suspected sinus node dysfunction. If a patient has an artificial pacemaker, the risk is eliminated and antidepressant therapy is perfectly safe (Alexopoulos and Frances, 1980). It must be noted that in all these conduction conditions, the severity of the pre-existing condition is a more important determinant of the risk than is the particular tricyclic used.

Two foci of frequent concern are heart rate and heart rhythm. For both, the risk with a tricyclic antidepressant is probably dramatically less than has generally been perceived. Tricyclics, although they vary a little from one drug to another, do tend to increase heart rate; but this propensity is rarely of clinical significance. For many years it had been thought that tricyclic drugs were contraindicated in patients with ventricular arrhythmia; it is now clear that this was a misunderstanding. Although, like quinidine, these drugs can cause ventricular irritability at higher plasma levels, the tricyclics at therapeutic levels are antiarrhythmic drugs and markedly decrease ventricular ectopic beats (Giardina et al., 1979).

One of the more complex questions about the tricyclic antidepressants is whether they are harmful to patients with impaired left ventricular function. Early data suggested that these drugs further impaired the contractility of the heart (Burckhardt et al., 1978; Taylor and Braithwaite, 1978; Burgess et al., 1979). It is now clear that this is not true and that these early observations were plagued by methodological problems. Recent studies using radionuclide technology at therapeutic tricyclic levels (Veith et al., 1982) and catheter investigations (Langou et al., 1980; Thorstrand, 1974) in overdose have shown unequivocally that tricyclics do not impair left ventricular function. Nevertheless, in patients with pre-existing left ventricular impairment imipramine has proven to be far from harmless (Glassman et al., in press). Although left ventricular function is not further impaired, these patients seem to be at extraordinary risk for severe orthostatic hypotension. At present it is not clear which drug is safe to use in these patients or what characteristics leave them vulnerable to this effect.

Orthostatic Hypotension

Probably the most important cardiovascular effect of the tricyclics is their propensity to produce orthostatic hypotension. As the most commonly serious side effect, orthostatic hypotension deserves special attention in the elderly patient and in patients with pre-existing cardiovascular disease. Muller compared a patient population older than 60 years of age having cardiovascular disease and a matched group of patients less than 60 years free of cardiovascular disease (Muller et al., 1961). The older patients with cardiovascular disease developed clinically significant postural hypotension three times more often than the younger patients who were free of cardiovascular disease. Although Muller attributed two acute myocardial infarctions to orthostatic hypotension, it is not clear that tricyclic-induced orthostatic hypotension can cause myocardial infarction. Indeed, in France the tricyclics have been used to treat angina assumedly without an apparent increase in infarction rate. But whether they can cause infarction or not, there is no question that tricyclic-induced orthostatic hypotension does result in serious injuries secondary to falls (Glassman et al., 1979). Glassman has shown that the magnitude of orthostatic hypotension does not vary primarily as a function of age, but that it is associated with increasing illness and the increasing use of a variety of medications (Glassman et al., in press). Obviously both physical illness and the use of drugs increase markedly in the elderly. Glassman has also shown that the orthostatic drop in blood pressure occurs at blood levels of tricyclics far below those that are therapeutic in treating severe depressions. Thus, a patient on imipramine can develop orthostatic hypotension on much smaller doses than those necessary for therapeutic efficacy. If the patient has a serious fall or develops large postural pressure drops, imipramine may not be usable.

Of all the adverse effects seen with the tricyclic drugs, orthostatic hypotension will probably be the most common reason for discontinuing the drug. Orthostatic hypotension has been well studied for imipramine (Muller et al., 1961; Glassman et al., 1979; Hayes et al., 1977) and nortriptyline (Freyschuss et al., 1970; Ziegler et al., 1977; Vohra et al., 1975), but there is significantly less information available on the other drugs in this class. Amitriptyline, desmethylimipramine, and doxepin, to a large extent, share similar effects with imipramine (Hayes et al., 1977; Veith et al., 1982). Freyschuss et al. (1970), using nortriptyline, found no effect on lying or standing blood pressure in a group of young patients. Although not done as elegantly, work by both Vohra et al.

(1975) and Ziegler et al. (1977) would suggest that Freyschuss is correct. However, all three of these workers examined only younger patients. Roose has recently demonstrated that nortriptyline causes less orthostasis than imipramine in a group of elderly patients (Roose et al., 1981). Although nortriptyline did produce modest drops in blood pressure, the difference between imipramine and nortriptyline was not only statistically significant, it was a clinically important and useful difference. From the available published literature, nortriptyline does appear to cause less orthostatic hypotension than imipramine and has the best documented record for safety in regard to orthostatic hypotension of any tricyclic presently available. In patients for whom postural blood pressure falls are dangerous, such as the elderly, this is a significant advantage.

Although the mechanism of tricyclic-induced orthostatic hypotension is unknown, there is no question that reduced blood volume places a patient at greater risk for this adverse event. Patients who are on fluid- or salt-restricted diets, those taking diuretics, or those who are poorly hydrated for whatever reason should be closely monitored if a tricyclic drug is to be started. Rehydration prior to beginning therapy is often useful. Florinef, a salt retaining corticosteroid, has been used to reduce orthostatic hypotension. However, this approach carries a significant risk, especially in a geriatric patient population where hypertension or impaired left ventricular function is common.

Hypertension

When a patient becomes depressed, pre-existing illness or its therapy may complicate the treatment of the depression. Although it is neither practical nor desirable to list individual conditions and enumerate ways in which they or their treatment might interact with the antidepressant drugs, such an approach probably is warranted for hypertension. This is so both because hypertension is extremely common and because the interactions among hypertension, depression, and antidepressant and antihypertensive drugs are so complex.

Hypertension is estimated to occur in 40% of elderly Americans. Several of the treatments for hypertension have been implicated as causal factors in depression. Reserpine causes depression in about 15% of the patients on chronic medication (Simpson, 1973). Methyldopa (Aldomet) has been implicated in causing depression as well. Paykel reviewed the incidence of psychiatric side effects among patients receiving antihypertensive drugs and estimated that patients receiving methyldopa have a depression incidence of 3.6% (Paykel et al., 1982). It is unclear how much this is in excess of the incidence of depression that could be expected in a similarly aged population not on medication. Certainly methyldopa-associated depression is not as frequent as reserpine-associated depression. The incidence of depression with clonidine (Catapres), guanethidine (Ismelin) and propranolol (Inderal) is only one to two percent. Since all data were collected in a similar way, this would suggest that there is an excess incidence of depression with methyldopa and a marked excess with reserpine as compared to the other drugs. Unfortunately, patients are frequently treated for hypertension with preparations containing reserpine in combination with other drugs (Diupres, Unipres, Ser-Ap-Es, etc.). Although propranolol has been implicated as a cause of depression, Paykel's review does not offer much support for that assertion (Paykel et al., 1982). It is clear that patients with significant hypertension and a history of depression require careful management. From a psychiatric point of view, they are probably best treated with a beta blocking agent, a diuretic and/or hydralazine, though even these preparations have their problems.

In addition to the difficulties that antihypertensive medications cause for patients with a history of depression, the antidepressant drugs themselves can diminish the efficacy of antihypertensive compounds. Both guanethidine (Mitchell et al., 1970) and clonidine (Briant et al., 1973) will have a reduced effect if given concomitantly with most antidepressant medication.

Just as tricyclics may interfere with the treatment of hypertension and antihypertensives may trigger depression, antihypertensive medication has a propensity to complicate the use of antidepressant drugs. Diuretics, probably the most commonly used drugs for the treatment of hypertension, cause patients to become relatively volume-depleted, and thereby increase the likelihood that orthostatic hypotension will develop as an effect of tricyclic drug treatment. As a matter of fact, strict salt-controlled diets for either hypertension or heart failure can, by themselves, volume-depleted patients and make them more susceptible to postural hypotension.

In a patient with both serious hypertensive disease and recurrent depression, interactions of the above sort can cause major difficulties. One potential involves the use of MAO inhibitors. Although this paper does not attempt to review carefully their contribution, it does point out that they do have certain advantages in the hypertensive patient. These drugs are themselves hypotensive agents. One monoamine oxidase inhibitor, pargyline, is, as a matter of fact, marketed for the treatment of hypertension (PDR). Unfortunately the MAO inhibitors do cause significant orthostatic hypotension and, as with the tricyclics, this can be troublesome (Kronig et al., in press). Although there is much less known about the interactions between MAO inhibitors and the antihypertensive drugs, than about the interaction between antihypertensives and tricyclics, MAO inhibitors are probably worth considering in the hypertensive patient for whom tricyclic antidepressants may lead to difficulties.

DRUG–DRUG INTERACTIONS

Even in younger patients the tricyclic antidepressants are particularly prone to interact with other drugs (Glassman and Perel, 1973). This is so because they are very heavily metabolism-dependent drugs; as such, any substance or process that influences the hepatic microsomal enzyme systems can potentially affect their clearance from the body. In an elderly population the potential for drug-drug interactions is greatly increased because of the greater number of drugs these patients take. As in younger people, those drugs that stimulate microsomal enzymes will decrease the plasma level of the antidepressant drug. The most common enzyme inducer is still probably cigarette smoking. Other substances known to stimulate hepatic enzymes include barbiturates, carbamazepine (Tegretol), glutethimide (Doriden) (Med. Lett., 1981a,b), and alcohol. In addition rifampin and griseofulvin are also known hepatic enzyme inducers (Bint and Burtt, 1980). Enzyme inhibitors decrease hepatic microsomal levels, with an associated decrease in the clearance of tricyclics and an increase in plasma levels. The drugs that most often will produce this interaction in a psychiatric population are the phenothiazines and haloperidol (Kragh-Sorensen et al., 1981). Other drugs that can cause inhibition of the microsomal enzymes include ritalin, cimetidine, disulfiram, oral hypoglycemics, phenytoin, allopurinol, chloramphenicol, PAS, isoniazid, and sulfonamide.

Not all of the drug-drug interactions seen with the tricyclics are brought about via hepatic enzymes. For example, the increased likelihood of orthostatic hypotension among patients receiving concomitant tricyclic antidepressant treatment and diuretics, and the interaction of tricyclics with clonidine in the treatment of hypertension are drug-drug interactions that are unrelated to alterations in metabolism. Such reactions are referred to as pharmacodynamic rather than pharmacokinetic interactions.

The large number of drugs that a geriatric population is likely to be exposed to make it difficult to anticipate exactly what alterations in drug clearance will occur. As a result it is extremely helpful, in any population receiving multiple drugs, to use plasma level measurements of tricyclic drugs to estimate the effect, if any, these multiple drug therapies have on tricyclic drug clearance. Certainly it is easiest to do this in drugs for which the therapeutic plasma concentration range has been well established. This is true for imipramine and nortriptyline and probably so for desmethylimipramine (Gram and Kragh-Sorensen, 1981). If we consider the newer antidepressant compounds, practically nothing is known about the relationship of plasma concentrations to efficacy; in many instances, even the metabolic pathways have been only partially clarified. As a result we have little ability to anticipate drug-drug interactions, a situation which argues for using more familiar and well-understood compounds in a geriatric population.

SUMMARY

The use of a tricyclic antidepressant in a geriatric population is, in many ways, much more complicated than in younger, healthier patient groups. On the other hand, there are probably more frequent indications for the use of an antidepressant drug in a geriatric population than in a younger group. Certainly the presence of a major affective disorder with a typical vegetative syndrome that persists for any reasonable length of time, with even moderate severity, is a clearcut indication for tricyclic drugs. If the patient has characteristics that place him at special risk, he should be seen by a physician with special experience using these drugs. Only rarely will it prove unwise to medicate such patients and in these circumstances, ECT remains a dependable treatment. The vast majority of the time the benefits of drug treatment will outweigh the risks. In milder illness or in patients whose depression is a symptom rather than a syndrome, the situation becomes more complex. Because a drug response becomes less certain and a placebo response probably more likely, one must very carefully balance the risks involved against the likely benefits of specific antidepressant treatment. But if the patient is healthy, the drug is probably safe and the trial worthwhile. By and large the tricyclics are safe drugs and only in a population with pre-existing conduction disease, far advanced cardiovascular disease, or in a group of patients on multiple other drugs are the risks of tricyclic treatment high. Even in the elderly, if the patient is relatively healthy, the tricyclics are generally safe compounds.

ACKNOWLEDGMENTS

This study was supported in part by Grant MH 32592, The National Institute of Mental Health and from The Taub Foundation.

REFERENCES

Alexopoulos, G.S., and Frances, R.J. ECT and cardiac patients with pacemakers. *Am. J. Psychiatry* 137:1111–1112, 1980.

Bint, A.J., and Burtt, I. Adverse antibiotic drug interactions. *Drugs* 20:57–68, 1980.

Branconnier, R.J., and Cole, J.O. Effects of acute administration of trazodone and amitriptyline on cognition, cardiovascular function, and salivation in the normal geriatric subject. *J. Clin. Psychopharmacology* 1(6, Suppl.): 82S–88S, 1981.

Briant, R.H., Reid, J.L., and Dollery, C.T. Interaction between clonidine and desipramine in man. *Br. Med. J.* 1:522–523, 1973.

Burckhardt, D., Raeder, E., Muller, V., Imhof, P., and Neubauer, H. Cardiovascular effects of tricyclic and tetracyclic antidepressants. *JAMA* 239(3): 213–216, 1978.

Burgess, C.D., Montgomery, S., Wadsworth, J., and Turner, P. Cardiovascular effects of amitriptyline, mianserin, zimelidine and nomifensine in depressed patients. *Postgrad. Med. J.* 55:704–708, 1979.

Freyschuss, U., Sjoqvist, F., Tuck, D., and Asberg, M. Circulatory effects in man of nortriptyline, a tricyclic antidepressant drug. *Pharmacol. Clin.* 2:68–71, 1970.

Giardina, E.G., Bigger, J.T., Jr., Glassman, A.H., Perel, J.M., and Kantor, S.J. The electrocardiographic and antiarrhythmic effects of imipramine hydrochloride at therapeutic plasma concentrations. *Circulation* 60:1045–1052, 1979.

Glassman, A.H., and Perel, J.M. The clinical pharmacology of imipramine. *Arch. Gen. Psychiatry* 28:649–653, 1973.

Glassman, A.H., Bigger, J.T., Jr., Giardina, E.V., Kantor, S.J., Perel, J.M., and Davies, M. Clinical characteristics of imipramine-induced orthostatic hypotension. *Lancet* 1:468–472, March, 1979.

Glassman, A.H., Bigger, J.T., Jr. Cardiovascular effects of therapeutic doses of tricyclic antidepressants: A review. *Arch. Gen. Psychiatry* 38:815–820, 1981.

Glassman, A.H., Walsh, B.T., and Roose, S.P. Factors influencing orthostatic hypotension with tricyclic antidepressants. Accepted for publication in *J. Clin. Psychiatry*.

Goldberg, H.L., Rickels, K., and Finnerty, R. Treatment of neurotic depression with a new antidepressant. *J. Clin. Psychopharmacol.* 1(No. 6 Suppl.): 35S–38S, 1981.

Gram, L.F., and Kragh-Sorensen, P. Pharmacokinetics and plasma level/effect relationships of tricyclic antidepressants: an update. In: *Clinical Pharmacology in Psychiatry*. E. Usdin, S.G. Dahl, L.F. Gram, and O. Lingjaerde, eds. MacMillan (London), 1981, pp. 241–251.

Hayes, J.R., Born, G.F., and Rosenbaum, A.H. Incidence of orthostatic hypotension in patients with primary affective disorders treated with tricyclic antidepressants. *Mayo Clin. Proc.* 52:509–512, 1977.

Klerman, G.L. Age and clinical depressions: Today's youth in the twenty-first century. *J. Gerontol.* 31:318–323, 1976.

Kragh-Sorensen, P., Gram, L.F., and Larsen, N.E. Routine use of plasma concentration measurement of tricyclic antidepressant drugs; Indications and limitations. In: E. Usdin, ed. *Clinical Pharmacology in Psychiatry*. Elsevier North Holland, New York, 1981, pp. 287–300.

Kronig, M.H., Roose, S.P., Walsh, B.T., Woodring, S., and Glassman, A.H. Blood pressure effects of phenelzine. Submitted for publication.

Langou, R.A., Van Dyke, C., Tahan, S.R., and Cohen, L.S. Cardiovascular manifestations of tricyclic antidepressant overdose. *Am. Heart J.* 100:458–464, 1980.

Medical Letter: Adverse interactions of drugs. *Med. Lett. Drugs Ther.* 23(5):17–28, 1981a.

Medical Letter: Interactions of drugs with alcohol. *Med. Lett. Drugs Ther.* 23(7):33–36, 1981b.

Mitchell, J.R., Cavanaugh, J.H., Arias, L., and Oates, J.A. Guanethidine and related agents. III. Antagonism by drugs which inhibit the norepinephrine pump in man. *J. Clin. Invest.* 49:1596–1604, 1970.

Muller, O.F., Goodman, N., and Bellet, S. The hypotensive effect of imipramine hydrochloride in patients with cardiovascular disease. *Clin. Pharmacol. Ther.* 2:300–307, 1961.

Newton, R. The side effect profile of trazodone in comparison to an active control and placebo. *J. Clin. Psychopharmacology* 1(6, Suppl.):89S–93S, 1981.

Pfeiffer, E., and Busse, E.W. Mental disorders in later life, affective disorders, paranoid, neurotic and situational reactions. In: E.W. Busse and E. Pfeiffer, (eds.) *Mental Illness in Later Life,* Washington, D.C., American Psychiatric Assn., 1973.

Physicians' Desk Reference, Oradell, N.J., Medical Economics Company, 1981.

Rickels, K., Csanalosi, I., Chung, H.R., Case, W.G., Pereira-Ogan, J.A., and Downing, R.W. Amitriptyline in anxious-depressed outpatients: A controlled study. *Am. J. Psychiatry* 131:25–30, 1974.

Rickels, K., Case, W.G., Werblowsky, J., Csanalosi, I., Schless, A., and Weise, C.C. Amoxapine and imipramine in the treatment of depressed outpatients: A controlled study. *Am. J. Psychiatry* 138:20–24, 1981.

Roose, S.P., Glassman, A.H., Siris, S.G., Walsh, B.T., Bruno, R.L., and Wright, L.B. Comparison of imipramine- and nortriptyline-induced orthostatic hypotension: A meaningful difference. *J. Clin. Psychopharmacology* 1(5): 316–319, 1981.

Simpson, F.O. Editorial: Hypertension and depression and their treatment. *Aust. N.Z. J. Psychiatry* 7:133–137, 1973.

Taylor, D.J. and Braithwaite, R.A. Cardiac effects of tricyclic antidepressant medication: A preliminary study of nortriptyline. *Br. Heart J.* 40:1005–1009, 1978.

Thorstrand, C. Cardiovascular effects of poisoning with tricyclic antidepressants. *Acta Med. Scand.* 195:505–514, 1974.

Veith, R.C., Raskind, M.A., Caldwell, J.H., Barnes, R.F., Gumbrecht, G., and Ritchie, J.L. Cardiovascular effects of tricyclic antidepressants in depressed patients with chronic heart disease. *N. Engl. J. Med.* 306:954–959, 1982.

Vohra, H., Burrows, G.D., and Sloman, G. Assessment of cardiovascular side effects of therapeutic doses of tricyclic antidepressant drugs. *Aust. N.Z. J. Med.* 5:7–11, 1975.

Ziegler, V.E., Co, B.T., and Biggs, J.T. Plasma nortriptyline levels and ECG findings. *Am. J. Psychiatry* 134:441–443, 1971.

3

The Use of Antidepressant Medication in Children and Adolescents

Barry D. Garfinkel

INTRODUCTION

Antidepressant medication has been used in child psychiatry for four main disorders: depression, enuresis, attention deficit disorders (hyperactivity), and separation anxiety/school phobia. It is surprising that antidepressants are claimed to be effective in such diverse conditions as these four. Nevertheless, there are significant numbers of clinical reports suggesting their efficacy for these disorders. In order to establish the utility of antidepressant medication for children, diagnostic and nosological problems must initially be addressed. This review critically evaluates the literature concerning childhood depression and whether there is support for the role of antidepressant medication in the treatment of children with depression and other conditions.

The first issue to be discussed is whether depression exists as a disease or syndrome in children. The presence of depression in this age group has been a controversial issue in child psychiatry. Kraepelin (1921) and Kanner (1948) described depression in children as an uncommon occurrence. Anthony (1960) assumed that prepubertal manic-depressive illness was an exceedingly rare phenomenon, accounting for a very small proportion of affective disorders in children. Traditional psychoanalytic theory (Rie, 1966) postulated that children, because of limited superego development, could not experience the self-reproach and guilt characteristic of adult depression. The existence of childhood depression was made more obscure with the advent of concepts of "anaclitic depression" (Spitz and Wolf, 1946), "masked depression (Glaser, 1967) and

31

depressive equivalents" (Malmquist, 1971). Anaclitic depression was reviewed by Rutter (1972) and his conclusions were that it likely results from an absence of adequate stimulation, contact and handling in the first two years of life. Marked developmental delays, viral infections and a high mortality rate were observed. There is no evidence that this condition is related to depressive states in later childhood or adult life. It was likely mislabeled as a variant of depression.

Masked depression, like depressive equivalents, is a concept which proposes that children are unable to exhibit the signs or verbally relate the symptoms of depression. This concept assumes that children primarily express themselves indirectly through their behavior. The examiner's interpretation of the child's behavior becomes the primary factor in making the diagnosis of an underlying depression.

Criteria of childhood depression have been proposed by Cytryn and McKnew (1974), Frommer (1971), Weinberg et al. (1973), Puig-Antich (1978) and Carlson and Cantwell (1980). The development of a classification system for childhood depression is important so that a group of children who are potentially responsive to antidepressant medication may be identified. Furthermore, distinguishing childhood depression from other syndromes, in particular Attention Deficit Disorder and Conduct Disorders, has led to a greater diagnostic clarity and a precision in the administration of medication for all children.

ARE THERE DEPRESSED CHILDREN?

There is good evidence (Carlson and Strober, 1978; Poznanski et al., 1976; Ossofsky, 1974) that depression as a clinical state exists in childhood. Four major observations as to the origin of affective disorders have evolved. Affective disorders may be regarded as arising de novo in adolescence and persisting into adulthood; they may be related to various childhood disorders that empirically appear different from depression [i.e., enuresis, hyperactivity (attention deficit disorder), conduct disorders and school phobia]; they may arise in childhood and persist as a "forme fruste" or more severe form of adult affective disorder. Finally, they may exist in children, but the expression of symptoms is modified by the child's developmental state.

Most authors agree that childhood "depressive states" are recognizable in prepubertal children. As Carlson and Cantwell (1980) and Puig-Antich (1982) have demonstrated, a recurring problem has been the separation of childhood depression from conduct disorders. There may indeed be a childhood disorder that meets the criteria for both conditions. Similarly, Shaffer and Greenhill (1979) have identified a broad overlap between conduct-disordered children and attention deficit disorder (ADD). Wender et al. (1981) has described particular affective symptoms as a major component of ADD. There is, therefore, a commonality of the presenting affective symptoms among these three conditions (Figure 1).

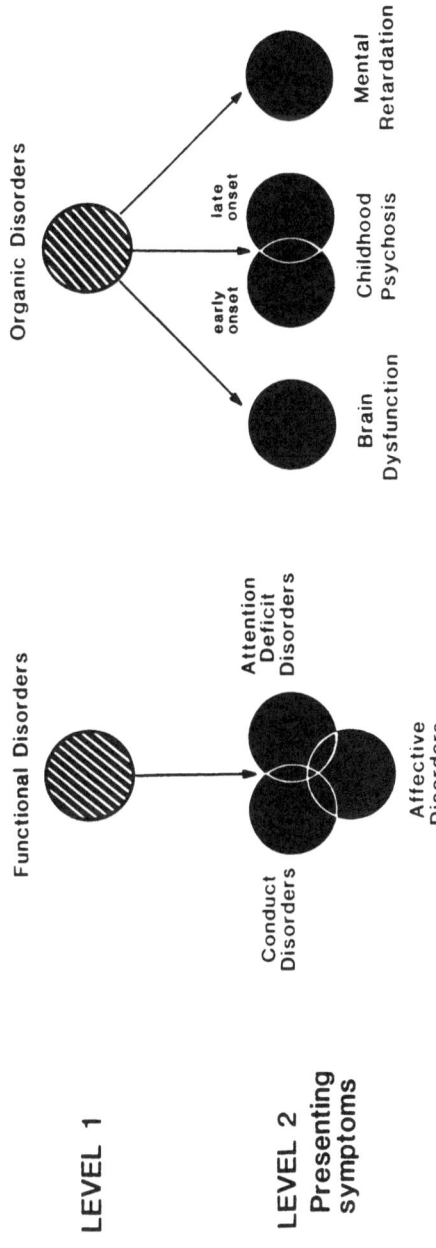

Figure 1. Classification of childhood disorders: The overlap of conduct disorders, affective disorders, and attention deficit disorders.

Approximately one-third of those children with a depressive state meet the criteria for a conduct disorder (Puig-Antich, 1982). As Carlson and Cantwell (1980) suggest, the dysphoric mood may or may not be secondary to the behavioral problems. This research is supported by Cytryn and McKnew (1972) who developed the concept of "masked depression" as one of their three forms of depression (acute, chronic, and masked). Children with masked depression often had conduct disorder symptoms and depression. By 1980, however, the concept of masked depression was dropped, although most of the children exhibited both behavioral problems and depression. Currently there is sufficient evidence to suggest that some children may be equally conduct-disordered and depressed.

A major problem has been establishing the validity of the criteria for the diagnosis of a depressive syndrome. Although there is an overlap of symptoms among Cytryn et al.'s (1980) criteria and those of Weinberg et al. (1973) and Brumback et al. (1974), the major criticism, however, of these classification systems, as well as Frommer's (1971) is that they are too inclusive. Rates of depression diagnosed by their criteria seem unrealistically high. Therefore, the validity of these criteria is questioned even though there is insufficient data on the construct validity of the criteria. Another error in these systems is to identify children as being depressed when they exhibit symptoms that are not unique to depression. For example, according to the Weinberg et al. (1973) criteria, a child with depression must have dysphoric mood, self-depreciation but may also be aggressive and doing poorly in school. The child with these four symptoms would receive the diagnosis of depression. Other nonspecific symptoms are diminished socialization, change in school attitude, loneliness, restlessness and sulkiness. In Weinberg et al.'s original report, as many as 58% of the original sample of children with school-related problems met criteria for depression. Depression in children according to the Weinberg criteria shows a high false positive rate compared to DSM-III criteria (Carlson and Cantwell, 1982).

The most inclusive classification system is that of Frommer (1971). Depression, according to Frommer, is of three types: enuretic and encopretic, phobic, and pure depression. A large number of children responded to various antidepressants, suggesting to Frommer that they were depressed. Drug responsivity alone is obviously an unacceptable way to make a diagnosis of depression, especially since children with various other diagnoses respond to antidepressants. Frommer's classification assumes that depression coexists with other psychological and somatic symptoms, which are themselves not specific to depression.

Puig-Antich et al. (1980), Cantwell and Carlson (1979) and Robbins et al. (1982) have established that depressive symptoms may be elicited when sought. These authors indicated that adult DSM-III criteria and Feighner et al. (1972) adult research diagnostic criteria apply equally well to prepubertal children. The failure to recognize depression in the past likely reflects that the signs and symptoms were not systematically illicited during clinical interviews of children.

THE CRITERIA OF CHILDHOOD DEPRESSION

Current research has revealed four symptom clusters of childhood depression (Table 1). The first is a mood disorder with symptoms of dysphoria, sadness, tearfulness, irritability, unhappiness and sulkiness. Disturbance of self-perception is the second criterion and is represented by low self-esteem, self-depreciation, helplessness and hopelessness. McConville et al. (1973) have noted that these disturbances of mood and self-perception occur within specific age groups. Psychomotor symptoms are the third cluster of symptoms observed, and these include loss of interest, psychomotor retardation, decreased concentration, aggressivity, and restlessness. The fourth type of symptoms are vegetative, and

Table 1. Symptom Clusters of Depressive States[a]

1. Mood
   + a) dyphoria
     b) tearfulness
     c) loss of pleasure
   + d) sadness
   + e) irritability
     f) sulkiness

2. Self-perception
     a) low self-esteem
   + b) guilt
     c) helplessness/hopelessness
   + d) self-reproach

3. Psychomotor
   + a) psychomotor retardation/agitation
   + b) loss of energy/fatigue
     c) restlessness
   + d) decreased concentration
     e) loss of interest
   + f) aggressivity

4. Vegetative
   + a) sleep disturbance
     b) somatic complaints
     c) appetite change
   + d) weight loss/gain
     e) enuresis/encopresis

[a]Mood symptoms and at least 4 of the remaining symptoms must be present nearly every day for at least a two week duration.

+Found in DSM-III.

they include: sleep disturbance, enuresis, encopresis, anorexia, and somatic complaints. Most authors agree that these symptoms must occur for a specific period of time, anywhere from one week to one month, and do not merely represent fluctuations in mood and functioning over hours or days. Cytryn and McKnew's (1972) criteria for the duration of symptoms persisting several months is unduly long and is overly restrictive. By limiting the diagnosis of depression to children with symptoms in these four areas for a specific duration, the clinical state of depression can be successfully identified.

Cantwell and Carlson (1979), however, have drawn attention to the absence of studies establishing the disorder of depressive illness in children. Unlike adult research into affective disorders, the delineation of childhood depression stops with the cross-sectional state. There are no studies of family history, biological markers associated with color blindness and blood groups, and biochemistry. These studies have been made difficult or impossible by the lack of appropriate, reliable diagnostic criteria. Two follow-up studies by Poznanski et al., (1976) and Herjanic (1976) on a limited number of patients have shown that depression continues in about 50% of those originally diagnosed as depressed. The finding that depression in children was more permanent over time provides limited support to the validity of the depressive disorder. Response to pharmacological treatment is still equivocal. Therefore, there is no conclusive evidence to indicate the existence of a syndrome in children with the same degree of certainty as for adults.

THE EVALUATION OF THE DEPRESSED CHILD

It is currently possible to evaluate a child for depression using standardized and reliable techniques (Kazdin, 1981). The diagnosis is based on five methods of clinical investigation. They include: structured interviews, rating scales (self-report, parent, and clinician), personality inventories, dexamethasone suppression test, and clinical pharmacological trials. Chambers et al. (1978) had demonstrated the utility of the KIDDIE–SADS. This structured interview has successfully identified children with major depression according to Research Diagnostic Criteria (Endicott and Spitzer, 1978), and who responded to antidepressant medication. The Children's Depression Inventory (CDI) (Kovacs and Beck, 1978) has been shown to be effective and is a simple self-report method of identifying depression in children between seven and seventeen years of age. There is a Short Children's Depression Inventory (SCDI) (Carlson and Cantwell, 1979) which is a modification of the CDI. The Children's Depression Scale (CDS) (Lang and Tisher, 1978) is a 48-item card-sorting task which addresses symptoms that are most-to-least like the patient. These techniques have both a high false positive and a false negative error rate but are found to compliment the structured interview.

The Children's Depression Rating Scale (CDRS) was developed by Poznanski et al. (1979) to be used following an interview by clinicians to rate the child according to items similar to those in the Hamilton Rating Scale of Adults. The Montgomery–Asberg Depression Rating Scale (1979) has also been used by clinicians following an interview with children. Parent rating of children by the Personality Inventory for Children (Wirt et al., 1977) has been useful in detecting depression.

Poznanski et al. (1982) has reported on the use of the dexamethasone suppression test in prepubertal children meeting criteria for major depression. Five of the nine children showed cortisol non-suppression following the administration of 0.5 mg of dexamethasone. In a recent study it was positive in 45 to 55% of those children with major depression and had a specificity of about 90%. This method of investigating depression must be further studied to determine the sensitivity and specificity for children. The last method of investigation is a clinical trial of antidepressant medication. A positive response, however, is much less conclusive in children as there are conditions other than depression that show a therapeutic response to tricyclic antidepressants.

THE EFFICACY OF ANTIDEPRESSANTS FOR CHILDHOOD DEPRESSION

Table 2 summarizes the reviewed literature on pharmacological management of affective disorders in children. This literature has been reviewed as to methodology, design and controls of the research, the instruments of evaluating improvement, the degree of improvement, duration of treatment and side effects. There have been twenty-six published reports describing drug treatment of childhood affective disorders. In general, the methodology is limited to seventeen case reports where no experimental control was implemented. Characteristically, these studies did not have a placebo phase, patient or clinician blindness, or objective review of therapeutic response. In most of these seventeen studies, the diagnostic criteria for inclusion were not rigidly described. The duration of the studies is also a significant factor, with six studies not recording length of treatment, five studies for one to three weeks, and only eight studies utilizing tricyclic antidepressants for longer than four weeks.

There were only five double blind studies. After excluding Frommer's (1967) study because of diagnostic imprecision, the remaining four double blind studies included fourteen children receiving imipramine, one child with amitriptyline and four with lithium carbonate. DeLong's (1978) study of four children receiving lithium carbonate had a double blind crossover with a placebo phase. Puig-Antich et al. (1979) conducted a crossed double blind study with a placebo phase. This study accounted for seven patients. Kashani et al. (1980) and Petti and Unis (1981) each had one patient who was in a double blind placebo-controlled crossover study.

Table 2. **Pharmacological Treatment of Affective Disorders**

Author (year)	N	Drug	Daily dosage	Duration of drug trial	Use of pla-cebo	Design
Frommer (1967)	32	Phenelzine Chlordiazepoxide Phenobarbitane	30 mg 20 mg 60 mg	2+ weeks	yes	Crossed
Annell (1969)	8	Amitriptyline and/or Lithium carbonate	30 mg 300 mg 600 mg	varied	no	Uncrossed/ case reports
Frommer (1971)	200	Amitriptyline	NR	NR	no	Uncrossed/ retrospective
Kuhn and Kuhn (1971)	100	Imipramine Desmethyl- imipramine Clomipramine Opipramol	NR	NR	no	Uncrossed/ 50% received IMI only, 50% received two or more
Stack (1971)	116	Opipramol Amitriptyline Imipramine	50 mg 2–5 mg 10 mg	4 weeks to 2 years	no	Uncrossed/ case reviews
Stack (1971)	75	Nortriptyline Amitriptyline Opipramol Phenelzine	30 mg 5–25 mg 50–150 mg NR	NR	no	Uncrossed/ case reviews
Stack (1971)	64	Phenelzine	NR	NR	no	Uncrossed/ case reviews
Stack (1971)	150	Nortriptyline Imipramine	75 mg 75 mg	NR	no	Uncrossed/ case reviews
Stack (1971)	85	Opipramol Amitriptyline	100–150 mg 75 mg	NR	no	Uncrossed/ case reports

Double blind	Diagnosis	Assessment procedures	Improvement	Side effects
yes	Affective/ depression	Clinical impression	88% combination of phenelzine and chlordiazepoxide	NR[a]
no	Affective/ manic depression	Parent, teacher, and clinician's impressions	100%	NR
no	Affective/ depression	Clinical impression	67%	NR
no	Affective/ phasic, chronic depression	NR	76%	Nausea, vomiting, dizziness, headaches, gastric upset
no	Affective/ depression (pre-school)	NR	Imipramine especially effective	Drowsiness; fatigue with opipramol and amitriptyline
no	Affective/ depression (school age)	NR	80%	Drowsiness; fatigue with opipramol and amitriptyline
no	Affective/ phobic ob- session with depressive states	NR	94%	NR
no	Affective/ mixed depression	NR	67%	NR
no	Affective/ depression related psychosis	NR	57%	Drowsiness; fatigue with opipramol and amitriptyline

(continued)

Table 2. (Continued)

Author (year)	N	Drug	Daily dosage	Duration of drug trial	Use of placebo	Design
Polvan and Cebiroglu (1971)	29	Pyrithioxin and amitriptyline, or nortriptyline and levomepromazine	According to age and weight	8 weeks	no	Uncrossed
Berg et al. (1974)	1	(Amitriptyline) Lithium carbonate	2400 mg/ 1mEq/1	1 year	no	Uncrossed/ case report prior medication ineffective
Sovner (1975)	1	(Haloperidol, mesoridazine) Lithium carbonate	2400 mg/ 1mEq/1	18+ days	no	Uncrossed/ case report prior medication ineffective
Warneke (1975)	1	(Haloperidol, doxepin) Lithium carbonate	1800 mg/ 1.2mEq/1	3 weeks	no	Uncrossed/ case report prior medication ineffective
Petti and Campbell (1975)	1	Imipramine	75 mg	20 days	no	Uncrossed/ case report
Horowitz (1977)	8	Lithium carbonate	1500– 2400 mg/ 0.5–1.2 mEq/1	2 weeks to 3 months	no	Uncrossed/ case reports/ serum levels attained
Brumback, et al. (1977)	19	Imipramine or amitriptyline	25–125 mg	4 weeks	no	Uncrossed
White and O'Shanick (1977)	1	(Haloperidol) Lithium carbonate	1200 mg/ 1mEq/1	6 weeks	no	Uncrossed/ prior medication ineffective
Brumback and Weinberg (1977)	6	Lithium carbonate	30–40 mg/kg/ 0.6–1.2 mEq/1	5–110 days	no	Uncrossed

Double blind	Diagnosis	Assessment procedures	Improvement	Side effects
no	Affective/ depression	NR	90%	NR
no	Affective/ bipolar, manic depressive psychosis	Clinical impression	Caused switch from depression to hypomania	NR
no	Affective/ manic depression	WAIS[b] Bender-Gestalt Test	Dramatic improvement	NR
no	Affective/ manic depression	Clinical impression	Marked improvement	NR
no	Affective/ manic depression	Clinical impression, EEG	Seizures occurred, IMI discontinued	Extensive seizures
no	Affective/ manic depression	Clinical impression	Marked improvement	NR
no	Affective/ depression	Clinical impression	95%	NR
no	Affective/ manic depression	Clinical impression	Marked improvement	NR
no	Affective/ manic depression	Clinical impression	33%	Nausea, anxiety, increased depression, EEG abnormalities

(continued)

Table 2. (Continued)

Author (year)	N	Drug	Daily dosage	Duration of drug trial	Use of pla-cebo	Design
DeLong (1978)	4	Lithium carbonate	450–1200 mg	6–32 months	yes	Crossed
Engstrom et al. (1978)	1	Lithium carbonate	2100–2400 mg/ 1.0–1.5 mEq/1	2+ weeks	no	Uncrossed/ case report
Puig-Antich et al. (1978)	8	Imipramine	3–5 mg/kg	6–8 weeks	no	Uncrossed
Davis (1979)	4	Lithium carbonate	0.8–1.0 mEq/1 serum level	6 months	no	Uncrossed/ case reports
Puig-Antich et al. (1979)	6 7	Imipramine	4 mg/kg	5 weeks	yes yes	Uncrossed Crossed
Kupfer et al. (1979)	12	Imipramine	4.3 mg/kg	3 weeks	no	Uncrossed
Mayo et al. (1979)		Lithium carbonate	NR	2 years	no	Uncrossed/ family (12) study
Pallmeyer and Petti (1979)	2	Imipramine	3.5–5 mg/kg	13 weeks	no	Uncrossed/ case reports
Kashani et al. (1980)	1	Amitriptyline	1.5 mg/kg	4 weeks	yes	Crossed/ case report

Double blind	Diagnosis	Assessment procedures	Improvement	Side effects
yes	Affective/ manic depression	Conner's PSQ[c]	Behaviorally effective	Minimal hand tremors, increased urination, blunted motivation
no	Affective/ manic depression	Clinical impression	Marked improvement	NR
no	Affective/ depression	RDC[d] CPRS[e]	75%	(Elicited interview) nausea, constipation somnolent tachycardia anorexia
no	Affective/ manic depression	Parental symptom assessment	Marked improvement	NR
no yes	Affective/ major depression	Kiddie-SADS[f] RDC	Plasma levels indicated good response	NR
no	Affective/ depression	EEG, sleep observation, clinical assessment	REM suppression	Sleep disturbance
no	Affective/ bipolar manic depression	RDC, CGI,[g] CPRS	Substantial decrease in stress events during treatment	NA[h]
no	Affective/ depression	CBI[i]	Anger and hostility increased with IMI	Hostility, anger
yes	Affective/ depression	Clinical impression	Hypomanic reaction (dose reduced)	Hypomanic side effects

(continued)

Table 2. (Continued)

Author (year)	N	Drug	Daily dosage	Duration of drug trial	Use of pla- cebo	Design
Petti et al. (1980)	1	Imipramine	5 mg/kg	40 days	no	Prior psycho- therapy ineffective/ uncrossed
Petti and Unis (1981)	1	Imipramine	5 mg/kg	1 week	yes	Crossed/ case report
Weller et al. (1982)	11	Imipramine	5 mg/kg	20 days	no	Uncrossed

[a]NR – not reported.
[b]WAIS – Wechsler Adult Intelligence Scale
[c]Conner's PSQ – Conner's Parent Symptom Questionnaire
[d]RDC – Research Diagnostic Criteria
[e]CPRS – Children's Psychiatric Rating Scale
[f]Kiddie-SADS – Schedule for Affective Disorders and Schizophrenia for School Age Children
[g]CGI – Clinical Global Impression Scale
[h]NA – not applicable
[i]CBI – Children's Behavior Inventory
[j]SoSAD – Scale of School Age Depression

Clinical improvement was measured in twelve studies by nonspecific clinician judgement alone, in seven by an unspecified method, and in nine studies by a combination of rating scales, clinical judgement and serial psychometric tests. With the above-mentioned limitations in mind, the reported efficacy for tricyclic antidepressants and monoamine oxidase inhibitors was between 57 and 100% with a mean of 85%. Puig-Antich (1979) and Weller (1982) have unequivocally demonstrated that serum levels of desmethylimipramine and imipramine were correlated with therapeutic efficacy, and that only with levels within the 150–300 ng/ml range will a positive therapeutic response be observed. Because these studies have been reported in a total of only twenty-four subjects, more subjects should be studied in order to replicate these preliminary reports.

Side effects observed were hypomania and aggression (Berg et al., 1974; Pallmeyer and Petti, 1979; Kashani et al.. 1980) and REM suppression (Kupfer

Double blind	Diagnosis	Assessment procedures	Improvement	Side effects
no	Affective/ depression	CBI, SoSAD[j]	Behavioral symptoms improved	NR
no	Affective/ depression borderline psychosis	Clinical and parent assessment PALS-C	Marked improvement	NR
no	Affective/ major depression	Plasma IMI levels, CGI rating scales	100%	Minimal— tachycardia syncope diaphoresis

et al. 1978). Puig-Antich et al. (1978) have documented cardiac arrythmias as a function of tricyclic antidepressant dosage. Monitoring for EKG abnormalities when one exceeds 3.5 mg/kg is mandatory as first degree heart blocks are common beyond this dosage.

ANTIDEPRESSANTS AND LITHIUM IN THE TREATMENT OF ATTENTION DEFICIT DISORDER

Twenty studies have been reviewed in which children with behavioral problems, specifically ADD, have been treated with antidepressants or Lithium (Table 3). The research examined the question of tricyclic antidepressant efficacy alone, and in comparison to the established standard of treatment,

Table 3. Pharmacological Treatment of Attentional Deficit Disorders/Hyperactivity

Author (year)	N	Drug	Daily dosage	Duration of drug trial	Use of placebo	Design
Rapoport (1964)	41	(d-amphetamine) Imipramine	5–30 mg	6 months 2 years	no	Uncrossed/ transferred to IMI when available
Krakowski (1965)	50	Amitriptyline	40 mg	30 days	yes	Uncrossed
Huessy and Wright (1971)	52	Imipramine	50 mg	2+ weeks	no	Uncrossed
Winsberg et al. (1972)	32	Imipramine d-amphetamine	150 mg 15–30 mg	7–10 days	yes	Counter balanced order
Greenhill et al. (1973)	9	d-amphetamine Lithium carbonate	10 mgs .8–1.2 mEq/1 serum level	3 weeks	yes	Crossed
Gross (1973)	259	d-amphetamine Methylphenidate Imipramine	3–10 mg 6–20 mg 20–100 mg	1 week	yes	Crossed/ retrospective
Brown et al. (1973)	3	Imipramine	150–225 mg	3 weeks	no	Uncrossed
Saraf et al. (1974)	102 (37 placebo)	Imipramine	132 mg	4 weeks	yes	Uncrossed
Waizer et al. (1972)	19	Imipramine	173 mg	8 weeks	yes	IMI/placebo, crossed

Double blind	Diagnosis	Assessment procedures	Improvement	Side effects
no	Behavior disorder/ learning problems	Achievement test, Rorschach, Bender–Gestalt	80.5%	Dry mouth, constipation
yes	ADD/ hyper-activity	Clinical impression, observation	72.3%	Drowsiness, perspiration, mydriasis
no	ADD/ hyper-activity	Parent and teacher impressions, report cards	67%	Irritability, constipation, dry mouth, hypertension
yes	ADD/ hyper-activity, aggressive	Conners' BRS[b]	69% (IMI responders) 44% (d-amph. responders)	NR[a]
yes	ADD/ hyper-activity	Conners' PSQ[c] Conners' TRS[d]	33%	Seizures, hyperthy-roidism, drowsiness
yes	MBD	Parent/ teacher rating	d-amphetamine, 21%; Methylphenidate, 26%; Imipramine, 21%	Anorexia, insomnia
no	ADD/ hyper-activity	Clinical impression	Seizures associated with imipramine	Seizures
no	ADD/ hyper-activity, school phobic	Checklist from inter-view of child and parent	Side effects in 43%	Dry mouth, nausea, tremors, sweating
no	ADD/ hyper-activity	CPRS,[e] CGI,[f] Conners' PSQ, Conners' TRS	IMI effective in reducing hyper-activity	Anorexia, insomnia

(continued)

Table 3. (Continued)

Author (year)	N	Drug	Daily dosage	Duration of drug trial	Use of placebo	Design
Rapoport et al. (1974)	76	Imipramine Methylphenidate	80 mg 20 mg	6 weeks	yes	Uncrossed
Greenberg et al. (1975)	47	Imipramine Methylphenidate	6.5 mg/kg 3.6 mg/kg	6 days	yes	Crossed
Winsberg et al. (1975)	7	Imipramine	5 mg/kg	4 weeks	no	Uncrossed
Gross (1976)	100	Methylphenidate d-amphetamine Imipramine	34 mg 16 mg 82 mg	5 years	yes	Uncrossed/ retrospective
Fras and Karlavage (1977)	3	Methylphenidate Imipramine	10–20 mg 25 mg	3 days	no	Uncrossed
Yepes et al (1977)	22	Amitriptyline Methylphenidate	92 mg 39.1 mg	2 weeks	yes	Crossed/ counter- balanced order
Gulatieri and Staye (1979)	1	(Methylphenidate) Amitriptyline	30 mg/ml	7 months	no	Uncrossed/ prior medication ineffective
Linnoila et al. (1979)	5	Imipramine Desipramine	67.7 mg	7 days	no	Crossed
Werry et al. (1980)	30	Methylphenidate Imipramine	.4 mg 1–2 mg	4 weeks	yes	Crossed

Double blind	Diagnosis	Assessment procedures	Improvement	Side effects
yes	ADD/hyper-activity	Conners' TRS, Conners' PSQ	Improvement relatively equal in IMI and methylphenidate	Constipation, drowsiness, increased diastolic blood pressure
yes	ADD/hyper-activity	Home and classroom inventories	Methyl/placebo different, IMI/placebo not different	Appetite loss, sleep disturb-ance
no	ADD/hyper-activity	EKG	NR	EKG abnor-malities
no	ADD/hyper-activity	Growth measure-ments	Less than expected growth rate due to medication is overcome with time	Growth rate diminution
no	Tourette's	Clinical observation	Deterioration with both drugs	Exacerbation of symptoms
yes	ADD/hyper-activity	CPT,[g] WWPAS[h] Conners' BRS	Comparably effective in both drugs	Anorexia, insomnia, headache
no	ADD/hyper-activity	Withdrawal symptoms	Limited success	Nausea, vomiting abdominal cramps, dehydration
yes	ADD/hyper-activity	Conners' PTQ,[i] WWPAS, CPT	Therapeutic response with low IMI plasma and RBC level	NR
yes	ADD/hyper-activity	CGI, CPT, Conners' PTQ	Imipramine more effective than methylphenidate	Weight loss, heart rate, blood pressure increase

(continued)

Table 3. (Continued)

Author (year)	N	Drug	Daily dosage	Duration of drug trial	Use of placebo	Design
Winsberg et al. (1980)	10	Imipramine	3.7 mg/kg	2 weeks	yes	Crossed
Dvoredsky and Stewart (1981)	2	Lithium carbonate	NR	NR	no	Uncrossed/ case reports

[a]NR – not reported
[b]Conners' BRS – Conners' Behavior Rating Scale
[c]Conners' PSQ – Conners' Parent Symptom Questionnaire
[d]Conners' TRS – Conners' Teacher Rating Scale
[e]CPRS – Children's Psychiatric Rating Scale
[f]CGI – Clinical Global Impression Scale
[g]CPT – Continuous Performance Task
[h]WWPAS – Werry-Weiss-Peters Activity Scale
[i]Conners' PTQ – Conners' Parent-Teacher Questionnaire

methylphenidate. Of the twenty studies, twelve had placebo comparisons, and of these, eight were a crossed or counter-balanced design. There was a total of ten double blind studies. No antidepressant serum levels were done in these studies so that appropriate dosage cannot be evaluated. In only four reports was improvement judged by clinical or parent/teacher impression. Otherwise, therapeutic efficacy was assessed by psychometric tests, rating scales and clinical interviews. In general, the methodology appears more precise than that used for depressed children, so that the conclusions may be more objectively derived and generalized.

Improvement was judged to be within the 65 to 70% range. Rapoport et al. (1974), Winsberg et al. (1972), Greenberg et al. (1975), Yepes et al. (1977), Linnoila (1979) and Werry et al. (1980) showed a positive therapeutic response over a brief study period (one to six weeks). Only two short-term controlled studies (Greenberg et al. 1975; Winsberg, 1980) demonstrated a lower efficacy than stimulants, whereas Winsberg et al. (1972), Rapoport et al. (1974), Yepes et al. (1977), and Werry et al. (1980) showed equal or superior effects of the tricyclic antidepressants compared to stimulants. Quinn and Rapoport (1975) subsequently demonstrated that very few ADD children treated with imipramine over a long period continued to show a positive therapeutic response.

Double blind	Diagnosis	Assessment procedures	Improvement	Side effects
yes	ADD/ hyper- activity	Conners' BRS, WWPAS, CPT	No significant therapeutic effect	Anorexia, dry mouth, insomnia, heart rate increase
no	ADD/ hyper- activity	Clinical observation	Good response	NR

Overall, side effects have been more severe than those with sympathomimetic medication. Winsberg et al. (1980) and Saraf et al. (1974) demonstrated a dose dependent cardiotoxicity with greater than 3.7 mg/kg. A first degree heart block, prolongation of the P-R interval, was observed. Second degree heart blocks have also been observed. Seizures were noted to be associated with imipramine use (Brown et al., 1973). In general, the short-term efficacy demonstrates the amelioration of attentional and conduct problems not associated with affective disturbance. If treatment outcome is one method of addressing classification, the finding that the long-term effects are poor, supports the diagnostic separation of Attention Deficit Disorder from depressed children.

TRICYCLIC ANTIDEPRESSANTS FOR ENURESIS

Table 4 summarizes recent reports on tricyclic antidepressant use in enuresis, six of which were double blind placebo-controlled crossover studies. These six studies review the efficacy of imipramine, chlordiazepoxide, desipramine, scopolamine, amphetamine, emopronium, and/or ephedrine over a two to

Table 4. Pharmacological Treatment of Enuresis

Author (year)	N	Drug	Daily dosage	Duration of drug trial	Use of pla-cebo	Design
Shaffer et al. (1968)	58	Imipramine	50–75 mg	1 month	yes	Crossed
McConaghy (1969)	60	Imipramine Amphetamine	10–75 mg 7.5 mg	12 weeks	yes	Uncrossed
Alderton (1970)	9	Imipramine	50 mg	4 weeks	yes	Crossed
Kunin et al. (1970)	30	Imipramine Ephedrine	25–50 mg 7.5–15 mg	28 days	no	Crossed
Peterson et al. (1973)	69	Imipramine Imipramine-N-oxide Emopronium	50 mg	4 weeks	yes	Crossed
Martin and Zaug (1975)	27	Imipramine	25–75 mg	2 months	no	Uncrossed
Werry et al. (1975)	20	Imipramine Chlordiazepoxide	50 mg 10 mg	3 weeks	yes	Crossed
Werry et al. (1975)	21	Imipramine	50 mg	3 weeks	yes	Crossed/counter-balanced
Rapoport et al. (1980)	40	Imipramine Desipramine Methscopolamine	75 mg 75 mg 6 mg	2 weeks	yes	Crossed

[a]NR – not reported
[b]Conners' PTQ – Conners' Parent–Teacher Questionnaire
[c]CGI – Clinical Global Impression Scale.

Double blind	Diagnosis	Assessment procedures	Improvement	Side effects
yes	Enuresis	Enuretic report	86 %	Constipation, dry mouth
no	Enuresis	Enuretic report	IMI−54%; amphetamine ineffective	Insomnia, Anorexia
yes	Enuresis	Enuretic report	More dry nights	NR[a]
yes	Enuresis	Enuretic report	IMI−51% ephedrine ineffective	NR
yes	Enuresis	Enuretic report	IMI−55%; N-oxide−74%; emopronium ineffective	NR
no	Enuresis	Enuretic report, EKG	60%	NR
yes	Enuresis	Enuretic report, Conners' PTQ,[b] CGI[c]	IMI decreased frequency; Chlordiazepoxide ineffective	Increased heart rate, weight loss
yes	Enuresis	Enuretic report	More dry nights	Sedation, stomach ache, anorexia
yes	Enuresis	Parental assessment	IMI and DMI superior to methscopolamine	Dry mouth

Table 5. Pharmacological Treatment for School Phobia

Author (year)	N	Drug	Daily dosage	Duration of drug trial	Use of placebo	Design
Gittelman-Klein and Klein (1973)	35	Imipramine	150 mg	6 weeks	yes	Uncrossed
Berney et al. (1981)	46	Clomipramine	75 mg	12 weeks	yes	Uncrossed

[a]CBQ – Children's Behavior Questionnaire
[b]PIRF – Psychiatric Interview Rating Form
[c]NR, not reported

four week period. The children studied in these controlled reports showed marked improvement by having more dry nights as compared to when they received placebo or other drugs. The three limitations of these reports are that they do not address the long-term efficacy, the relapse rate following drug cessation, and a comparison to behavioral modification programs of known efficacy. It is significant that only a modest dosage was administered. A maximum dose of 75 mg was used. Side effects were minimal or not reported. Of all the research with tricyclic antidepressants in children, this group of studies is clearly the most supportive of the role of pharmacology in the child's overall management. At present, more studies are needed comparing medication to behavior modification techniques. In addition, a further exploration of the neurochemical substrate by which tricyclic antidepressants exert their antienuretic effects would be useful.

THE TREATMENT OF SCHOOL PHOBIA

Table 5 reviews two articles that report tricyclic antidepressant treatment of school phobia/separation anxiety. Saraf et al. (1974) also describe the side effects in one group of children. Imipramine efficacy was studied in primates documenting its efficacy for separation anxiety (Suomi, 1978).

Interestingly, the two clinical reports present conflicting findings. Gittleman-Klein and Klein (1973) showed in a double blind, placebo controlled, uncrossed study, a high response rate to approximately 150 mg of imipramine in thirty-five school phobic children. The duration of the drug trial was approximately six

Double blind	Diagnosis	Assessment procedures	Improvement	Side effects
yes	School phobia	School attendance, CBQ,[a] PIRF[b]	School return in 70%	Dry mouth, constipation, dizziness, tremor
yes	School phobia	Clinical impression/ assessment	Significant improvement with Clomipramine	NR[c]

weeks, with 70% returning to school with the others showing an incomplete decrease in their school phobic symptoms. [In a recent study by the same authors (1980), 88% of forty-five school phobics improved and returned to school.] Berney et al. (1981) in a double blind uncrossed study lasting twelve weeks, described forty-six school phobic children who received 75 mg of clomipramine. The tricyclic antidepressant could not be differentiated from the placebo. There is criticism of both studies. Both were open studies and showed high spontaneous remission or placebo rate of improvement. In the earlier study, patients were selected by their failure to respond to psychotherapy. The second study has been criticized because of the low dosage, and the greater likelihood of diagnostic heterogeneity of this sample of school phobic children. Although these initial results are very promising, this area of tricyclic antidepressant usage requires more study under controlled conditions.

CONCLUSIONS

There have been two significant developments in the area of childhood depression and its treatment. First, research has focused on the identification of the depressive syndrome and the disease depression. Unlike studies of adult depression, there are no family studies, biological markers, neuroendocrine, neurochemical, neurophysiological investigations, or longitudinal studies. Currently, the diagnosis of the cross-sectional state of depression can be made reliably through structured psychiatric interviews, clinical rating scales and psychometric tests. Also, there is a need for the recognition of diverse symptom presentation resulting from developmental factors. Interestingly, there is a sub-group of depressed children who meet DSM-III and RDC criteria for major depression and conduct disorder.

There has been, however, little progress in the delineation of a depressive disease. Most researchers agree that family studies, further biological research and longitudinal investigations will support the existence of this syndrome. Promising results have been obtained with the dexamethasone suppression test. Its specificity and sensitivity may be similar to that observed with adults. The routine use of this test with prepubertal children is warranted.

Winokur et al. (1982) has shown an incidence of major depression of 10 to 14% in family members of patients with bipolar affective illnesses. This group of children may be the appropriate at-risk population to study further for the description of the disease. Follow-up studies, like that of Poznanski et al. (1976) should be repeated on a larger sample of depressed children with or without con-duct disorders. The outcome research to date on conduct-disordered children (Vaillant, 1981; Robins, 1966) has not found that this disorder is associated with a higher incidence of adult depression.

The second area reviewed was the efficacy of antidepressant medication. The studies that were most vigorously controlled and have the least equivocal results are for disorders other than depression. Tricyclic antidepressants are the pharmacological treatment of first choice for enuresis. Comparisons with placebo are unanimously in favor of tricylic antidepressants. At this time, further comparisons between tricyclics and behavioral modification procedures such as completed by McConaghy (1969), as well as studies of the relapse rate following drug cessation, are necessary. A second paradoxical finding concerns the high efficacy with very low doses. Future research should include serum levels of tricyclic antidepressants needed to ameliorate enuresis as compared with serum levels effective for other conditions.

The treatment of school phobia is still a controversial area. There are two major studies with known methodological limitations. Because of different drugs (clomipramine vs. imipramine), different doses (50–75 vs 150 mg), different samples (all school phobics vs. psychotherapy treatment failures), generaliza-tions cannot be made about tricyclic antidepressant efficacy at this time. This would be an exceedingly worthwhile area to study further in a systematic manner.

The ADD studies are an example of more precise methodology. The short-term efficacy is equal to or greater than that of sympathomimetic medication. It will be important to determine the reason for the drop-off of efficacy with pro-longed use. Future research must include serum levels, objective ratings of drug efficacy and crossover design with placebo, sympathomimetic medication, and behavioral modification phases.

Drug research into the treatment of affective disorders in children and adolescents is confounded by imprecise methodology. Case reports of open clinical trials is what is commonly reported. Double blind, placebo controlled, crossover studies with precise inclusion criteria are exceedingly rare. Serum levels with objective clinical rating is also necessary. With these controls, the question concerning the efficacy of tricyclic antidepressant medication for the treatment of depression in children can ultimately be answered.

REFERENCES

Alderton, H.R. Imipramine in childhood enuresis: Further studies on the relationship of time of administration to effect. *Can. Med. Assoc. J* 102: 1179–1180, 1972.

Annell, A.L. Manic-depressive illness in children and effect of treatment with lithium carbonate. *Acta. Paedopsychiatrica. (Basel)* 36(8/9/10):292–301, 1969.

Anthony, E.J., and Scott, P. Manic-depressive psychosis in childhood. *J Child. Psychol. Psychiatry* 1:53–72, 1960.

Berg, I., Hullin, R., Allsopp, M., O'Brien, P., and MacDonald, R. Bipolar manic-depressive psychosis in early adolescence: A case report. *Br. J. Psychiatry* 125:416–417, 1974.

Berney, T., Kolvin, I., Bhate, S.R., Garside, R.F., Jeans, J., Kay, B., and Scarth, L. School phobia: A therapeutic trial of clomipramine and short-term outcome. *Br. J. Psychiatry* 138:110–118, 1981.

Brown, D., Winsberg, B.G., Bialer, I., and Press, M. Imipramine therapy and seizures: Three children treated for hyperactive behavior disorders. *Am. J. Psychiatry* 130(2):210–212, 1973.

Brumback, R.A., Dietz-Schmidt, S.G., and Weinberg, W.A. Depression in children referred to an educational diagnostic center: Diagnosis and treatment and analysis of criteria and literature review. *Dis. Nerv. Sys.* 38:529–534, 1977.

Brumback, R.A., and Weinberg, W.A. Mania in childhood: II. Therapeutic trial of lithium carbonate and further description of manic-depressive illness in children. *Am. J. Dis. Child.* 131:112–126, 1977.

Cantwell, D.P., and Carlson, G. Problems and prospects in the study of childhood depression. *J. Nerv. Ment. Dis.* 167(9):522–529, 1979.

Carlson, G.A., and Cantwell, D.P. A survey of depressive symptoms in a child and adolescent psychiatric population: Interview data. *J. Am. Acad. Child. Psychiatry* 18(4):587–599, 1979.

Carlson, G.A., and Cantwell, D.P. A survey of depressive symptoms, syndrome and disorder in a child psychiatric population. *J. Child. Psychol. Psychiatry* 21:19–25, 1980.

Carlson, G.A., and Cantwell, D.P. Unmasking masked depression in children and adolescents. *Am. J. Psychiatry* 137(4):445–449, 1980.

Carlson, G.A., and Cantwell, D.P. Diagnosis of childhood depression: a comparison of the Weinberg and DSM-III Criteria. *J. Am. Acad. Child. Psychiatry* 21:247–250, 1982.

Carlson, G.A., and Strober, M. Manic-depressive illness in early adolescence: A study of clinical and diagnostic characteristics in sex cases. *J. Am. Acad. Child. Psychiatry* 17(1):138–153, 1978.

Chambers, W.J., Puig-Antich, J., Tabrizi, M.A. The ongoing development of the Kiddie-SADS (Schedule for Affective Disorders and Schizophrenia for School-age Children). Read at the American Academy of Child Psychiatry Annual Meeting, San Diego, Calif., 1978.

Cytryn, L., and McKnew, D.H. Proposed classification of childhood depression. *Am. J. Psychiatry* 129(2):63–69, 1972.

Cytryn, L., and McKnew, D.H. Factors influencing the changing clinical expression of the depressive process in children. *Am. J. Psychiatry* 131(8):879–881, 1974.

Cytryn, J., McKnew, D.H., Bunney, W.E. Diagnosis of depression in children. A reassessment. *Am. J. Psychiatry* 137(1):22–25, 1980.

Davis, R.E. Manic-depressive variant syndrome of childhood: A preliminary report. *Am. J. Psychiatry* 136(5):702–705, 1979.

DeLong, G.R. Lithium carbonate treatment of select behavior disorders in suggesting manic-depressive illness. *J. Pediatrics* 93(4):689–694, 1978.

Dvoredsky, A.E., and Stuart, M.A. Hyperactivity followed by manic-depressive disorder: Two case reports. *J. Clin. Psychiatry* 42(5):212–214, 1981.

Endicott, J., and Spitzer, R.L. Use of the Research Diagnostic Criteria and the Schedule for Affective Disorders and Schizophrenia for School-age Children. *Am. J. Psychiatry* 136:52–56, 1979.

Engstrom, F.W., Robbins, D.R., and May, J.G. Manic-depressive illness in adolescence. *J. Am. Acad. Child Psychiatry* 17(3):514–520, 1978.

Feighner, J.P., Robins, E., Guze, S.B., Woodruff, R.A., Winokur, G., and Munoz, R. Diagnostic criteria for use in psychiatric research. *Arch. Gen. Psychiatry* 26:57–63, 1972.

Fras, I., and Karlavage, J. The use of methylphenidate and imipramine on Gilles de la Tourette's disease in children. *Am. J. Psychiatry* 134(2):195–197, 1977.

Frommer, E.A. Treatment of childhood with antidepressant drugs. *Br. Med. Journal* 1:729–732, 1967.

Frommer, E.A. Indications for antidepressant treatment with special reference to depressed preschool children. In: *Depressive States in Childhood and Adolescence*. Proc. 4th U.E.P. Congress, Stockholm: Almquist & Wiksell, 1971, pp. 449–454.

Gittleman-Klein, R., and Klein, D.F. Separation anxiety in school refusal and its treatment wtth drugs. In: *Out of School*, L. Hersov and I. Berg, eds. New York: Wiley & Sons, 1980, 321–340.

Glaser, K. Masked depression in children and adolescents. *Am. J. Psychotherapy* 21:565–574, 1967.

Greenberg, L.M., Yellin, A.M., Spring, C., and Metcalf, M. Clinical effects of imipramine and methylphenidate in hyperactive children. *Intl. J. Mental Health* 4:144–155, 1975.

Greenhill, U., Rieder, R.O., Wender, P.H., Buchsbaum, H., and Zahn, T.P. Lithium carbonate in the treatment of hyperactive children. *Arch. Gen. Psychiatry* 28:636–640, 1973.

Gross, M.D. Imipramine in the treatment of minimal brain dysfunction in children. *Psychosomatics* 14:283–285, 1973.

Gross, M.D. Growth of hyperkinetic children taking methylphenidate, dextroamphetamine or imipramine/desipramine. *Pediatrics* 58(3):423–431, 1976.

Gualtieri, C.T., and Staye, J. Withdrawal symptoms after abrupt cessation of amitriptyline in an eight-year-old boy. *Am. J. Psychiatry* 136(4A):457–458, 1979.

Herjanic, B. Follow-up study of 200 children given a discharge diagnosis of depression. St Louis Children's Hospital. Presented at the American Psychiatric Association Meeting, Miami, Florida, 1976.

Horowitz, H.A. Lithium and the treatment of adolescent manic-depressive illness. *Dis. Nerv. Sys.* 38(6):480–483, 1977.

Huessey, H.R., and Wright, A.L. The use of imipramine in children's behavior disorders. *Acta. Paedopsychiatrica. (Basel)* 37:194–199, 1971.

Kanner, L. *Child Psychiatry* (2nd edition), Springfield, Illinois: CC Thomas, 1948.

Kashani, J.H., Hodges, K.K., Shekim, W.O. Hypomanic reaction to amitriptyline in a depressed child. *Psychosomatics* 21(10):867–872, 1980.

Kazdin, A.E. Assessment techniques for childhood depression: A critical appraisal. *J. Am. Acad. Child Psychiatry* 20(2):358–375, 1981.

Kovacs, M., and Beck, A.T. An empirical clinical approach toward the definition of childhood depression. In: *Depression in Childhood*, J.G. Schulterbrandt and A. Raskin, eds. New York: Raven Press, pp. 1–25, 1977.

Kraepelin, E. *Manic-Depressive Insanity and Paranoia*, Livingstone, Edinburgh, pp. 167–170, 1921.

Krakowski, A.J. Amitriptyline in treatment of hyperkinetic children. *Psychosomatics* Sept-Oct, 355–360, 1965.

Kuhn, V., and Kuhn, R. Drug therapy for depression in children: Indications and methods. In: *Depressive States in Childhood and Adolescence*, Proc. 4th U.E.P. Congress, Stockholm: Almquist and Wiksell, pp. 455–459, 1971.

Kunin, S.A., Limbert, D.J., Platzker, A.C.G., and McGinley, J. The efficacy of imipramine in the management of enuresis. *J. Urol.* 104:612–615, 1970.

Kupfer, D.J., Cable, P., Kane, J., Petti, T., and Conners, C.K. Imipramine and EEG sleep in children with depressive symptoms. *Psychopharmacology* 60:117–123, 1979.

Lang, M., and Tisher, M. *Children Depression Scale*. Victoria, Australia, The Council for Educational Research, 1978.

Linnoila, M., Gualtieri, T., Jobson, K., and Staye, J. Characteristics of the therapeutic response to imipramine in hyperactive children. *Am. J. Psychiatry* 136(9):1201–1205, 1979.

Malmquist, C.P. Depression in childhood and adolescence. *N. Eng. J. Med.* 284:887–893, 1971.

Martin, G.L., and Zaug, P.J. Electrocardiographic monitoring enuretic children receiving therapeutic doses of imipramine. *Am. J. Psychiatry* 132(5):544–551, 1975.

McConaghy, N. A controlled trial of imipramine, amphetamine, pad-and-bell conditioning and random awakening in the treatment of nocturnal enuresis. *Med. J. Australia* 2:237–239, 1969.

McConville, B.J., Boag, L.C., and Purohit, A.P. Three types of childhood depression. *Can. Psychiatr. Assoc. Journal* 18:133–137.

Montgomery, S.A., and Asberg, M. A new depression scale designed to be sensitive to change. *Br. J. Psychiatry* 134:382–389, 1979.

Ossofsky, H.J. Endogenous, depression in infancy and childhood. *Comprehensive Psychiatry* 15:19–25, 1974.

Pallmeyer, T.P., and Petti, T.A. Effects of imipramine on aggression and dejection in depressed children. *Am. J. Psychiatry* 136(11):1472-1473, 1979.

Peterson, K.E., Andersen, O.O., and Hansen, T. The mode of action of imipramine and related drugs and their value in the treatment of different categories of nocturnal enuresis. *Eur. J. Clin. Pharmacol* 7:187-194, 1973.

Petti, T.A. Depression in hospitalized child psychiatry patients: Approaches to measuring depression. *J. Am. Acad. Child Psychiatry* 17(1):49-59, 1978.

Petti, T.A., Bornstein, M., Delameter, A., and Conners, C.K. Evaluation and multimodality treatment of a depressed prepubertal girl. *J. Am. Acad. Child Psychiatry* 19(4):690-702, 1980.

Petti, T.A., and Campbell, M. Imipramine and seizures. *Am. J. Psychiatry* 132(5): 538-539, 1975.

Petti, T.A., and Unis, A. Imipramine treatment of borderline children's case reports with a controlled study. *Am. J. Psychiatry* 134(4):516-518, 1981.

Polvan, O., and Cebiroglu, R. Treatment with psychopharmacologic agents in childhood depressions. In: *Depressive States in Childhood and Adolescence*, Proc. 4th U.E.P. Congress, Stockholm: Almquist and Wiksell, 467-472, 1971.

Poznanski, E.O., Carroll, B.J., Banegas, M.C., Cook, S.C., and Grossman, J.A. The dexamethasone suppression test in prepubertal depressed children. *Am. J. Psychiatry* 139(3):321-324, 1982.

Poznanski, E.O., Cook, S.C., and Carroll, B.J. A depression rating scale for children. *Pediatrics* 64:442-450, 1979.

Poznanski, E.O., Krahenbuhl, V., and Zrull, J.P. Childhood depression: A longitudinal perspective. *J. Am. Acad. Child Psychiatry* 15:491-501, 1976.

Puig-Antich, J. Affective disorders in childhood. *Psychiatric Clinics of North America* 3(3):401-424, 1980.

Puig-Antich, J. Major depression and conduct disorder in prepuberty. *J. Am. Acad. Child Psychiatry* 21(2):118-128, 1982.

Puig-Antich, J., Blau, S., Marx, N., Greenhill, L.L., and Chambers, W. Prepubertal major depressive disorder. *J. Am. Acad. Child Psychiatry* 17:695-707, 1978.

Puig-Antich, J., Perel, J.M., Lupatkin, W., Chambers, W.J., Shea, C., Tabrizi, M.A., and Stiller, R.L. Plasma levels of imipramine (IMI) and desmethylimipramine (DMI) and clinical response in prepubertal major depressive disorders. *J. Am. Acad. Child Psychiatry* 18(4):616-627, 1979.

Quinn, P.O., and Rapoport, J.L. One-year follow-up of hyperactive boys treated with imipramine or methylphenidate. *Am. J. Psychiatry* 132(3):241-245, 1975.

Rapoport, J. Childhood behavior and learning problems treated with imipramine. *Intl. J. Neuropsychiatry* Nov-Dec: 635-642, 1965.

Rapoport, J.L., Mikkelson, E.J., Zavadil, A., Nee, L., Gruenau, C., Mendelson, W., and Gillin, J.C. Childhood enuresis II. Psychopathology, tricyclic concentration in plasma and antienuretic effect. *Arch. Gen. Psychiatry* 37: 1149-1152, 1980.

Rapoport, J.L., Quinn, P.O., Bradbard, G., Riddle, D., and Brooks, E. Imipramine and methylphenidate treatment of hyperactive boys. *Arch. Gen. Psychiatry* 30(6):789-793, 1974.

Rie, H.E. Depression in childhood. *J. Am. Acad. Child Psychiatry* 5:653-685, 1966.

Robbins, D.R., Alessi, N.E., Cook, S.C., Poznanski, E.O., and Yanchyshyn, G. H. The use of the research diagnostic criteria (RDC) for depression in adolescent psychiatric inpatients. *J. Am. Acad. Child Psychiatry* 21:251-255, 1982.

Robins, L.N. *Deviant Children Grown up: A Sociological and Psychiatric Study of Sociopathic Personality*, Baltimore: Williams and Wilkins, 1966.

Rutter, M. Maternal deprivation reconsidered. *J. Psychosom. Research* 16:241-250, 1972.

Saraf, K.R., Klein, D.F., Gittleman-Klein, R., and Groff, S. Imipramine side effects in children. *Psychopharmacologia (Berel)* 37:265-274, 1974.

Shaffer, D., Costello, A.J., and Hill, I.D. Control of enuresis with imipramine. *J. Dis. Childhood* 43:665-671, 1968.

Shaffer, D., and Greenhill, L. A critical note on the predictive validity of the "hyperkinetic syndrome". *J. Child Psychol. Psychiatry* 20:61-72, 1979.

Sovner, R. The diagnosis and treatment of manic depressive illness in childhood and adolescence. *Psychiatric Opinion* 12(9):37-42, 1975.

Spitz, R.A., Wolf, K.M. Anaclitic depression. *Psychoanalytic Study of the Child* 2:313-342, 1946.

Stack, J. J. Chemotherapy in childhood depression. In: *Depressive States in Childhood and Adolescence*. Proc. 4th U.E.P. Congress, Stockholm: Almquist and Wiksell, pp. 460-466, 1971.

Suomi, S.J., Seaman, S.F., Lewis, J.K., DeLizio, R.D., and McKinncy, W.T. Effects of imipramine treatment of separation-induced social disorders in rhesus monkeys. *Arch. Gen. Psychiatry* 35:321-325, 1978.

Vaillant, G.E., and Vaillant, C.O. Natural history of male psychological health. X:Work as a predictor of positive mental health. *Am. J. Psychiatry* 138(11): 1433-1440, 1981.

Waizer, J., Hoffman, S.P., Polizos, P., and Engelhardt, D.M. Outpatient treatment of hyperactive school children with imipramine. *Am. J. Psychiatry* 131(5):587-591, 1974.

Warneke, L. A case of manic-depressive illness in childhood. *Can. Psychiatr. Assoc. Journal* 20:195-200, 1975.

Weinberg, W., Rutman, J., Sullivan, L., Penick, E., and Dietz, S. Depression in children referred to an educational diagnostic center: Diagnosis and treatment/preliminary report. *J. Pediatrics* 83:1065-1072, 1973.

Weller, E.B., Weller, R.A., Preskorn, S.H., and Glotzbach, R. Steady state plasma imipramine levels in prepubertal depressed children. *Am. J. Psychiatry* 139(4):506-508, 1982.

Welner, Z. Childhood depression: An overview. *J. Nerv. Ment. Dis.* 166(8):588-593, 1978.

Wender, P.H., Reimherr, F.W., and Wood, D.R. Attention deficit disorder (minimal brain dysfunction) in adults. *Arch. Gen. Psychiatry* 38:449-456, 1981.

Werry, J.S., Aman, M.G., and Diamond, C. Imipramine and methylphenidate in hyperactive children. *J. Child Psychiatry* 21:27-35, 1980.

Werry, J. S., Aman, M.G., Dowrick, P., and Lampen, E.L. Imipramine and chlordiazepoxide in enuresis. *Psychopharmacology Bull.* 13:38-39, 1977.

Werry, J.S., Dowrick, P.W., Lampen, E.L., and Vamos, M.J. Imipramine in enuresis: psychological and physiological effects. *J. Child Psychol. Psychiatry* 16:289-299, 1975.

White, J.H., O'Shanick, G. Juvenile manic-depressive illness. *Am. J. Psychiatry* 134(9):1035–1036, 1977.

Winokur, G., Tsuang, M.T., and Cross, R.R. The Iowa 500: Affective disorders in relatives of manic and depressed patients. *Am. J. Psychiatry* 139(2):209–212, 1982.

Winsberg, B.G., Bialer, I., Kupietz, S., and Tobias, J. Effects of imipramine and *d*-amphetamine on behavior of neuropsychiatrically impaired children. *Am. J. Psychiatry* 128(11):1425–1431, 1972.

Winsberg, B.G., Goldstein, S., Yepes, L.E., and Perel, J.M. Imipramine and electrocardiographic abnormalities in hyperactive children. *Am. J. Psychiatry* 132(5):542–545, 1975.

Winsberg, B.G., Kupietz, S.S., and Yepes, L.E. Ineffectiveness of imipramine in children who fail to respond to methylphenidate. *J. Aut. Devel. Ass.* 10(2):129–137, 1980.

Wirt, R.D., Lachar, D., Klinedinst, J.K., and Seat, P.D. *Multidimensional Description of Child Personality: Personality Inventory for Children*, WPS Publishers: Calif., 1977.

Yepes, L.E., Balka, E.B., Winsberg, B.G., and Bialer, I. Amitriptyline and methylphenidate treatment of behaviorally disordered children. *J. Child Psychol. Psychiatry* 18:39–52, 1977.

4

Mechanisms and Interventions in Tricyclic Antidepressant Overdoses

SHELDON H. PRESKORN AND THOMAS A. KENT

Most physicians will encounter patients seriously poisoned by tricyclic anti-depressants (TCAs). These potentially life-threatening poisonings occur in three ways: (a) accidental ingestion in children, (b) suicide attempts, and (c) unintentional overdosage by the prescribing physician (Dawn Quarterly Report, 1977). Despite the magnitude of the problem, many physicians are not familiar with the mechanisms underlying the adverse effects of these drugs on the cardiovascular and central nervous systems. Moreover, treatment of TCA overdosage differs from other drug overdoses and recovery may well depend on this knowledge. Finally, the development of assays capable of measuring TCA plasma concentrations has provided a means of avoiding inadvertent toxicity. The purpose of this paper is to discuss: (a) factors which increase the risk of inadvertent toxicity, (b) use of plasma monitoring to reduce such risk, and (c) the drug metabolism, pathophysiology, and treatment of TCA overdoses.

RISK FACTORS

Pharmacologic Considerations

TCA toxicity is concentration-dependent. The high risk of serious toxicity is the result of their low therapeutic index (median toxic concentration divided by median effective concentration). While 2-4 mg/kg orally is a therapeutic dose, 20 mg/kg is potentially lethal (Bickel, 1975; Alexanderson and Sjoqvist,

63

1971; Carr and Hobson, 1977). Hence, as little as four 75 mg tablets for a 15 kg child or a typical two weeks prescription for an adult can be lethal.

Some patients experience serious toxicity when taking routine doses. Such toxicity occurs because of the large interindividual variability in TCA elimination rates (Alexanderson and Sjoqvist, 1971). A 40-fold difference in steady-state concentrations can occur between fast and slow metabolizers receiving the same dose. In a sample of 330 patients taking routine doses, 5-10% achieved levels in excess of 400 ng/ml, and some in excess of 1000 ng/ml (Figure 1). Hence, iatrogenic toxicity due to slow metabolism occurs periodically when these drugs are administered on the basis of dosage alone. For example, of 100 patients receiving routine doses of amitriptyline TCA-induced delirium occurred

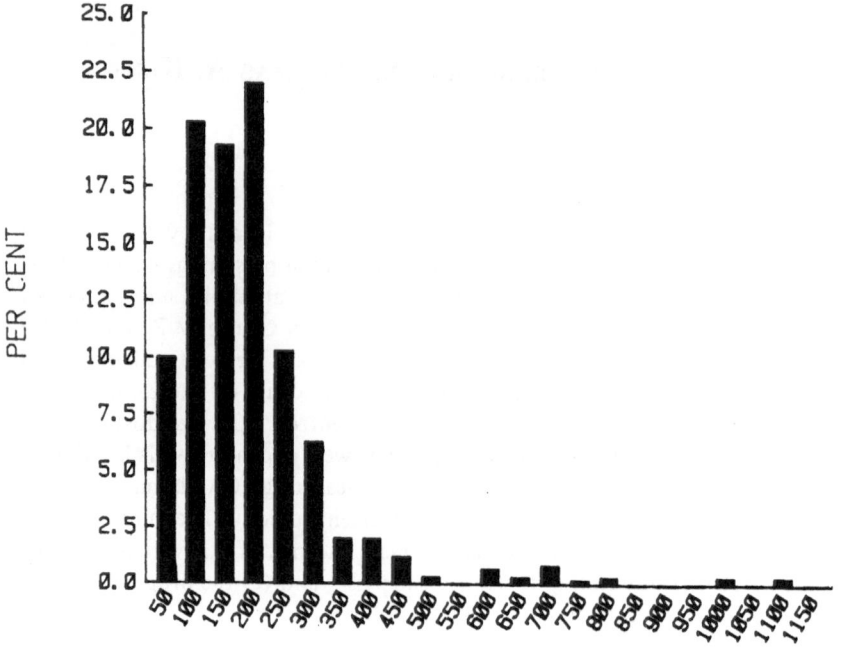

TOTAL PLASMA CONCENTRATION

Figure 1. Percentage of patients (n = 330) achieving different steady-state plasma levels (ng/ml) of amitriptyline + nortriptyline on routine doses. All patients were receiving amitriptyline for treatment of their depressive disorder and in no case did the dose exceed 300 mg/day. All plasma levels were drawn: (a) after the patients had been on a stable dose for at least 7 days, and (b) 10-12 hours after the last dose was administered. Approximately 45% of these patients achieved plasma levels below 150 ng/ml which is generally considered the lower limit for optimal therapeutic response. Over 5% of patients achieved levels in excess of 400 ng/ml putting them at increased risk for adverse effects.

in 6 of the 7 patients who achieved steady-state plasma levels of amitriptyline
and its major metabolite, nortriptyline, in excess of 450 ng/ml (Preskorn and
Simpson, 1982). Slow metabolism is genetically determined but metabolism can
be further impaired by: (a) hepatic or renal disease, (b) reduced hepatic blood
flow, and (c) concomitant use of drugs (e.g., neuroleptics) which interfere with
the metabolism of TCAs. Such problems can be detected by monitoring the
steady-state plasma concentration of the drug (Preskorn and Biggs, 1978). The
physician can then adjust the dose to titrate the patient within a safe but effective concentration range.

Other Risk Factors

Additional risk factors are: (a) advanced age, (b) pre-existing cardiac problems, and (c) potentiation of TCA toxicity by drugs with similar actions (Carr
and Hobson, 1977; Kantor, Glassman, and Bigger, 1978; Coull et al., 1970).
Higher mortality rates have been observed for cardiac patients on TCAs when
compared to age-matched cardiac patients not receiving these drugs (Coull et al.,
1970; Moir, Dingwall-Fordyce, and Weir, 1973). There has also been reports of
sudden death—principally in elderly patients and cardiac patients—associated
with therapeutic administration of TCAs (Sloman, 1978). These reports and
studies were conducted before plasma monitoring was feasible; however, such
monitoring may well have implicated slow metabolism as one factor increasing
the mortality rates.

METABOLISM

In considering intervention in overdose patients, both the pharmacokinetics and the pharmacodynamics of the ingested drug must be considered.
TCAs are rapidly and completely absorbed from the small bowel. Before being
excreted via the kidneys, the drugs must be converted to polar metabolites. This
metabolism occurs in the liver by three major pathways: (a) N-demethylation,
(b) N-oxidation, and (c) aromatic hydroxylation (Bickel, 1975). While the lipophilic metabolites move easily into cells and across the blood-brain barrier, the
polar metabolites are limited to extracellular spaces—plasma, bile, urine, and
feces. Gastric and bilary secretion of TCAs accounts for as much as 30% of the
ingested dose (Gard et al., 1973, Manoguerra, 1977). However, fecal excretion of
these drugs is negligible since most is reabsorbed prolonging the overdose and
causing greater morbidity (Bickel, 1975).

TCAs are highly lipophilic and demonstrate high protein binding affinity.
These properties account for their extensive distribution. TCAs accumulate in
parenchymal tissue, at 40 to 50 times the plasma level (Bonaccorsi et al., 1977;

Bianchetti et al., 1977). The plasma concentration at steady-state conditions accurately reflects the myocardial and brain tissue concentrations (Glotzbach and Preskorn, 1982). This relationship forms the basis for the usefulness of plasma monitoring during routine treatment because TCAs have different pharmacological effects depending upon the tissue concentration.

However, the usefulness of such monitoring in evaluating the severity of an acute overdose is limited because a single sample does not indicate whether absorption is complete. Moreover, there is insufficient data to use such plasma level results to predict complications or the need for specific antidotes. Rather, such levels are useful to document the nature of the overdose and to avoid discharging patients who may be asymptomatic with high plasma levels.

Knowledge of pharmacokinetics helps explain the difficulty of attempting to facilitate clearance of these drugs once ingested. Forced diuresis, peritoneal dialysis, and hemodialysis are ineffective ways of speeding drug elimination (Manoguerra, 1977). This lack of success is not surprising. Due to the tissue:plasma distribution ratio, little drug is accessible in plasma for elimination bv these techniques.

MECHANISMS OF TOXICITY

In TCA overdose, the central nervous system and the circulatory system are the organ systems principally affected. The impairment of the central nervous system presents as convulsions, coma, and depression of respiratory centers. TCAs directly impair myocardium, causing: (a) slowing of impulse conduction leading to heart block and serious arrhythmias, and (b) depression of myocardial contractility (Bonaccorsi et al., 1977; Bianchetti et al., 1977; Barth and Muscholl, 1974; Jandhyala et al., 1977). Clinically, the former effect is much more important than the latter which rarely is severe enough to warrant treatment. In addition, cardiovascular collapse can occur in seriously overdosed patients due to TCA-induced peripheral adrenergic receptor blockade which results in: (a) vasodilatation, (b) relative intravascular hypovolemia, and (c) decreased cardiac output (Langou et al., 1980). In overdosed patients, TCAs can also cause seizures and/or respiratory depression which results in hypoxia and hence further compromised myocardial function (Crome and Newman, 1979). The severity of cardiac impairment depends upon drug concentration achieved, rate of elimination, and prior cardiac status. Based on studies of overdoses, virtually all patients having TCA plasma levels >1000 ng/ml experience impaired intracardiac conduction as detectable on a routine EKG by QRS durations >100 msec (Spiker et al., 1975).

Such QRS prolongation can be used to assess the seriousness of TCA overdose with two reservations. First, toxicity manifested by other electrocardiograph (EKG) alterations, heart failure, or sudden death has been reported at plasma concentrations under 1000 ng/ml (Kantor, Bigger, and Glassman, 1975; Reed et al., 1980; Manoguerra, 1977; Spiker and Biggs, 1976). Second, patients may have pre-existing cardiac dysfunction causing QRS prolongation without being toxic from TCAs. Despite these reservations, a baseline EKG is useful for initial evaluation of the overdose patient. The clinician can monitor recovery by repeated tracings, realizing this procedure is neither sensitive nor specific.

Before deciding upon intervention, the multiple effects of TCAs should be considered: (a) cholinergic antagonism, (b) catecholamine reuptake blockage, (c) direct membrane stabilization, and (d) adrenergic receptor blockade. Only the first two are commonly considered. Most attempts at pharmacologic intervention involve cholinergic agonism with physostigmine. However, limited research exists to support general use of this agent as an antidote for TCA-induced cardiotoxicity.

Controversy surrounds treatment of these overdoses. While mechanisms have been elucidated in laboratory animal experimentation, conclusions drawn from such studies have not been systematically tested in the clinical situation. For a variety of reasons, findings in laboratory preparations may not be directly relevant to the clinical situation.

Unfortunately, despite the frequency and magnitude of the problem, reports on overdose patients are generally deficient in several respects: (a) small sample size, (b) pooling patients whose overdoses vary greatly in terms of amount ingested and hence severity, (c) nonsystematic application of various treatment modalities, and (d) no controlled comparisons of specific interventions. Hence, our present knowledge is incomplete and treatment recommendations must be based on a synthesis of laboratory findings and clinical reports as discussed below.

TCAs can exert either beneficial or adverse cardiac effects depending upon their tissue concentration (Ziegeler, Co, and Biggs, 1977; Bianchetti et al., 1977; Bonaccorsi et al., 1977; Franco et al., 1976; Baum et al., 1976; Babulova et al., 1973; Thorstrand, Bergstrom, and Castenfors, 1976; Elonen, 1974; Elonen, Mattila, and Saarnivaara, 1974; Langslet et al., 1971). At low concentrations, TCAs exert positive inotropic effects increasing myocardial contractility and consequently systemic blood pressure (Laddu and Somani, 1969). As concentration increases, both negative inotropic effects and intracardiac conduction defects can occur. However, the conduction defects are more clinically important than the negative inotropic effects. The positive effects at low concentrations are adrenergically mediated, while the adverse effects at high concentrations result from the direct membrane actions of these drugs.

PHYSIOLOGICAL INTERVENTION

The first step in reducing the risk of serious toxicity in a TCA overdose patient is to block the absorption of the drug. TCAs delay gastric emptying thus significant quantities can be recovered many hours following ingestion (Bickel, 1975; Gard et al., 1973; Munksgaard, 1969; Work, 1969). Activated charcoal instilled into the stomach can bind these drugs further reducing absorption (Crome et al., 1975; Gard et al., 1973; Manoguerra, 1977).

Once absorbed, a means of speeding elimination would be desirable. TCAs are avidly extracted from portal blood by hepatocytes, and excreted into the bilary system. This process can result in up to 50% of the dose collecting in the gallbladder within hours of ingestion. However, a significant portion of this amount will be reabsorbed when emptied back into the small bowel and will eventually reach the central compartment to be distributed to the tissues. Instillation of charcoal, or possibly resins such as cholestyramine can interrupt such enterohepatic recirculation (Bickel, 1975).

Theoretically feasible but unproven means of speeding elimination include: prolonged administration of charcoal or resins, and hemoperfusion. TCAs are secreted across the gastrointestinal wall. Normally, the amount is substantial but rapidly reabsorbed. By binding the drugs in the intestine, the rate of elimination may be significantly increased. This process has been successfully tested with chemically similar toxins. The same might be true for hemoperfusion which has been attempted with variable results (Iverson, Willassen, and Bakke, 1978). However, any benefits from this latter procedure must be carefully weighed against its risks: lysis of red and white blood cells and platelets and disturbances in electrolytes and blood gases.

Alkalanization appears to be an effective and safe means to reverse toxicity once absorption has occurred (Hoffman and McElroy, 1981). The mechanism is unknown, but is thought to involve changing the binding characteristics of the TCA and thus altering distribution within tissue compartments. Such alkalinization can be accomplished by either hyperventilation and/or the administration of sodium bicarbonate (Kingston, 1979). These procedures should be pursued as one of the initial steps to reversing toxicity once antiabsorption methods have been instituted. Whether it is better to achieve a venous pH of 7.4 or to achieve alkalosis is not known.

Vigorous oxygenation of arterial blood and correction of fluid status should be simultaneously implemented. A large series of over 100 fatal TCA overdoses reported that the single most correctable cause of fatality was insufficient attention to maintenance of adequate respiration via mechanical support (Crome and Newman, 1979).

PHARMACOLOGICAL INTERVENTION

Physostigmine has been widely recommended as being the "antidote" for TCA poisoning (Aquilonus and Hedstrand, 1978). This anticholinesterase drug increases the amount of acetylcholine at the receptor by inhibiting its degradatory enzyme. However, consideration of its pharmacologic effects and pharmacokinetics suggests the efficacy of physostigmine in TCA overdosed patients is limited to reversing TCA-induced tachycardias and the central anticholinergic syndrome.

The central anticholinergic syndrome is a TCA-induced delirium which can occur in the absence of cardiotoxicity. Parenthetically, a variety of anticholinergic drugs can cause this syndrome. Physostigmine, unlike some anticholinesterase agents, readily crosses the blood–brain barrier and can antagonize central atropine-like effects of TCAs (Burks et al., 1974). These central depressant effects are not life-threatening when vigorous respiratory support is pursued and remit when the anticholinergic drug is eliminated.

While physostigmine can reverse TCA-induced delirium and coma, this use must be weighted against several limitations. First, repeated doses may be required to maintain improvement since physostigmine has a duration of action of only 30 to 60 minutes (Burks et al., 1974). Second, physostigmine can induce seizures in TCA overdose cases when administrated too rapidly (Aquilonus and Hedstrand, 1978; Tobis and Das, 1976). This clinical finding has been confirmed in laboratory animals (Vance et al., 1977). When recurrent TCA-induced seizures occur, treatment with intravenous diazepam or phenytoin is preferable to either physostigmine (because of the increased risk of further seizures) or barbiturates (because of the increased risk of further respiratory depression).

Of all the cardiac effects of TCAs, only the tachycardia appears to be due to the anticholinergic actions of these drugs (Taylor and Braithwaite, 1978; Thorstrand, Bergstrom, and Castenfors, 1976). Under experimental conditions, TCA-induced tachycardias can be blocked by either physostigmine or propranolol (Tobis and Aronow, 1980). Counteracting this adverse effect, however, should not markedly reduce either morbidity or mortality except for patients who are unable to tolerate a sustained tachycardia due to pre-existent ischemic heart disease.

With regard to the more serious problems of TCA-induced impairment in cardiac conduction and myocardial contractility, there are retrospective, uncontrolled case reports purporting that physostigmine can reverse widened QRS complexes, atrioventricular block, and arrhythmias (Tobis and Das, 1976). While the myocardium does contain muscarinic receptors, stimulation of these receptors impairs intracardiac conduction and depresses myocardial function (Wei and

Sulake, 1978). Hence, physostigmine can aggravate TCA-induced impairment in myocardial contractility by indirectly stimulating these receptors. This mechanism may be responsible for the fall in blood pressure which occurs in TCA poisoned patients following physostigmine administration (Newton, 1975; Nattel, Bayne, and Ruedy, 1979). Moreover, administration of physostigmine has reportedly produced profound bradycardia and even asystole in some TCA overdose patients (Pentel and Peterson, 1980). Taken together, the improvement in consciousness induced by physostigmine is transient, usually not critical to patient care, and occurs at the risk of increasing the likelihood of seizures, systemic hypotension and asystole with little beneficial effect on cardiac status. Given these problems, this drug should be used cautiously and administered slowly. Moreover, the usefulness of physostigmine appears to be limited to reversing TCA-induced tachycardias and serving as a test to confirm the diagnosis of the central anticholinergic syndrome. However, a controlled study of its place in the management of TCA overdoses is long overdue.

Propranolol has purportedly corrected TCA-induced conduction defects restoring sinus rhythm (Freeman and Loughead, 1973). The rationale is that propranolol is an antiarrhythmic and an adrenergic blocker which can block the indirect adrenergic agonism of TCAs. However, the catecholaminergic action of TCAs improves rather than worsens myocardial contractility and occurs at concentrations well below those which are toxic. The conduction defects and reduced myocardial contractility caused by high concentrations of TCAs are the result of the potent membrane stabilizing properties of these drugs (Elonen, 1974; Elonen, Mattila, and Saarnivaara, 1974; Bianchetti et al., 1977; Bonaccorsi et al., 1977). Of importance, propranolol itself has membrane stabilizing properties and can decrease nodal conduction velocity and myocardial contractility causing profound hypotension (Franco et al., 1976; Freeman and Loughead, 1973; Nymark and Rasmussen, 1966). In several laboratory animal studies, propranolol increased the cardiotoxicity of TCA (Laddu and Somani, 1968; Thorstrand, Bergstrom, and Castenfors, 1976). However, these adverse effects of propranolol are rare in the clinical setting unless there is preexistent cardiomyopathy. Still, the use of propranolol as an antidote for TCA poisoning is open to question and as with physostigmine a controlled study of its usefulness is needed.

Antiarrhythmic drugs have been used to treat TCA overdoses. However, there are no controlled studies of agents such as lidocaine despite its widespread use in intensive care units. Both imipramine and lidocaine are direct membrane stabilizers. Each causes concentration-dependent impairment in intracardiac conduction and myocardial contractility (Bigger and Heissenbuttel, 1969). When administered concomitantly in animals, lidocaine potentiates TCA-induced cardiotoxicity (Langslet et al., 1971). Additionally, lidocaine can produce the same central nervous system toxicity as do TCAs (Bigger and Heisenbuttel, 1969).

Despite the risk of potentiating TCA-induced central and cardiac toxicity, three factors mitigate for the safety of lidocaine in such overdoses: (a) when given intravenously, lidocaine is rapidly cleared having a half-life of two hours, (b) at therapeutic concentrations, it does not depress intracardiac conduction as does quinindine or procainamide, and (c) it does not impair myocardial contractility (Bigger and Mandel, 1970). Indeed, lidocaine is commonly used to prophylactically suppress ventricular premature beats in patients with recent myocardial infarction precisely because at appropriate concentrations it will not depress the myocardium. When cautiously administered, lidocaine can be used with reasonable safety to control TCA-induced ventricular arrhythmias which are recurrent, life-threatening, and refractory to other therapy.

Another agent which has been reported to successfully treat TCA-induced arrhythmias is phenytoin (Hagerman and Hanashiro, 1981). This drug has several theoretical benefits over other antiarrhythmics. First, it shortens rather than prolongs intracardiac conduction. Second, it is devoid of peripheral cardiovascular effects. Third, it may reduce the risk of seizures without further compounding respiratory depression. Thus, lidocaine or phenytoin may be the agents of choice but only when nonpharmacologic treatment (alkalinization/fluid restoration/respiratory support) has failed. A controlled comparison of the usefulness of these two drugs would be helpful in making more definitive recommendations.

Cardiac glycosides reverse experimental TCA-induced heart failure in laboratory animals (Nymark and Rasmussen, 1966). Similar results have been reported clinically. However, careful monitoring of the patient's cardiac status is necessary if cardiac glycosides are administered, Digitalis can increase myocardial automaticity and cause A-V block in toxic amounts. Varying degrees of conduction blocks and arrhythmias can occur with TCA overdoses. Due to the potential additive effects of digitalis and TCAs on nodal conduction, the use of digitalis in TCA overdose could result in complete heart block. Moreover, congestive heart failure is rarely a major problem in TCA overdoses. Instead, fatalities result from respiratory depression, intracardiac conduction disturbance, seizures, and systemic hypotension (Crome and Newman, 1979). Thus, cardiac glycosides are of limited usefulness and should be given only in combination with ventricular pacing.

While gaps exist in our knowledge of these drugs, research has provided useful information. Iatrogenic toxicity can be avoided by monitoring plasma concentrations and adjusting the dose accordingly. When an overdose occurs, treatment should include measures to decrease drug absorption such as gastric lavage and administration of activated charcoal to block enterohepatic recirculation. Continuous EKG monitoring is required for the patient who is: (a) comatose, (b) hypotensive, (c) having arrhythmias, (d) having prolongation of QRS interval >100 msec, or (e) above a postabsorption plasma concentration of

500 ng/ml. Vigorous respiratory care, alkalanization of the blood, and volume correction are the mainstays of acute intervention once steps at preventing drug absorption have been instituted. These steps will suffice for the vast majority of patients who do not require aggressive treatment.

Direct adrenergic agonists such as dopamine or norepinephrine may be efficacious in profound systemic hypotension and resultant cardiac failure which has been refractory to fluid replacement. However, prolonged or overly aggressive use of peripheral vasoconstrictors, should be avoided because they may precipitate or worsen arrhythmias and can result in peripheral ischemia including renal failure. Physostigmine should be avoided unless tachycardia is a significant problem. Arrhythmias should be treated conservatively and lidocaine or phenytoin used only for refractory or severe arrhythmias. In the patient with recurrent arrhythmias or cardiac failure, intracardiac pacing is indicated. If congestive heart failure occurs, cardiac glycosides are the treatment choice. In such rare cases, ventricular pacing eliminates the concern that cardiac glycosides could potentiate the A–V nodal conduction defect. In these cases, fluids should be carefully monitored to avoid the development of pulmonary edema.

Finally, the optimum length of intensive cardiac monitoring remains controversial. Early case reports of late-occurring sudden death and severe arrhythmias prompted the current practice of intensive care unit (ICU) monitoring for 72 hours. However, these earlier case reports involved patients who had prior cardiac disease, or had ongoing cardiovascular, central nervous system or pulmonary complications (Masters, 1967, Sunshine and Yaffee, 1963). A more rational approach, then, may be to discontinue ICU monitoring when the patient has been asymptomatic for 12 to 24 hours without active treatment (Fasoli and Glauser, 1981; Pentel and Sioris, 1981).

ACKNOWLEDGEMENTS

Supported in part by NIMH Research Scientist Development Awards MH-00272 and MH-36739, and NINCDS grant NS-17252 to Dr. Preskorn, and clinical pharmacology fellowship to Dr. Kent from the Pharmaceutical Manufacturers Association Foundation. The authors warmly thank Ms. Adelaide Lumary for manuscript preparation.

REFERENCES

Alexanderson, B., and Sjoqvist, F. Individual differences in the pharmacokinetics of monomethylated tricyclic antidepressants: Role of genetic and environmental factors and clinical importance. *Ann. N.Y. Acad. Sci.* 179:739–751, 1971.

Auilonus, S., and Hedstrand, U. The use of physostigmine as an antidote in tricyclic antidepressant intoxication. *Acta. Anaesth. Scand.* 22:40–45, 1978.

Babulova, A., Bareggi, S., Bonaccorsi, A., et al. Correlation between desipramine levels and (-)-noradrenaline uptake and chronotropic effect in isolated atria of rats. *Br. J. Pharmacol.* 48:464–474, 1973.

Barth, N., and Muscholl, E. The effects of the tricyclic antidepressants: Desipramine, doxepin, and iprindole on the isolated perfused rabbit heart. *Naunyn-Schmiedeberg Arch. Pharmacol.* 284:215–232, 1974.

Baum, T., Peters, J., Butz, F., et al. Tricyclic antidepressants and cardiac conduction: Changes in ventricular automaticity. *Eur. J. Pharmacol.* 39:323–329, 1976.

Bianchetti, G., Bonaccorsi, A., Chiodaroli, A., et al. Plasma concentrations and cardiotoxic effects of desipramine and protriptyline in the rat. *Br. J. Pharmacol.* 60:11–19, 1977.

Bickel, M. Poisoning by tricyclic antidepressant drugs. *Int. J. Clin. Pharmacol.* 11:145–176, 1975.

Bigger, J. T., and Heisenbuttel, R.H. Use of procainamide and lidocaine in the treatment of cardiac arrhythmias. *Prog. Cardiovasc. Dis.* 11:515–534, 1969.

Bigger, J.T., and Mandel, W.J. Effects of lidocaine on conduction in canine Purkinje fibers and at the ventricular musclePurkinje fiber. *J. Pharmacol. Exp. Therap.* 172:239, 1970.

Bonaccorsi, A., Franco, R., Garattini, S., et al. Plasma nortriptyline and cardiac responses in young and old rats. *Br. J. Pharmacol.* 60:21–27, 1977.

Burks, J., Walker, J., Rumack, B., et al. Tricyclic antidepressant poisoning: Reversal of coma, choreoathetosis, and myoclonus by physostigmine. *J.A.M.A.* 230:1405–1407, 1974.

Carr, A., and Hobson, R. High serum concentrations of antidepressants in elderly patients. *Br. Med. J.* 2:1151, 1977.

Coull, D., Crooks, J., Dingwall-Fordyce, I., et al. A method of monitoring drugs for adverse reaction II: Amitriptyline and cardiac disease. *Eur. J. Clin. Pharmacol.* 3:51–55, 1970.

Crome, P., and Newman, B. Fatal tricyclic antidepressant poisoning. *J. R. Soc. Med.* 72:649–653, 1979.

Crome, P., Dawling, S., Braithwaite, R.A., et al. Effect of activated charcoal on absorption of nortriptyline. *Br. Med. J.* 4:705, 1980.

Dawn Quarterly Report (1977) July–September (Contract number DEA-77-11) IMS America, Lt.

Elonen, E.L. Correlation of the cardiotoxicity of tricyclic antidepressants to their membrane effects. *Med. Biol.* 52:415–423, 1974.

Elonen, E., Mattila, M., and Saarnivaara, L. Cardiovascular effects of amitriptyline, nortriptyline, and doxepin in conscious rabbits. *Eur. J. Pharmacol.* 28:178–188, 1974.

Fasoli, R.A., and Glauser, F.L. Cardiac arrhythmias and ECT abnormalities in tricyclic antidepressant overdose. *Clin. Toxicol.* 18:155–163, 1981.

Franco, R., Bonaccorsi, A., Caastelli, K., et al. Relationship between chronotropic effect, 1-^{3}H-noradrenaline uptake and tissue concentrations of desipramine, protriptyline, and doxepin in rat isolated atria. *Acta. Int. Pharmacodyn.* 224:55–65, 1976.

Freeman, J., and Loughead, M. Beta blockade in the treatment of tricyclic antidepressant overdosages. *Med. J. Aust.* 1:1233–1235, 1973.

Gard, H., Knapp, D., Walle, T., et al. Qualitative and quantitative studies on the disposition of amitriptyline and other tricyclic antidepressant drugs in man as it related to the management of the overdosed patient. *Clin. Toxicol.* 6: 561–584, 1973.

Glassman, A.H., and Perel, J.M. The clinical pharmacology of imipramine. *Arch. Gen. Psychiatry* 28:649–653, 1973.

Glotzbach, R.K., and Preskorn, S.H. Brain concentrations of tricyclic antidepressants: Single-dose kinetics and relationship to plasma concentrations in chronically dosed rats. *Psychopharmacology*, in press.

Hagerman, G.A., and Hanashiro, P.K. Reversal of tricyclic antidepressant-induced cardiac conduction abnormalities by phenytoin. *Ann. Emerg. Med.* 10: 82–86, 1981.

Hoffman, J.R., and McElroy, C.R. Bicarbonate therapy for dysrhythmia and hypotension in tricyclic antidepressant overdose. *West. J. Med.* 134: 60–64, 1981.

Inverson, B.M., Willassen, Y., and Bakke, O.M. Charcoal haemoperfusion in nortriptyline poisoning. *Lancet* 1:388–389, 1978.

Jandhyala, B., Steenberg, M., Perel, J., et al. Effects of several tricyclic antidepressants on the hemodynamics and myocardial contractility of anaesthetized dogs. *Eur. J. Pharmacol.* 42:403–410, 1977.

Kantor, S., Bigger, J., Glassman, A., et al. Imipramine-induced block: A longitudinal case study. *J.A.M.A.* 231:1364–1366, 1975.

Kantor, S., Glassman, A., Bigger, J., et al. The cardiac effects of therapeutic plasma concentration of imipramine. *Am. J. Psychiatry* 15:534–548, 1978.

Kingston, M.E. Hyperventilation in tricyclic antidepressant poisoning. *Crit. Care Med.* 7:550–551, 1979.

Laddu, A., and Somani, P. Desipramine toxicity and its treatment. *Toxicol. Appl. Pharmacol.* 15:287–394, 1969.

Langou, R.A., Dyke, C.V., Tahan, S.R., et al. Cardiovascular manifestations of tricyclic antidepressant overdose. *Am. Heart J.* 100:458–463, 1980.

Langslet, A., Johansen, W., Ryg, M., et al. Effects of dibenzepine and imipramine on the isolated rat heart. *Eur. J. Pharmacol.* 14:333–339, 1971.

Manoguerra, A. Poisoning with tricyclic antidepressant drugs. *Clin. Toxicol.* 10: 149–158, 1977.

Masters, A.B. Delayed death in imipramine poisoning. *Br. Med. J.* 3:866–867, 1967.

Moir, D., Dingwall-Fordyce, L., and Weir, R. Medicine evaluation and monitoring group: A follow-up study of cardiac patients receiving amitriptyline. *Eur. J. Clin. Pharmacol.* 6:98–101, 1973.

Munksgaard, E. Concentrations of amitriptyline and its metabolites in urine, blood, and tissue in fatal amitriptyline poisoning. *Acta. Pharmacol. et Toxicol.* 27:129–134, 1969.

Nattel, S., Bayne, L., Ruedy, J. Physostigmine in coma due to drug overdose. *Clin. Pharm. Ther.* 25:96–102, 1979.

Newton, R. Physostigmine salicylate in the treatment of tricyclic antidepressant overdosage. *J.A.M.A.* 229:941–943, 1975.

Nymark, M., Rasmussen, J. Effect of certain drugs upon amitriptyline induced electrocardiographic changes. *Acta. Pharmacol. et Toxicol.* 24:148–156, 1966.

Pentel, P., Peterson, D.C. Asystole complicating physostigmine treatment of tricyclic antidepressant overdose. *Ann. Emerg. Med.* 9:588–590, 1980.

Pentel, P., and Sioris, L. Incidence of late arrhythmias following tricyclic antidepressant overdose. *Clinical Toxicology* 18:543–545, 1981.

Preskorn, S., and Biggs, J. Use of tricyclic antidepressant blood levels. *N. Eng. J. Med.* 298:166, 1978.

Preskorn, S., and Simpson, S. Tricyclic antidepressant-induced delirium: A function of plasma drug concentration. *Am. J. Psychiatry* 39:822–823, 1982.

Reed, K., Smith, R., Schoolar, J., et al. Cardiovascular effects of nortriptyline in geriatric patients. *Am. J. Psychiatry* 137:986–988, 1980.

Sloman, L. Myocardial infarction during imipramine treatment of depression. *Can. MAJ* 82:20–22, 1978.

Spiker, D., and Biggs, J. Tricyclic antidepressants: Prolonged plasma levels after overdose. *J.A.M.A.* 236:1711–1712, 1976.

Spiker, D., Weiss, A., Chang, S., et al. Tricyclic antidepressant overdose: Clinical presentation and plasma levels. *Clin. Pharmacol. Ther.* 18:539–546, 1975.

Sunshine, P., and Yaffee, S.J. Amitriptyline poisoning. *Am. J. Dis. Child.* 106:501–506, 1963.

Taylor, D.J., and Braithaite, R.A. Cardiac effects of tricyclic antidepressant medication. *Br. Heart J.* 40:1105–1109, 1978.

Thorstrand, C., Bergstrom, J., and Castenfors, J. Cardiac effect of amitriptyline in rats. *Scand. J. Clin. Lab. Invest.* 36:7–15, 1976.

Tobis, J., and Arnonow, W. Effects of amitriptyline antidotes on repetitive extrasystole threshold. *Clin. Pharm. Ther.* 27:602–606, 1980.

Tobis, J., and Das, B. Cardiac complications in amitriptyline poisoning: Successful treatment with physostigmine. *J.A.M.A.* 235: 1474–1746, 1976.

Vance, M., Ross, S., Millington, W., et al. Potentiation of tricyclic antidepressant toxicity by physostigmine in mice. *Clin. Tox.* 11:413–421, 1977.

Wei, J., and Sulakhe, P. Regional and subregional distribution of myocardial muscarinic cholinergic receptors. *Eur. J. Pharmacol.* 52:235–238, 1978.

Work, K. Fatal amitriptyline poisoning: Determination of the drug in forensic-chemical material. *Acta. Pharmacol. Toxicol.* 27:439–444, 1969.

Ziegeler, V., Co, B., and Biggs, J. Plasma nortriptyline levels and ECG findings. *Am. J. Psychiatry* 134:441–443, 1966.

5

Recent Developments Regarding the Use of Monoamine Oxidase Inhibitors in Psychopharmacology

Dennis L. Murphy,
Laurence B. Guttmacher, and Robert M. Cohen

INTRODUCTION

The first effective antidepressant drugs were a series of inhibitors of monoamine oxidase (MAO) developed during the late 1950s. Their use was superceded by that of the tricyclic antidepressants, which appeared more generally effective and lacked the dangerous side effect of hypertensive crises. In the last few years, there has been a spate of articles and editorials suggesting that the MAO-inhibiting drugs are underutilized, that there are subgroups of patients who respond preferentially to them, and that they are generally safe (Robinson et al., 1978; Editorial, 1976; Quitkin et al., 1979).

The re-emergence of these drugs as an important adjunct in the pharmacotherapy of depression seems based on several research findings: (a) studies of the clinical pharmacology of phenelzine revealed that many earlier investigations, including the influential British Medical Research Council (1965) trial, used phenelzine doses which were too low to achieve sufficient MAO inhibition to lead to optimum clinical responses (Robinson et al., 1978; Davidson et al., 1978a); (b) recent work highlighting the antianxiety effects of MAO-inhibitors (Paykel et al., 1979; Ravaris et al., 1980; Murphy et al., 1981a) as well as the efficacy of MAO-inhibitors in panic disorder (Sheehan et al., 1980) have helped to target more specific patient populations for treatment with these agents;

(c) hypertensive crises were found to be generally related to the ingestion of tyramine or certain sympathomimetic drugs; avoidance of these substances using dietary guidelines essentially eliminated this risk (Raskin, 1972; Robinson et al., 1973); and (d) recent research on the biochemistry of MAO and the pharmacological properties of MAO inhibitors has generated a new understanding of their clinical effects (Singer, Von Korff, and Murphy, 1979; Youdim and Paykel, 1981).

We survey a number of current clinical and laboratory developments relevant to the recent upsurge of interest in the MAO-inhibitors in psychiatry. In the space available, it will not be possible to review the general clinical use of these drugs; this information is readily available in a number of comprehensive reviews of their clinical efficacy, behavioral and physiological effects, and side effects (Kupfer and Detre, 1978; Quitkin et al., 1979; Squires, 1978; Murphy, 1977).

MAO AND MAO INHIBITORS: BASIC ASPECTS RELEVANT TO THE USE OF MAO INHIBITORS IN PSYCHOPHARMACOLOGIC TREATMENT

MAO is an outer mitochondrial membrane protein whose active form is a dimer consisting of two subunits, each having a molecular weight of approximately 60,000 daltons. The enzyme active site contains flavin adenine dinucleotide (FAD) as a cofactor and also depends upon the availability of sulfhydryl groups and lipids for full activity (see Singer, Von Korff, and Murphy, 1979, for references).

Clinically used MAO inhibitors (Table 1) all act by irreversibly inactivating the enzyme. The cyclopropylamines, such as tranylcypromine, alkylate a sulfhydryl group at the catalytic site, thereby blocking access of oxygen to the reduced flavin and preventing its reoxidation (Paech et al., 1979). Acetylenic inhibitors such as pargyline, clorgyline and deprenyl covalently bind the 8α-5-cysteine FAD cofactor at the active site. Hydrazines such as phenylhydrazine and phenelzine appear to form an irreversible adduct with the flavin in addition to alkylating sulfhydryl groups (Kenney et al., 1979; Maycock et al., 1976). It is of interest that all of these "suicide" inhibitors are actually substrates for the enzyme, and initially react competitively before forming the irreversible, covalent linkage.

New experimental work on MAO-inhibitors has been in three areas: (a) Several compounds which are potent reversible inhibitors of the enzyme (Table 1) are being evaluated in animals and man in the anticipation that dose-by-dose control of their effects, and also their toxicities, including tyramine

Table 1. MAO-Inhibitors

A. Clinically-available irreversible MAO-inhibitors:
    phenelzine, tranylcypromine, isocarboxazid

B. Clinically-studied, substrate-selective, irreversible MAO-inhibitors:
    MAO-A inhibitors: Clorgyline, Lilly 51641
    MAO-B inhibitors: Deprenyl, Pargyline

C. Clinically-studied, substrate-selective reversible MAO-A inhibitors:
    Cimoxatone (MD 780515), FLA 336(+), Ro 11-1163,
    CGP 11305

potentiation, may yield a safer drug; (b) other reversible MAO-inhibitors with amine uptake-inhibiting properties which may result in a wider spectrum of action among depressed patient subgroups and fewer side effects are also being investigated; the ability of these drugs to block the uptake of tyramine into noradrenergic nerve endings, thereby preventing the release of accumulated norepinephrine stores, should reduce the risk of hypertensive crises; and (c) the largest body of recent experimental work has been directed towards the explication of the properties of substrate-selective, irreversible MAO-inhibiting drugs (Table 1) (Singer, Von Korff, and Murphy, 1979; Youdim and Paykel, 1981; Beckmann and Reiderer, 1983).

MAO consists of two major subtypes, MAO-A and MAO-B, which very recent evidence suggests may be different proteins (Denney et al., 1982; Cawthon et al., 1981). MAO-A is preferentially inhibited by clorgyline, Lilly 51641, and harmaline, as well as by some of the new reversible inhibitors mentioned above; it selectively deaminates serotonin, norepinephrine, epinephrine and, in rodents, dopamine (Fowler et al., 1978, Murphy, 1978). MAO-B is somewhat selectively inhibited by deprenyl and to a lesser extent by pargyline and Lilly 54761; it selectively deaminates phenylethylamine, tele-methyl-histamine, benzylamine, phenylethanolamine, ortho-tyramine and, in primates, dopamine. It should be noted that the comonly used MAO-inhibitors such as phenelzine, tranylcypromine and isocarboxazid demonstrate no selectivity towards MAO-A or MAO-B, and also that a number of amines such as tyramine and tryptamine are metabolized nearly equally as well by either enzyme subtype. As noted below, the clinical interest in these substrate-selective inhibitors stems from their possible use in delineating which amine systems are involved in the clinical effects of the MAO inhibitors, as well as in the possibility that substrate selective inhibition might yield better therapeutic effects or fewer side effects.

MAO INHIBITORS: NEW INFORMATION ON THEIR MECHANISM
OF ACTION FROM ANIMAL AND IN VITRO STUDIES

Numerous animal studies have demonstrated rapid changes in brain nor-adrenergic and serotonergic functional activity in response to monoamine oxidase inhibitor antidepressants. The ability to inhibit oxidative deamination and produce elevations in cellular biogenic amine concentrations corresponds most closely to the behavioral effects of this drug group (Pletcher et al., 1966). It should be noted, however, that certain of these drugs produce effects other than inhibition of MAO, such as effects on amine uptake and release (as well as other pharmacologic properties, some of which are amine-selective, associated with different behavioral responses in animals and most likely in man).

For many years, the pharmacological and behavioral effects of MAO in-hibitors in animals were studied almost exclusively following acute, high-dosage drug administration. A delay of two or more weeks, however, is generally observed before the onset of both antidepressant efficacy as well as some promi-nent side effects such as orthostatic hypotension. These temporal discrepancies have led to studies of the adaptive changes that take place in the noradrenergic and serotonergic systems during the continued administration of MAO-inhibitors in animals and man.

In rats, the daily administration of the selective MAO-A inhibiting anti-depressant, clorgyline, leads to a rapid increase in brain serotonin concentration which, however, returns towards pretreatment levels at the end of the third week of drug administration; brain norepinephrine levels remain elevated for three weeks (Campbell et al., 1979b). Similarly, phenelzine and tranylcypromine given for six weeks result in a peak in rat brain norepinephrine, dopamine and sero-tonin concentrations during the first week of treatment, followed by a gradual decline to control levels. These decrements in brain amine concentrations are not explained by reductions in brain tryptophan hydroxylase or tyrosine hydroxy-lase activities (Campbell et al., 1979a).

After several weeks treatment with MAO-inhibitors, a reduction in α_2-adrenoreceptor numbers and in β-adrenoreceptor numbers and functional activity—as measured by norepinephrine stimulated cyclic-AMP formation—as well as in serotonin receptor numbers, have been observed in several studies (Sulser et al., 1978; Savage et al., 1980; Peroutka and Snyder, 1980; Sallinger-Barnette et al., 1980; Kellar et al., 1981; Cohen et al., 1982a). These changes are observed with both nonselective MAO-inhibitors (nialamide and phenelzine) and the selective MAO-A inhibitor clorgyline at low doses, but occur only at high, probably nonselective doses of the partially selective MAO-B inhibitor, pargyline. These neurochemical alterations induced by MAO-A inhibition are accompanied by a decrease in the firing rate of noradrenergic neurons in the locus ceruleus and a reduction in the sensitivity of cortical neurons to iontophoretically-applied

norepinephrine and serotonin, presumably reflecting the changes in amine receptor numbers and function reviewed above (Campbell et al., 1979a; Olpe, 1981;
Olpe and Schellenger, 1980). These adaptive neurochemical changes also appear
to be reflected in behavioral changes in animals, as chronic, but not acute clorgyline treatment leads to an attenuation of the changes in locomotor activity
produced by the α_2-adrenergic agonist clonidine (Cohen et al., 1982b;
Aulakh, Cohen, Pradhan, and Murphy, in press). Clonidine's effects under
these circumstances are believed to be mediated through an α_2-adreno-
receptor presynaptic inhibitor system. These latter results in rodents are in agreement with findings from a recent clinical study indicating that clonidine's hypotensive effects, which are also believed to involve α_2-adrenoreceptors, are significantly reduced after treatment with clorgyline for 21 days, but not 3 days, in
depressed patients (Siever et al., 1981).

CLINICAL PHARMACOLOGY OF THE MAO INHIBITORS: CORRELATIONS WITH CLINICAL RESPONSE, AND POSSIBLE MECHANISMS OF ACTION

Possible associations between the biological consequences of MAO-inhibitor
administration and the behavioral responses to these drugs have been explored in
a number of ways. Unlike the situation for many drugs, including the tricyclic
antidepressants, little useful information has been accrued from measurement of
the plasma concentrations of these drugs. As noted above, the currently used
MAO-inhibitors are irreversible inhibitors of this enzyme which, in brain, has a
half-life of approximately 12 days (Nelson et al., 1979), while the drugs themselves are quite rapidly cleared from plasma, with half-lives measured in hours
(Campbell et al., 1979c; Robinson et al., 1980). Thus, there is no necessary
association between the amount of MAO inhibition present in cellular mito-
chrondria and concentrations of the MAO inhibitor in plasma. Similarly, possible
individual differences in the metabolism of the hydrazine MAO-inhibitors via
acetylation, although originally reported to correlate with clinical response, have
subsequently been found to neither correspond to drug plasma levels nor the
amount of platelet MAO inhibition nor the clinical response to phenelzine
administration, according to three recent studies (Robinson et al., 1978, 1980;
Yates and Loudon, 1979; Tyrer et al., 1980). The predominant current view is
that phenelzine's clinical use is not aided by the determination of whether an
individual is a slow or fast acetylator.

Measurement of platelet MAO inhibition, in contrast, has provided evidence that higher phenelzine doses, on the order of 60-75 mg/day (or 1 mg/kg),
yield greater than 80-85% enzyme inhibition (Robinson et al., 1978). This level
of inhibition is associated with significantly greater antideprssant and antianxiety

efficacy than lesser amounts of platelet MAO inhibition (Davidson et al., 1978a; Ravaris et al., 1980). No general association between pretreatment platelet MAO activity and response to phenelzine has been observed. It should be noted that the association between reductions in platelet MAO activity and clinical response has only been studied for phenelzine, and does not hold for a selective MAO-A inhibitor with antidepressant properties like clorgyline, as the platelet contains only MAO-B, and it is possible to achieve greater than 85% inhibition of MAO-A (as reflected in changes in urinary amine metabolites) with negligible reductions in platelet MAO-B in clorgyline-responsive depressed patients (Lipper et al., 1979; Murphy et al., 1979). On the other hand, very low doses of pargyline and deprenyl, which have not been demonstrated to consistently lead to antidepressant effects, produce over 95% inhibition of platelet MAO activity in a matter of a few hours (Murphy et al., 1979; Eisler et al., 1981). Similarly tranylcypromine, and to a lesser extent isocarboxazid, yield marked platelet MAO inhibition at clinically sub-therapeutic doses (Giller and Loeb, 1980; Giller et al., 1982).

As discussed earlier, there is good evidence that the clinical responses to MAO-inhibiting agents result primarily from the delayed biochemical consequences of reduced oxidative deamination of biogenic amines, rather than some other property of these drugs. Some individual pharmacologic properties of these drugs may contribute, however, to differences in their clinical consequences, such as the reportedly greater stimulant properties of tranylcypromine, which seem related to its amphetamine-like amine releasing properties (Simpson and Cabot, 1976). However, neither this effect, nor the norephinephrine uptake-inhibiting effect of the (-)-isomer os tranylcypromine, are as important as MAO inhibition for the antideprssant action of the clinically-available, racemic (+) tranylcypromine, since the (+)-isomer, which is a better MAO-inhibitor but poorer uptake inhibitor, is the more effective antidepressant (Reynolds et al., 1980; Moises and Beckmann, 1981).

The question of which of the amines affected by MAO inhibition is most likely to be involved in therapeutic responses to these agents has recently been approached in comparative studies using clorgyline, pargyline and deprenyl for their substrate-selective actions. The largest aggregation of evidence from these studies suggests that reductions in depressive symptoms during treatment with MAO-inhibitors are most closely correlated with norepinephrine neurotransmitter systems changes, as based on direct measurements of the plasma and cerebrospinal fluid concentration of norepinephrine and its metabolites and on a series of indirect measures of changes in noradrenergic function, such as blood pressure alterations, during MAO-inhibitor treatment (Murphy et al., 1981a; Murphy et al., 1981b). The data suggest that a reduction in a central noradrenergic output, dependent upon longer-term drug administration (rather than an acutely-produced norepinephrine increase), is most closely associated with clinical improvement (Murphy et al., in press-a).

The data from these studies with selective MAO-inhibitors argue against the existence of a disorder in phenylethylamine metabolism as an important component of depression, as depressed patients have no evident abnormality in phenylethylamine production (Murphy et al., 1983). Furthermore, the fifty-fold elevations in phenylethylamine observed in patients treated with pargyline were not associated with clinical improvement, while clorgyline treatment, which did not elevate phenylethylamine, was clinically effective. Dopamine and histamine changes seem unlikely to have a primary role in the antidepressant effects of MAO inhibitors, as their metabolism is also more affected by pargyline than by clorgyline (Major et al., 1979; Hough and Domino, 1979). A role for serotonin has not been clarified (Murphy et al., in press-a). Changes in tyramine sensitivity which are associated with clinical effectiveness seem not to be directly related to clinical change via any selective alteration in tyramine metabolism. Rather, the enhanced sensitivity to tyramine found with MAO inhibition seems to depend upon changes in tyramine-releasable norepinephrine stores in neurons (Pickar et al., 1981). The positive association between clinical antidepressant responses and changes in tyramine sensitivity thus serve to reinforce the conclusion that norepinephrine changes are most likely connected with clinical response.

MAO-INHIBITORS COMPARED TO TRICYCLIC ANTIDEPRESSANTS: SPECTRUM OF ACTION, AND THE EFFECTS OF COMBINED TREATMENT

While there have been numerous attempts to compare tricyclics and MAO-inhibitors, many of the earlier studies were flawed by mixed diagnostic populations and most especially by low, probably sub-therapeutic, doses. A recent study examining depressed outpatients compared phenelzine, 60 mg/day with amitriptyline, 150 mg/day (Ravaris et al., 1980). The two drugs were found to be equally effective with a similar range of side-effects. Interestingly, given the literature on MAO-inhibitors and anxiety, phenelzine was found to have a significantly greater effect than the tricyclic on both self-ratings and observer-ratings of anxiety. This is also consistent with the findings of Paykel and co-workers (1979) that anxiety subscores in a depressed population correlated with successful outcome of treatment with phenelzine. In our clorgyline study, significant antianxiety and antidysphoric effects on an array of both self and observer ratings equalled and in some cases exceeded in magnitude the changes in depression ratings (Lipper et al., 1979; Murphy et al., 1981a).

Rowan et al. (1981) found amitriptyline and phenelzine equally effective in depressed outpatients, many of whom had anxious and phobic features. Phenelzine was slightly more effective against anxiety symptoms. It might well be that the "atypical depressives" originally proposed as peculiarly responsive to

MAO-inhibitors (Sargant, 1961), were in fact those with significant anxiety. A recent review concluded that several studies have demonstrated that phenelzine is effective in neurotic or atypical depression, but that insufficient information is available regarding the antidepressant efficacy of phenelzine in patients with more endogenous features (Quitkin et al., 1979).

Few controlled studies of the antidepressant properties of tranylcypromine in different depressed patient subgroups are available; the available evidence suggests this drug is effective across several patient subtypes including neurotic and endogenous or involutional patients (Bartholomew, 1962; Quitkin et al., 1979). Our studies with clorgyline in a referral hospital setting suggested that this selective MAO-inhibitor led to antidepressant responses in patients with more endogenous-type features, including very high Hamilton depression scale ratings (Murphy et al., 1981a). It is possible that some of the conclusions regarding MAO-inhibitor efficacy in certain patient subgroups have been biased by the almost exclusive use of phenelzine in these investigations, and it may be that different MAO inhibitors preferentially benefit different patient subgroups, as we have suggested elsehwere (Murphy et al., 1981a; Murphy et al., 1981b).

MAO-Inhibitors Combined with Tricyclic Antidepressants

The use of monoamine oxidase inhibitors in conjunction with tricyclic antidepressants was common 20 years ago, accounting for five percent of antidepressant prescriptions (Ananth and Luchins, 1977). During this period a number of case reports of toxicities and fatalities appeared, leading the Food and Drug Administration to issue a warning against their combined use. Coprescription declined although reviewers repeatedly indicated that, if used judiciously, the two groups of drugs could be safely combined (Ananth and Luchins, 1977; Ponto et al., 1977; White and Simpson, 1981). While the dangers apparently had been overexaggerated, there have been very few controlled studies supporting the efficacy of combined use, although noncontrolled studies have repeatedly suggested their utility in individual patients nonresponsive to either class of drugs alone. The few controlled trials have been flawed and have failed to demonstrate any increase in efficacy for combined treatment.

Potential research questions concerning the combined use of tricyclic antidepressants and MAO-inhibitors center in three areas: Their mechanism of interaction, documentation of whether there is more toxicity with the combination than with either drug class alone, and the indications for use. There is some theoretical appeal to co-prescription of tricyclics and MAO-inhibitors as they have differing immediate mechanisms of action. A synergism is the most likely explanation for the suggested beneficial effects, yet to our knowledge no one has demonstrated that biogenic amine changes are greater with co-administration than with either drug alone, or that adaptive responses to longer-term drug administration, such as brain neurotransmitter receptor changes, are different with combined treatment.

There are currently no clear criteria for which patients, if any, should receive combined tricyclic-MAO-inhibitor therapy. The perception of the combination as hazardous has meant that most clinicians have limited its use to refractory patients, those who have not responded to more orthodox therapies. Three studies of efficacy have recently appeared, and a fourth is nearing completion (White and Simpson, 1981). Davidson and coworkers (1978a) compared low dose amitriptyline plus phenelzine to electroconvulsive therapy in 19 medication resistant depressed patients in a non-blind trial; ECT was found to be superior. White et al., (1980) ran a non-blind, three-cell pilot study with non-refractory depressed inpatients comparing amitriptyline, tranylcypromine, and the combination and using higher drug doses than Davidson et al. (1978b); the three treatments were found to yield equal antidepressant effects. Young et al. (1979) conducted a double-blind study with 135 outpatients, but the protocol was flawed by a low dosage (45 mg/day) of phenelzine; the tricyclic, trimipramine, given alone was found superior to phenelzine, isocarboxazid, or either MAO-inhibitor in conjunction with the tricyclic. In summary, it is becoming increasingly clear that MAO-inhibitors and tricyclics can be used safely in combination if the two are started concurrently, if parenteral use is avoided, if imipramine is avoided, and if dosage is kept at relatively modest levels. What is less clear is what patient group, if any, should receive the combination, and at what point in treatment.

MAO-Inhibitors in Conjunction with Other Drugs

In a study published several years ago, Himmelhoch and coworkers (1972) began 21 tricyclic-unresponsive depressed patients on lithium carbonate and then added tranylcypromine. Eleven had a complete remission, five were substantially better, and the remaining five improved initially, but developed hypomania. To date this has not been followed up with a double-blind study. The provocative findings suggesting possible synergism between triiodothyronine and tricyclics (Banki, 1977) might justify a trial with thyroid hormone and MAO-inhibitors. Three well designed double-blind trials have shown that tryptophan, when combined with an MAO-inhibitor, is superior to the MAO-inhibitor and placebo (Coppen et al., 1963; Glassman and Platman, 1969; Ayuso-Guttierez and Lopez-Iboralino, 1971).

Use of MAO-Inhibitors in Non-Depressed Patient Populations:
Neurologic Disorders

The striking ability of MAO-inhibitors to suppress rapid eye movement sleep makes them a logical therapy in narcolepsy. Phenelzine has been found to be an effective treatment, reducing the cataplexy, hypersomnia, and sleep paralysis for periods of over a year, yet side effects including orthostatic hypotension, edema, and sexual dysfunction were found to limit its long-term use (Wyatt et al., 1971). Treatment with deprenyl did not benefit narcoleptic patients (Schacter et al., 1979). This observation fits with recent data indicating that REM sleep suppression is a characteristic of MAO-A but not MAO-B inhibition (Cohen et al., 1982c); therapeutic trials with one of the new MAO-A inhibitors may thus be of interest in narcolepsy.

In Parkinson's disease, MAO-inhibitors had relatively little effect on symptoms when used alone, but in some studies decreased the necessary dose of levodopa, as well as prolonging its effects (Lees et al., 1977; Csanda et al., 1978; Schacter et al., 1980). MAO-inhibitors have been used both in the treatment and prophylaxis of migraine (Anthony and Lance, 1969). In patients with idiopathic orthostatic hypotension, MAO-inhibitors have been combined with tyramine to create a controlled "cheese reaction" with moderate effectiveness (Diamond et al., 1970; Nanda et al., 1976).

Other Psychiatric Disorders

MAO-inhibitors have been used in patients with anxiety-related disorders. Several double-blind trials have demonstrated their efficacy in treating patients with mixed phobias (Tyrer et al., 1973; Solyom et al., 1973) and patients with agoraphobia (Lipsedge et al., 1973). Sheehan and coworkers (1980) recently reported a trial of phenelzine compared to imipramine and placebo in patients with agoraphobia with panic disorder. Both drugs were significantly more effective than placebo, and there was a trend suggesting superiority for the MAO-inhibitor over the tricyclic. Single case reports have indicated marked improvement in patients with obsessive-compulsive disorder treated with phenelzine (Isberg, 1981) or tranylcypromine (Jeneke, 1981); a double-blind study of clorgyline, however, revealed that this drug was less effective than clomipramine in obsessive-compulsive patients (Insel, et al., in press). According to a recent review (Brenner and Shopsin, 1980), MAO-inhibitors have never been shown to be superior to placebo in double-blind use with chronic schizophrenics. In regard to treatment-resistant bipolar affective disorder patients, five rapidly cycling individuals who were unresponsive to lithium and other usual treatments were given clorgyline in addition to more conventional therapies. Four responded with more prolonged intervals of euthymia and decreased severity of manic-depressive cycling (Potter et al., 1982).

SIDE EFFECTS AND TOXICITY

Several recent reviews and studies have added new information regarding the side effects of drug-induced MAO-inhibition. Hypertensive crises due to foods containing tyramine or other pressor amines or due to sympathomimetic drugs have become quite uncommon according to several large studies involving over 100 patients each (Raskin, 1972; Robinson et al., 1978). While this reaction has been regarded as resulting from an impairment of tyramine metabolism together with an enhanced amount of norepinephrine stored in sympathetic nerve terminals available for release by tyramine, it now appears that it is the increased amount of stored norepinephrine resultant from MAO-A inhibition that is responsible for the altered sensitivity to tyramine (Pickar et al., 1981). The magnitude of inhibition of norepinephrine metabolism, as reflected in reduced plasma 3-methoxy, 4-hydroxyphenylglycol concentrations, was found to be highly correlated with the enhanced blood pressure responses to tyramine (Pickar et al., 1981). Use of the selective MAO-B inhibitor, deprenyl, which in low doses has only minimal effects on norepinephrine metabolism, has negligible tyramine potentiating actions (Pickar et al., 1981; Elsworth et al. 1978).

It now seems clear that the tyramine hypertensive response or "cheese reaction" is a peripheral sympathetic nervous system syndrome, which should be differentiated from another syndrome with prominent central nervous system involvement characterized by delirium often progressing to coma, seizures and other neurologic abnormalities, including hyperreflexia and dilated, fixed pupils; severe hyperpyrexia (with temperatures to 108°F); hypotension; and acute renal failure. This syndrome has most characteristically been described to follow the administration of a tricyclic antidepressant such as imipramine during or within a few days after a period of treatment with an MAO-inhibitor. Unlike the tyramine hypertensive crisis, which responds to adrenergic blocking agents such as phentolamine, reversal of the central syndrome has been described to follow treatment with barbiturates, chlorpromazine and massive support measures (White and Simpson, 1981).

Among other side effects, attention has been drawn to potential problems with other drug interactions (Stockley, 1973a,b; Blackwell, 1981); behavioral toxicities such as restlessness, agitation, insomnia and in bipolar patients, manic switches (Murphy, 1977; Pickar et al., 1982); orthostatic hypotension (Murphy et al., 1981b); and sexual dysfunction (Kupfer and Detre, 1978). In regard to sexual function, retarded ejaculation and anorgasmia with intact sexual interest and erectile function in men has most commonly been reported. The sexual function abnormalities may be another manifestation of the reduced sympathetic nervous system outflow which results in hypotension, and hence principally represent an MAO-A inhibitor-related consequence; they do not appear to be a problem with the selective MAO-B inhibitor, deprenyl (Knoll, 1981). Anorgasmia has been noted in a case report of a female patient (Barton, 1979), but its basis and frequency in women has not yet been studied. Other possible contributions to sexual dysfunction from MAO-inhibitors may result from neuroendocrine changes produced by these drugs (Squires, 1978).

BIBLIOGRAPHY

Ananth, J.D., and Luchins, D. A review of combined tricyclic and MAOI therapy. *Compr. Psychiatry* 18:221–230, 1977.

Anthony, M., and Lance, J.W. Monoamine oxidase inhibition in treatment of migraine. *Arch. Neurol.* 21:263–268, 1969.

Aulakh, C.S., Cohen, R.M., Pradhan, S.N., and Murphy, D.L. Self-stimulation responses are altered following long-term but not short-term treatment with clorgyline. *Brain Research*, in press.

Ayuso-Gutierrez, J.L., and Lopez-Iboralino, J.J. Tryptophan and an MAOI (Nialamide) in the treatment of depression. *Int. Pharmacopsych.* 6:92–97, 1971.

Banki, C.M. Cerebrospinal fluid amine metabolites after combined amitriptyline-triiodothyronine treatment of depressed women. *Eur. J. Clin. Pharm.* 11:311–315, 1977.

Bartholomew, A. An evaluation of tranylcypromine in the treatment of depression. *Med. J. Aust.* 1:655–662, 1962.

Barton, J.L. Orgasmic inhibition by phenelzine. *Am. J. Psychiatry* 136:1616–1617, 1979.

Beckmann, H., and Riederer, P. *Monoamine Oxidase and Its Selective Inhibitors: New Concepts in Therapy and Research*. Basel, Karger, 1983.

Blackwell, B. Adverse effects of antidepressant drugs. Part 1: Monoamine oxidase inhibitors and tricyclics. *Drugs* 21:201–219, 1981.

Brenner, R., and Shopsin, B. The use of monoamine oxidase inhibitors in schizophrenia. *Biol. Psychiatry* 15:633–647, 1980.

British Medical Research Council. Clinical trial of the treatment of depressive illness. *Br. Med. J.* 1:881–886, 1965.

Campbell, I.C., Murphy, D.L., Gallager, D.W., Tallman, J.F., and Marshall, E.F. Neurotransmitter-related adaptation in the central nervous system following chronic monoamine oxidase inhibition. In Singer, T.P., Von Korff, R.W., and Murphy, D.L., eds., *Monoamine Oxidase: Structure, Function, and Altered Functions*. New York, Academic Press, pp. 517–530, 1979a.

Campbell, I.C., Robinson, D.S., Lovenberg, W., and Murphy, D.L. The effects of chronic regimens of clorgyline and pargyline on monoamine metabolism in the rat brain. *J. Neurochem.* 32:49–55, 1979b.

Campbell, I.C., Shiling, D.J., Lipper, S., Slater, S., and Murphy, D.L. A biochemical measure of monoamine oxidase type A and type B inhibitor effects in man. *J. Psychiatry Res.* 15:77–84, 1979c.

Cawthon, R.M., Pintar, J.E., Haseltine, F.P., and Breakefield, X.O. Differences in the structure of A and B forms of human monoamine oxidase. *J. Neurochem.* 37:363–372, 1981.

Cohen, R.M., Campbell, I.C., Dauphin, M., et al. Changes in α- and β-receptor densities in rat brain as a result of treatment with monoamine oxidase inhibiting antidepressants. *Neuropharmacology* 21:293–298, 1982a.

Cohen, R.M., Aulakh, C.S., Campbell, I.C., and Murphy, D.L. Functional subsensitivity of alpha 2 adrenoreceptors accompanying reductions in yohimbine binding after clorgyline treatment. *Eur. J. Pharmacol.*, 81:145–148, 1982b.

Cohen, R.M., Pickar, D., Garnett, D., Lipper, S., Gillen, J.C., and Murphy, D.L. REM sleep suppression induced by selective monoamine oxidase inhibitors. *Psychopharmacology* 78:137–140, 1982c.

Coppen, S., Shaw, D.M., and Farrel, J.P. Potentiation of the antidepressive effect of a monoamine-oxidase inhibitor by tryptophan. *Lancet* 1:79–80, 1963.

Csanda, E., Antal, J., Anthony, M., and Csanaky, A. Experiences with l-deprenyl in Parkinsonism. *J. Neural Transm.* 43:263–269, 1978.

Davidson, J., McLeod, M., Law-Yone, B., and Linnoila, M. A comparison of electroconvulsive therapy and combined phenelzine-amitriptyline on refractory depression. *Arch. Gen. Psychiatry* 35:639–642, 1978a.

Davidson, J., McLeod, M.N., and White, H.L. Inhibition of platelet monoamine oxidase in depressed subjects treated with phenelzine. *Am. J. Psychiatry* 135:470–472, 1978b.

Denney, R.M., Fritz, R.M., Patel, N.T., and Abell, C.W. Human liver MAO-A and MAO-B separated by immunoaffinity chromatography with MAO-B-specific monoclonal antibody. *Science* 215:1400–1403, 1982.

Diamond, M.A., Murray, R.H., and Schmid, D.G. Idiopathic postural hypotension: Physiologic observations and report of a new mode of therapy. *J. Clin. Invest.* 49:1341–1348, 1970.

Editorial. New look at monoamine oxidase inhibitors. *Br. Med. J.* 2:69, 1976.

Eisler, T., Teravainen, H., Nelson, R., Knebs, H., Weise, V., Lake, C.R., Ebert, M.H., Whetzel, N., Murphy, D.L., Kopin, I.J., and Calne, D.B. Deprenyl in Parkinson disease. *Neurology* 31:19–23, 1981.

Elsworth, J.D., Glover, V., Reynolds, G.P., Sandler, M., Lees, A.J., Phuapradit, P., Shaw, K.M., Stern, G.M., and Kumar, P. Deprenyl administration in man: a selective monoamine oxidase B inhibitor without the "cheese effect." *Psychopharmacology* 57:33–38, 1978.

Fowler, C.J., Callingham, B.A., Mantle, T.J., and Tipton, K.F. Monoamine oxidase A and B: A useful concept? *Biochem. Pharmacol.* 27:97–101, 1978.

Giller, E., and Loeb, J. MAO inhibitors and platelet MAO inhibition. *Commun. Psychopharmacol.* 4:79–82, 1980.

Giller, E., Bialos, D., Riddle, M., Sholomskas, A., and Harkness, L. Monoamine oxidase inhibitor-responsive depression. *Psychiatry Res.* 6:41–48, 1982.

Glassman, A.H., and Platman, S.R. Potentiation of a monoamine oxidase inhibitor by tryptophan. *J. Psych. Res.* 7:83–88, 1969.

Himmelhoch, J.M., Defre, T., Kupfer, D.J., Swartzburg, M., and Byck, R. Treatment of previously intractable depression with tranylcypromine and lithium. *J. Nerv. Ment. Dis.* 155:216–220, 1972.

Hough, L.B., and Domino, E.F. Tele-methylhistamine oxidation by type B monoamine oxidase. *J. Pharmacol. Exp. Ther.* 208:422–428, 1979.

Insel, T.R., Murphy, D.L., Cohen, R.M., Alterman, I., Kilts, C., and Linnoila, M. Obsessive-compulsive disorder: A double-blind trial of clomipramine and clorgyline. *Arch. Gen. Psychiatry* (in press).

Isberg, R.A. A comparison of phenelzine and imipramine in an obsessive-compulsive patient. *Am. J. Psychiatry* 139:1250–1251, 1981.

Jeneke, M.A. Rapid response of severe obsessive-compulsive disorder to tranylcypromine. *Am. J. Psychiatry* 138:1249–1250, 1981.

Kellar, K.T., Cascio, C.S., and Butler, T.A. Differential effects of electroconvulsive shock and antidepressant drugs on serotonin-2-receptors in rat brain. *Eur. J. Pharmacol.* 69:515–518, 1981.

Kenney, W.C., Nagy, J., Salach, J.I., and Singer, T.P. In T.P. Singer, R.W. Von Korff, and D.L. Murphy, eds., *Monoamine Oxidase: Structure, Functions, and Altered Functions,* New York, Academic Press, 1979, pp. 25–38.

Knoll, J. The pharmacology of selective MAO inhibitors. In M.B.H. Youdim, and E.S. Paykel, eds. *Monoamine Oxidase Inhibitors: The State of the Art.* New York, John Wiley and Sons Ltd., 1981, pp. 45–61.

Kupfer, D.J., and Detre, T.P. Tricyclic and monoamine-oxidase-inhibitor antidepressants: Clinical use. In L.L. Iversen, S.D. Iversen, and S.H. Snyder, eds., *Handbook of Psychopharmacology. Affective Disorders: Drug Actions in Animals and Man,* vol. 14, New York, Plenum Press, 1978, pp. 199–232.

Lees, A.J., Shaw, K.M., Kohout, L.J., Stern, G.M., Elsworth, J.D., Sandler, M., and Youdim, M.B.H. Deprenyl in Parkinson's disease. *Lancet* 2:791–795, 1977.

Lipper, S., Murphy, D.L., Slater, S., and Buchsbaum, M.S. Comparative behavioral effects of clorgyline and pargyline in man: A preliminary evaluation. *Psychopharmacology* 62(2):123–128, 1979.

Lipsedge, J.S., Haijjoff, J., Huggins, P., Napier, L., Pearce, J., Pine, D.F., and Rich, M. The management of severe agoraphobia: A comparison of iproniazid and systematic desensitization. *Psychopharmacologia* 32:67–80, 1973.

Major, L.F., Murphy, D.L., Lipper, S., and Gordon, E. Effects of clorgyline and pargyline on deaminated metabolites of norepinephrine, dopamine and serotonin in human cerebrospinal fluid. *J. Neurochem.* 32:229–231, 1979.

Major, L.F., Lake, R.C., Lipper, S., Lerner, P., and Murphy, D.L. The central noradrenergic system and affective response to MAO inhibitors. *Prog. Neuro-Psychopharmacol.* 3:5–6, 1980.

Maycock, A.L., Abeles, R.H., Salach, J.I., and Singer, T.P. The structure of the covalent adduct formed by the interaction of 3-dimethy-amino-1-propyne and the flavine of mitochondrial amine oxidase. *Biochemistry* 15:114–125, 1976.

Moises, H.-W., and Beckmann, H. Antidepressant efficacy of tranylcypromine isomers: A controlled study. *J. Neural Transm.* 50:185–192, 1981.

Murphy, D.L. The behavioral toxicity of monoamine oxidase inhibiting antidepressants. *Adv. Pharmacol. Chemother.* 14:71–105, 1977.

Murphy, D.L. Substrate-selective monoamine oxidases: Inhibitor, tissue, species and functional differences. *Biochem. Pharmacol.* 27:1889–1893, 1978.

Murphy, D.L., Lipper, S., Slater, S., and Shiling, D. Selectivity of clorgyline and pargyline as inhibitors of monoamine oxidases A and B *in vivo* in man. *Psychopharmacology* 62(2):129–132, 1979.

Murphy, D.L., Pickar, D., Jimerson, D., Cohen, R.M., Garrick, N.A., Karoum, F., and Wyatt, R.J. Biochemical indices of the effects of selective MAO inhibitors (clorgyline, pargyline and deprenyl) in man. In E. Usdin, S. Dahl, L.F. Gram, and O. Lingjaerde, eds., *Clinical Pharmacology in Psychiatry,* London, MacMillan Press, 1981a, pp. 307–316.

Murphy, D.L., Roy, B., Pickar, D., Lipper, S., Cohen, R.M., Jimerson, D., Lake, C.R., Muscettola, G., Saavedra, J., and Kopin, I.J. Cardiovascular changes accompanying monoamine oxidase inhibition in man. In E. Usdin, N. Weiner, and C. Creveling, eds., *Function and Regulation of Monoamine Enzymes: Basic and Clinical Aspects.* London, MacMillan, 1981b, pp. 549–560.

Murphy, D.L., Cohen, R.M., Garrick, N.A., Siever, L.J., and Campbell, I.C. Utilization of substrate selective monoamine oxidase inhibitors to explore neurotransmitter hypotheses of the affective disorders. In R.M. Post, and J.C. Ballenger, eds., *Neurobiology of the Mood Disorders.* Baltimore, Williams and Wilkins Co., in press-a.

Murphy, D.L., Cohen, R.M., Siever, L.J., Roy, B., Karoum, F., Wyatt, R.J., Garrick, N.A., and Linnoila, M. Clinical and laboratory studies with selective monoamine oxidase inhibiting drugs: Implications for hypothesized neurotransmitter changes associated with depression and antidepressant drug effects. In H. Beckmann and P. Riederer, *Monoamine Oxidase and Its Selective Inhibitors: New Concepts in Therapy and Research.* Karger, Basel, 1983, pp. 287-303.

Nanda, R.N., Johnson, R.H., and Keogh, H.J. Treatment of neurogenic orthostatic hypotension with a monoamine oxidase inhibitor and tyramine. *Lancet* 2:1164-1167, 1976.

Nelson, D.L., Herbet, A., Glowinski, J., and Hamon, M. [³H]Harmaline as a specific ligand of MAO A–II. Measurement of the turnover rates of MAO A during ontogenesis in the rat brain. *J. Neurochem.* 32:1829-1836, 1979.

Olpe, H.-R., and Schellenberg, A. Reduced sensitivity of neurons to noradrenaline after chronic treatment with antidepressant drugs. *Eur. J. Pharmacol.* 63:7-13, 1980.

Olpe, H.-R. Differential effects of clomipramine and clorgyline on the sensitivity of cortical neurons to serotonin: Effect of chronic treatment. *Eur. J. Pharmco.* 69:375-377, 1981.

Paech, C., Salach, J.I., and Singer, T.P. In T.P. Singer, R.W. Von Korff, and D.L. Murphy, eds., *Monoamine Oxidase: Structure, Functions, and Altered Functions,* New York, Academic Press, 1979, pp. 39-50.

Paykel, E.S., Parker, R.R., Penrose, R.J.J., and Rassaby, E.R. Depressive classification and prediction of response to phenelzine. *Br. J. Psychiatry* 134: 572-581, 1979.

Peroutka, S., and Snyder, S.H. Long-term antidepressant treatment decreases spiroperidol labeled serotonin receptor binding. *Science* 210:88-90, 1980.

Pickar, D., Cohen, R.M., Jimerson, D.C., Lake, R.L., and Murphy, D.L. Tyramine infusions and selective MAO inhibitor treatment. II. Interrelationships among pressor sensitivity changes, platelet MAO inhibition and plasma MHPG reduction. *Psychopharmacology* 74:8-12, 1981.

Pickar, D., Murphy, D.L., Cohen, R.M., Campbell, I.C., and Lipper, S. Behavioral disturbances during the administration of selective and nonselective MAO inhibitors to depressed patients. *Arch. Gen. Psychiatry,* 39:535-548, 1982.

Pletscher, A., Gey, F.K., and Burkand, W.P. Inhibitors of monoamine oxidase and decarboxylase of aromatic amino acids. In *Handbook of Experimental Pharmacology* 19:593-735, 1966.

Ponto, L.B., Perry, P.J., Liskow, B.I., and Seaba, H.H. Drug therapy reviews: Tricyclic antidepressant and monoamine oxidase inhibitor combination therapy. *Am. J. Hosp. Pharm.* 34:954-961, 1977.

Potter, W.Z., Murphy, D.L., Wehr, T.A., Linnoila, M., and Goodwin, F.K. Clorgyline: A new treatment for refractory rapid cycling patients. *Arch. Gen. Psychiatry,* 1982.

Quitkin, F., Rifkin, A., and Klein, D.F. Monoamine oxidase inhibitors. A review of antidepressant effectiveness. *Arch. Gen. Psychiatry* 36:749-760, 1979.

Raskin, A. Adverse reactions to phenelzine: Results of a nine-hospital depression study. *J. Clin. Pharmacol.* 12:22-25, 1972.

Ravaris, C.L., Robinson, D.S., Ives, J.O., Nies, A., and Bartlett, D. Phenelzine and amitriptyline in the treatment of depression. *Arch. Gen. Psychiatry* 37:1075-1080, 1980.

Reynolds, G.P., Rausch, W.D. and Riederer, P. Effects of tranylcypromine stereo-
isomers on monoamine oxidation in man. *Br. J. Clin. Pharmacol.* 9:521–
523, 1980.

Robinson, D.S., Nies, A., Ravaris, L. and Lamborn, K.R. The monoamine oxidase inhibitor, phenelzine, in the treatment of depressive-anxiety states.
Arch. Gen. Psychiatry 29:407–413, 1973.

Robinson, D.S., Nies, A., Ravaris, C.L. Ives, J.O., and Bartlett, D. Clinical
pharmacology of phenelzine. *Arch. Gen. Psychiatry* 35:629–635, 1978.

Robinson, D.S., Nies, A., Ravaris, C.L., Ives, J.O., and Bartlett, D. Clinical
Psychopharmacology of phenelzine: MAO activity and clinical response. In
Lipton, M.A., DiMascio, A., and Killam, K.F., eds., *Psychopharmacology:
A Generation of Progress*, New York, Raven Press, 1978, pp. 961–973.

Robinson, D.S., Nies, A. and Cooper, T.B. Relationships of plasma phenelzine
levels to platelet MAO inhibition, acetylator phenotype, and clinical outcome in depressed outpatients. *Clin. Pharmacol. Ther.* 29:180, 1980.

Rowan, P.R., Paykel, E.S., Parkert, R.R., Gatehouse, J.M., and Rao, B.M. Tri-
cyclic anti-depressant and MAO inhibitor: Are there different effectsπ In
M.B.H. Youdim and E.S. Paykel, eds., *Monoamine Oxidase Inhibitors – The
State of the Art*, New York, John Wiley and Sons, 1981, pp. 125–140.

Sallinger-Barnette, M.M., Mendels, J., and Frazer, A. The effect of psychoactive
drugs on beta-adrenergic receptor binding sites in rat brain. *europharma-
cology* 19:447–454, 1980.

Sargant, W. Drugs in the treatment of depression. *Br. Med. J.* 1:225–227, 1961.

Savage, D.J., Mendels, J., and Frazer, A. Monoamine oxidase inhibitors and serotonin uptake inhibitors: Differential effects on [^{3}H] serotonin binding
sites in rat brain. *J. Pharmacol. Exp. Ther.* 212:259–263, 1980.

Schacter, M., Price, P.A. and Parkes, J.D. Deprenyl in narcolepsy. *Lancet* 1:831–
832, 1979.

Schacter, M., Marsden, C.D., Parkes, J.D., Jenner, P., and Testa, B. Deprenyl in
the management of response fluctuations in patients with Parkinson's
disease on levodopa. *J. Neurol. Neurosurg. Psychiatry* 43:1016–1021,
1980.

Sheehan, D.V., Ballenger, J., and Jacobsen, G. Treatment of endogenous anxiety
with phobic, hysterical, and hypochrondriacal symptoms. *Arch. Gen. Psychiatry* 37:51–59, 1980.

Siever, L.J., Cohen, R.M., and Murphy, D.L. Antidepressants and α_2-adrenergic
autoreceptor desensitization. *Am. J. Psychiatry* 138:681–682, 1981.

Simpson, L.L., and Cabot, B. Monoamine oxidase inhibitors. In Simpson, L.L.,
ed., *Drug Treatment of Mental Disorders*. New York, Raven Press, pp.
147–160, 1976.

Singer, T.P., Von Korff, R.W., and Murphy, D.L. *Monoamine Oxidase: Structure, Function and Altered Functions*, New York, Academic Press, 1979.

Solyom, L., Hesseltine, G.F.D., McClure, D.J., Solyom, C., Led-Widge, B., and
Steinberg, G. Behavior therapy versus drug therapy in the treatment of
phobic neuroses. *Can. Psych. Assoc. J.* 18:25–32, 1973.

Squires, R.F. Monoamine oxidase inhibitors: Animal pharmacology. In L.L.
Iversen, S.D. Iversen, and S.H. Snyder, eds., *Handbook of Psychopharma-
cology, Affective Disorders: Drugs Actions in Animals and Man*, vol. 14,
New York, Plenum Press, 1978, pp. 1–58.

Stockley, I.H. Monoamine oxidase inhibitors. Part I: Interactions with sympathomimetic amines. *Pharmaceutical J.* 210:590-594, 1973a.

Stockley, I.H. Monoamine oxidase inhibitors. Part 2: Interactions with antihypertensive agents, hypoglycaemics, CNS depressants, narcotics and anti-Parkinsonian agents. *Pharmaceutical J.* 210:95-98, 1973b.

Sulser, F., Vetulani, J., and Mobley, P. Mode of action of antidepressant drugs. *Biochem. Pharmcol.* 27:257-261, 1978.

Tyrer, P., Candy, J., and Kelly, D. Phenelzine in phobic anxiety: A controlled trial. *Psycho. Med.* 3:120-124, 1973.

Tyrer, P., Gardner, M., Lambourn, J., and Whitford, M. Clinical and pharmacokinetic factors affecting response to phenelzine. *Br. J. Psychiatry* 136: 359-365, 1980.

White, K., Pistole, T., and Boud, J.L. Combined monoamine oxidase inhibitor-tricyclic antidepressant treatment: a pilot study. *Am. J. Psychiatry* 137: 1422-1425, 1980.

White, K., and Simpson, G. Combined MAOI-tricyclic antidepressant treatment: A reevaluation. *J. Clin. Psychopharm.* 1:264-282, 1981.

Wyatt, R.J., Fram, D.A., Buchbinder, R., and Snyder, F. Treatment of intractable narcolepsy with a monoamine oxidase inhibitor. *N. Engl. J. Med.* 285: 987-991, 1971.

Yates, C.M., and Loudon, J.B. Acetylator status and inhibition of platelet monoamine oxidase following treatment with phenelzine. *Psychol. Med.* 9:777-779, 1979.

Youdim, M.B.H., and Paykel, E.S. *Monoamine Oxidase Inhibitors. The State of the Art.* New York, John Wiley and Sons, 1981.

Young, J.P.R., Lader, M.H., and Hughes, W.C. Controlled trial of trimipramine, monoamine oxidase inhibitors, and combined treatment on depressed outpatients. *Br. Med. J.* 2:1315-1317, 1979.

6

Lithium in Prophylaxis
and Maintenance of Affective Disorders

PER VESTERGAARD

INTRODUCTION

Long-term lithium treatment effectively prevents manic and depressive relapses in many patients with affective disorders. Recent comprehensive reviews have summarized the evidence for efficacy in bipolar (Schou, 1979a) as well as in unipolar patients (Schou, 1979b). However, lithium treatment is not effective in all patients with affective disorders and the treatment is not without inconveniences and at times even hazards. It is therefore important both to search for valid treatment alternatives to lithium and, if lithium treatment is indicated, to administer the treatment in the most effective way, possibly in connection with other treatment modalities.

ALTERNATIVES TO PROPHYLACTIC LITHIUM TREATMENT

Patients who present both depressions and manias (bipolar patients) are affected differently by psychotropic drugs than patients who have only recurrent depressive episodes (unipolar patients).

Bipolar Patients

In a recent Scandinavian multicenter investigation (Ahlfors et al., 1981) the efficacy with which flupenthixol decanoate prevented manic depressive replapses in patients with affective disorders was compared with that of lithium.

95

The authors found that treatment with flupenthixol decanoate in some patients was associated with significant reductions in the frequency of manic episodes and that flupenthixol did not prevent the recurrence of depressive episodes. However, the investigation suffered from many of the pitfalls inherent in multi-center trials as discussed by the authors. They concluded that it is not known whether flupenthixol decanoate is of value in the prevention of manic and depressive relapses, but they found the drug worth trying in patients whose disease is dominated more by manic than by depressive recurrences and who do not respond to lithium or who do not tolerate it or do not wish to take it. No other drug from the group of antipsychotics has been examined systematically for relapse-preventive properties in bipolar patients. Antidepressant drugs are less effective than lithium and occasionally these drugs precipitate manic episodes in bipolar patients (Bunney, 1978; Wehr and Goodwin, 1979). Of other drugs which have been tried recently, carbamazepine (Ballenger and Post, 1981) may have relapse-preventive properties, but the evidence is still scarce.

Unipolar Patients

Open and controlled trials with small patient groups have shown antidepressant drugs of both the tricyclic type and of their second generation to possess prophylactic efficacy which is either inferior or equal, but not superior to lithium (Schou, 1979b). In a preliminary report from a recent British multicenter trial (Medical Research Council, 1981) the relapse-preventive efficacy of lithium was compared with that of amitriptyline in unipolar depressed patients. The results of this study showed lithium and amitriptyline to be equal in efficacy and both active treatments were more effective than placebo. Antipsychotic drugs will not prevent relapses in unipolar depressed patients (Ahlfors et al., 1981). The efficacy of monoamine oxidase inhibitors (Larsen and Rafaelsen, 1980) and carbamazepine (Ballenger and Post, 1981) are not sufficiently proven.

Conclusion

For the majority of patients with bipolar affective disorders no effective prophylactic treatment alternative to lithium exists. For some patients with a unipolar course, long-term prophylaxis with antidepressants may prove effective. The cost/benefit ratio for long-term treatment of unipolar patients with antidepressants has not been established. These drugs, like lithium, have side effects. Such side effects are well known in acute treatments, some of them are serious, and long-term treatment with antidepressants may give rise to yet other side effect profiles, different from the ones known. It is reasonable to expect that at least for some years to come lithium will be the drug of choice for prevention of manic and depressive relapses in most patients with affective disorders regardless of their polarity.

MANAGEMENT OF LITHIUM PROPHYLAXIS

No agreement exists about what is the proper management with lithium for prophylaxis. The recent debate has especially centered around the criteria for selection of patients, the administration of lithium, the requirements for monitoring long-term treatment and the problems of noncompliance and drop-out from treatment.

Criteria for the Selection of Patients

It has been customary to select affective disorder patients for lithium prophylaxis on the basis of the frequency of recent manic or depressive episodes, e.g., two or more episodes within two years. Angst (1980) and Grof et al. (1979a) have shown that these commonly employed criteria may be too strict and lead to the omission of prophylactic treatment in patients for whom this is profitable, since many patients who do not fulfill the criteria mentioned still have frequent recurrences. On the other hand Angst (1980) also showed that about 40% of unipolar patients and about 20% of bipolar patients showed a favorable course with free intervals of more than five years duration with no prophylactic medication. Routine life-long lithium prophylaxis should definitely not be started in patients who have had only one episode. Angst has suggested as a practical rule-of-thumb that prophylactic lithium should be considered in bipolar patients after the second disease episode and in unipolar patients after the third episode. The indications for prophylactic treatment become stronger as the patients grow older and the intervals between the episodes shorter.

The frequency of previous episodes may predict the frequency of episodes to come but not which type of patients will respond to prophylactic lithium treatment. Predictor studies by Grof et al. (1979b) have shown that clinical characteristics such as the purity of the diagnosis (primary affective disorder), the quality of the free intervals between episodes (no psychopathology) and the number of recent episodes (absence of rapid cycling) may predict better than various biological variables which patients will show a favorable response to prophylactic lithium treatment.

Prediction of episode recurrences and treatment response provide good grounds for the selection of patients for lithium prophylaxis, but they can only be supplementary to the clinical assessment of the individual patient's case. Considerations of what would be the impact of a new episode on the patient's life circumstances, his job, and family relations are of importance, as is the psychological and physiological impact of the lithium treatment per se with the establishment of a sick-role, the binding to a hospital, the risk of side effects and so on. For some patients lithium prophylaxis may be considered after the first (manic) episode.

The question of how long lithium prophylaxis should be continued is also of importance. For young patients and for patients who have had only few episodes prior to the start of lithium, it is reasonable to consider after three to five years without relapses if lithium prophylaxis should be discontinued.

Administration of Lithium

The way in which the patient is exposed to lithium has two dimensions, a quantitative one expressed as the 12-hour serum lithium level (12h-SLi) and a qualitative one, illustrated by the shape of the 24-hour serum lithium concentration curve.

The Serum Lithium Level. Studies of side effects in patients given long-term lithium treatment have shown a dose (serum lithium concentration)-effect relationship between, on the one hand, the serum lithium concentration and, on the other, the renal concentrating ability (Vestergaard and Amdisen, 1981). Higher serum lithium concentrations are associated with lower renal concentrating ability and with the occurrence of side effects such as thirst, polyuria and nocturia and possibly weight gain and dehydration.

A similar relationship may exist between the serum lithium concentration and the development of other side effects such as lithium-induced tremor. Therefore, in prophylactic lithium treatment the concentration should be kept at the lowest effective level, if possible below 0.8 mmol/l. On the other hand, for prophylactic efficacy a lower limit of 0.5 mmol/l is suggested based on controlled studies by Hullin (1980) and reports from other clinics in which a satisfactory prophylactic efficacy has been obtained with average serum lithium concentrations in the range between 0.5 and 0.8 mmol/l. This range is lower than the usually recommended one which is between 0.6–0.7 and 1.0–1.2 mmol/l. Some patients may not show a satisfactory prophylactic response with an average serum lithium concentration between 0.5 and 0.8 mmol/l, and only for such patients should higher serum lithium concentrations be tried.

It has been customary to express the quantitative exposure to lithium as the 12h-SLi concentration. A study (Lauritsen et al., 1981) in which the serum lithium concentration was determined around the clock in patients treated with conventional tablets given once daily in the evening and in patients treated with slow-release tablets given twice daily in the morning and in the evening showed markedly different concentration curve shapes in the two groups. But calculations of the ratio of the mean serum lithium concentration over the 24-hour day to the serum lithium concentration in blood samples drawn 12 hours after the last intake of lithium showed the ratios to be similar in the two patient groups. This indicates that in the two patient groups mentioned, where lithium was administered in quite different ways, the 12h-SLi concentration represented the same amount of lithium in serum over 24 hours. However, it may also be inferred from this study that if lithium is administered in yet a different way, for instance as sustained-release lithium given *once a day* in the evening, a 12h-SLi concentration may represent a different amount of lithium in serum over the 24 hours. Thus, references in the literature to 12h-SLi concentrations, e.g., when recommendations are made about serum concentrations which offer optimum prophylaxis or which involve the risk of side effect development, should also include information about the type of lithium preparation and the number of daily doses.

The Shape of the 24-Hour Serum Lithium Concentration Curve. The shape of the 24-hour serum lithium concentration curve is determined by the properties of the lithium preparation, by the number of daily lithium doses, by the time of the day they are administered and by patient properties, including the renal lithium clearance, which shows a difference between night and day (Lauritsen et al., 1981). The shape of the curve has implications for the qualitative exposure to lithium as illustrated by the peaks and troughs of the curve. It has been suggested that curve peaks are undesirable, especially in connection with the development of side effects, and much effort has been put into the development of sustained-release lithium preparations which yield rather flat concentration curves. Recently an opposite suggestion has been forwarded (Plenge et al., 1981), namely that although peaks may be undesirable, the troughs of the serum lithium concentration curve could be beneficial, since they leave the cells of the organism time for regenerative processes to take place. In a study in which different lithium treatment regimens were compared (Schou et al., 1982), it was shown that distal water reabsorption was significantly less affected and polyuria less pronounced in patients given conventional tablets twice daily than in patients given slow-release tablets twice daily. Animal studies have shown similar differences in outcome when different ways of administering lithium were applied (Plenge et al., 1981). Speculations about the importance of the qualitative aspects of lithium exposure have led to considerations about drug holidays and to the question of whether lithium could be given every other day or possibly once a week and still be therapeutically effective but without side effects (Plenge et al., 1982).

Monitoring of Long-Term Lithium Treatment

The narrow therapeutic range of lithium and the treatment periods for many years make close monitoring of the treatment mandatory. However, not all patients need the same scrutiny. Some patients given long-term lithium treatment will tolerate the treatment well with only trivial side effects and derive the desired advantage from the treatment. These patients can be monitored at nonspecialized facilities with access to a minimal number of laboratory examinations. For other patients more elaborate control facilities are needed. Irrespective of the type of facilities the patient and his relatives must always be properly informed verbally about the benefits and problems of the treatment and preferably also informed from written sources (Schou, 1980). During the whole period of treatment laboratory control should also be supplemented with a clinical interview to detect slight symptoms of side effects and the early signs of relapses.

Regular Facilities. Patients who prior to the start of lithium treatment have shown no signs of renal or thyroid diseases or other serious somatic complications, who do not develop important side effects and who gain benefit from the treatment may be monitored by the general practitioner or by the practising psychiatrist. For this group of patients laboratory control, once steady-state lithium concentrations are obtained, may be confined to regular assessment of the serum lithium concentration and serum creatinine at intervals of 2-4 months and assessment of serum TSH at intervals of 6 months (Vestergaard et al., 1982).

Extended Facilities. Other patients who do not fulfill the criteria mentioned above should have their lithium treatment initiated at specialized facilities or have the possibility of being referred to special clinics. The staff at such facilities should be able to master the detection and treatment of lithium-induced side effects, alternative ways of administering lithium, the problems which arise when lithium is given together with other psychotropic drugs and with drugs for various somatic conditions. Such facilities must have a specially trained staff, access to medical expertise from other fields and access to laboratory facilities which, in addition to the above mentioned laboratory variables, can provide full-scale thyroid assessment and the assessment of renal function with the determination of glomerular filtration rate and renal concentrating ability.

Noncompliance

As many as 20 to 30% of patients who start lithium treatment may discontinue treatment before the prophylactic properties of lithium can be properly assessed (Van Putten and Jamison, 1980). Many drop-outs will occur during the first six months of treatment. Factors responsible for the discontinuation may be associated with the patient, his illness, the lithium preparation, the undesired effects of lithium, the treatment facilities in general, and the physician's attitude in particular. Side effects are probably the most common reasons for discontinuation, but more subtle psychological factors are also of importance.

Conclusion

Many questions regarding the optimum management of lithium prophylaxis are still unanswered or remain controversial. For many patients specialist care is necessary if an optimum ratio between the benefits and costs of lithium treatment shall be obtained. The specialist must serve two functions: One is the direct handling of patients who present complex treatment problems and the other is the administration of specialized facilities, lithium clinics, with the training of staff, research obligations and an advisory function for colleagues inside and outside the psychiatric institutions.

INTERACTION OF LITHIUM WITH OTHER TREATMENTS

Concomitant treatment with nonpsychotropic drugs (e.g., diuretics) may interfere adversely with lithium treatment; concomitant treatment with psychotropic drugs may at times be necessary and beneficial but can also be problematic (for review, see Jefferson et al., 1981). The interactions between lithium and various psychotherapies have so far attracted little attention.

Lithium and Other Psychotropic Drugs

Only recently have treatment combinations which involve lithium and other psychotropic drugs been studied systematically with regard to their prophylactic efficacy. The results did not favor the combination of lithium and antidepressants, when compared with either drug given alone; this was so for unipolar as well as for bipolar patients (Peselow et al., 1981, Quitkin et al., 1981). The prophylactic efficacy of lithium and antipsychotics administered concomitantly has not been studied systematically.

Some patients with incomplete effect of lithium prophylaxis may profit from the combination of lithium with other psychotropic drugs during episode recurrences. However, when figures for concomitant treatment with other psychotropic drugs in a large lithium-treated population reach levels as high as 60% (Vestergaard et al., 1979) it is reasonable to speculate if not some of the patients were better off with lithium alone or without lithium. When lithium is administered concomitantly with other psychotropic drugs, the propylactic efficacy of lithium cannot be properly assessed. Furthermore, additional treatment with tricyclic antidepressants may increase the number of patients who complain of tremor and may also increase the risk of mood instability, since antidepressant drugs may antagonize the stabilizing effect of lithium (Reginaldi et al., 1981). Additional treatment with neuroleptics has been claimed to add to the impairment of water metabolism and to the risk of neurological impairment, although evidence for both of these claims is debatable.

Lithium and Psychological Treatments

Systematic studies of the combined effect of lithium treatment and various forms of psychotherapy are few which is in a startling contrast to the large number of British and American studies on the combined effect of antipsychotics and psychotherapy for chronic schizophrenia (Schooler, 1978). In the prophylaxis and maintenance of patients with chronic schizophrenia it has been shown that the combination of antipsychotics with various forms of psychotherapy which are either supportive or directed at social skills is superior to either treatment given alone. Also for the acute treatment of depression the combination of antidepressant drugs with various forms of psychotherapy has received a great deal of attention, and carefully executed studies have shown that also for this condition may the combination of drug therapy and psychotherapy be superior to either treatment modality given alone (Weissman, 1979). As regards the prophylaxis and maintenance of patients with affective disorders only few studies have been published which examined these problems. Davenport et al. (1977) found that couples group therapy added significantly to the effect of lithium prophylaxis. Other authors (O'Connell and Mayo, 1981) have commented on the benefits of viewing lithium therapy in a biopsychosocial perspective, and both family therapy (Keith, 1980) and group therapy (Volkmar et al., 1981) have been advocated as a beneficial adjunct to lithium treatment.

Conclusion

In viewing the interactions of lithium with other treatment modalities the negative interactions so far have received the main part of attention; positive interactions, especially between lithium and various psychotherapies, have been explored only to a very limited degree. It is to be hoped that the addition of formalized psychotherapy, one type or another, will support the pharmacological treatment through increased patient motivation and that it may even lead to insight, if not in the dynamic aspects of the illness per se, at least in the type of life events which precipitate episodes or which are precipitated by the illness and the treatment.

VISTAS FOR FUTURE RESEARCH

Confirmation and refutation of present suppositions and the acquisition of new knowledge might come from an examination of the following questions: (a) Which patient or illness factors will most precisely predict the type of patient who will stay in lithium treatment and benefit from the treatment? (b) What is the optimum serum lithium level for prophylaxis and maintenance of the majority of patients with affective disorders? (c) Will the addition of psychotherapy in one form or another add beneficially to the outcome of long-term lithium treatment? (d) Are there valid treatment alternatives to lithium? (e) Does the treatment regimen (dosage pattern and tablet type) influence the outcome of the treatment?

BIBLIOGRAPHY

Ahlfors, U.G., Baastrup, P.C., Dencker, S.J., Elgen, K., Lingjaerde, O., Pedersen, V., Schou, M., and Aaskoven, O. Flupenthixol decanoate in recurrent manic-depressive illness. A comparison with lithium. *Acta Psychiat. Scand.* 64:226-237, 1981.

Angst, J. Verlauf unipolar depressiver, bipolar manisch-depressiver und schizoaffektiver Erkrankungen und Psychosen. Ergebnisse einer prospektiven Studie. *Fortschr. Neurol. Psychiat.* 48:3-30, 1980.

Ballenger, J.C., and Post, R.M. Carbamazepine in manic-depressive illness: A new treatment. *Am. J. Psychiat.* 137:782-790, 1980.

Bunney, W.E., Jr. Psychopharmacology of the switch process in affective illness. In M.A. Lipton, A. DiMascio, and K.F. Killam, eds., *Psychopharmacology: A Generation of Progress.* New York: Raven Press, 1978.

Davenport, Y.B., Ebert, M.H., Adland, M.L., and Goodwin, F.K. Couples group therapy as an adjunct to lithium maintenance of the manic patient. *Am. J. Orthopsychiatry* 47(3):495-502, 1977.

Grof, P., Angst, J., Karasek, M., and Keitner, G. Patient selection for long-term lithium treatment in clinical practice. *Arch. Gen. Psychiatry* 36:894-897, 1979a.

Grof, P., Lane, J., MacCrimmon, D., Werstiuk, E., Blajchman, M., Daigle, L., and Varma, R. Clinical and laboratory correlates of the response to long-term lithium treatment. In M. Schou and E. Strömgren, eds., *Origin, Prevention and Treatment of Affective Disorders.* London: Academic Press, 1979b.

Hullin, R.P. Minimum serul lithium levels for effective prophylaxis. In F. Neil Johnson, ed., *Handbook of Lithium Therapy.* Lancaster: MTP Press, 1980.

Jefferson, J.W., Greist, J.H., and Baudhuin, M. Lithium: interactions with other drugs. *J. Clin. Psychopharmacol.* 1(3):124-134, 1981.

Keith, D.V. Family therapy and lithium deficiency. *J. Marital Family Ther.* January:49-53, 1980.

Larsen, J.K., and Rafaelsen, O.J. Long-term treatment of depression with isocarboxazide. *Acta Psychiat. Scand.* 62:456-463, 1980.

Lauritsen, B.J., Mellerup, E.T., Plenge, P., Rasmussen, S., Vestergaard, P., and Schou, M. Serum lithium concentrations around the clock with different treatment regimens and the diurnal variation of the renal lithium clearance. *Acta Psychiat. Scand.* 64:314-319, 1981.

Medical Research Council Drug Trials Subcommittee. Continuation therapy with lithium and amitriptyline in unipolar depressive illness: a controlled clinical trial. *Psychol. Med.* 11:409-416, 1981.

O'Connell, R.A., and Mayo, J.A. Lithium: a biopsychosocial perspective. *Comprehens. Psych.* 22:87–93, 1981.

Peselow, E.D., Dunner, D.L., Fieve, R.R., Gulbenkian, G., Deutsch, S.I., and Kaufmann, M. Maintenance treatment of unipolar depression. *Psychopharmacol. Bull.* 17:53–56, 1981.

Plenge, P., Mellerup, E.T., and Nørgaard, T. Functional and structural rat kidney changes by peroral or parenteral lithium treatment. *Acta Psychiat. Scand.* 63:303–313, 1981.

Plenge, P., Mellerup, E.T., Bolwig, T.G., Brun, C., Hetmar, O., Ladefoged, J. Larsen, S., and Rafaelsen, O.J. Lithium treatment: Does the kidney prefer one daily dose instead of two? *Acta Psychiat. Scand.* 66:121–128, 1982.

Putten, T. Van and Jamison, K.R. Rejection of lithium maintenance therapy by the patient. In F. Neil Johnson, ed., *Handbook of Lithium Therapy*. Lancaster: MTP Press, 1980.

Quitkin, M., Kane, J., Rifkin, A., Ramos-Lorenzi, J.R., and Nayak, D.V. Prophylactic lithium carbonate with and without imipramine for bipolar 1 patients. *Arch. Gen. Psychiatry* 38:902–907, 1981.

Reginaldi, D., Tondo, L., Floris, G., Pignatelli, A., and Kukopulos, A. Poor prophylactic lithium response due to antidepressants. *Int. Pharmacopsychiatry* 16:124–128, 1981.

Schooler, N.R. Antipsychotic drugs and psychological treatment in schizophrenia. In M.A. Lipton, A. DiMascio, and K.F. Killam, eds., *Psychopharmacology: A Generation of Progress*. New York: Raven Press, 1978.

Schou, M. Lithium prophylaxis: Is the honeymoon over? *Aust. N.Z. J. Psychiatry* 13:109–114, 1979a.

Schou, M. Lithium as a prophylactic agent in unipolar affective illness. Comparison with cyclic antidepressants. *Arch. Gen. Psychiatry* 36:849–851, 1979b.

Schou, M. *Lithium Treatment of Manic-Depressive Illness: A Practical Guide.* Basel, München, Paris, London, New York, Sydney: Karger, 1980.

Schou, M., Amdisen, A., Thomsen, K., Vestergaard, P., Hetmar, O., Mellerup, E.T., Plenge, P., and Rafaelsen, O.J. Lithium treatment regimen and renal water handling. The significance of dosage pattern and tablet type examined through comparison of results from two clinics with different treatment regimens. *Psychopharmacology* 77:387–390, 1982.

Vestergaard, P., and Amdisen, A. Lithium treatment and kidney function. A follow-up study of 237 patients in long-term treatment. *Acta Psychiat. Scand.* 63:333–345, 1981.

Vestergaard, P., Amdisen, A., Hansen, H.E., and Schou, M. Lithium treatment and kidney function. A survey of 237 patients in long-term treatment. *Acta Psychiat. Scand.* 60:504–520, 1979.

Vestergaard, P., Schou, M., and Thomsen, K. Monitoring of patients in prophylactic lithium treatment. As assessment based on recent kidney studies. *Br. J. Psychiatry* 140:185–187, 1982.

Volkmar, F.R., Bacon, S., Shakir, S.A., and Pfefferbaum, A. Group therapy in the management of manic-depressive illness. *Am. J. Psychother.* 35:226–233, 1981.

Weissman, M.M. The psychological treatment of depression. Evidence for the efficacy of psychotherapy alone, in comparison with, and in combination with pharmacotherapy. *Arch. Gen. Psychiatry* 36:1261–1269, 1979.

Wehr, T.A. and Goodwin, F.K. Rapid cycling in manic-depressives induced by tricyclic antidepressants. *Arch. Gen. Psychiatry* 36:555–559, 1979.

7

Somatic Side Effects
of Long-Term Lithium Treatment

PAUL GROF AND KARL O'SULLIVAN

INTRODUCTION

In recent years, the side effects of long-term lithium treatment have attracted increasing attention for two main reasons. Firstly, as the recurring nature of most affective disorders is now well recognized, there has been a shift in emphasis from treatment of acute conditions to prevention of recurrences by long-term treatment. Secondly, as lithium treatment has become widely used for extended periods of time, the side effects of long-term treatment have become an important clinical issue.

For practical purposes, it is useful to make a distinction between early and late side effects of lithium therapy. Early side effects occurring in the first few weeks of treatment may be similar in manifestation to those developing months or years after long-term lithium administration. In spite of these similarities, their frequency and clinical relevance may differ greatly depending on time of occurrence. In addition, there are qualitative differences in side effects occurring early and late in treatment.

This volume is concerned with practical guidelines for the use of psychoactive drugs and thus this paper focuses mainly on selected issues which are practical and clinically important. Space does not allow a comprehensive coverage of the extensive literature on side effects. However, the reader is referred to several excellent reviews for details (Schou, 1968; Shopsin, 1973; Brown, 1976; Vacaflor, 1975; Amdisen and Schou, 1978, 1979, 1980; Reisenberg and Gershon, 1979; Vestergaard et al., 1980). In addition, selected references are quoted in each section of the paper, to avoid fragmentation of the text and to stress that it is not the intention of this manuscript to be comprehensive. For similar reasons, we do not discuss a number of important issues such as factors modifying the nature and severity of side effects, the complex issues of lithium's impact on psychological functioning, the underlying mechanisms of side effects, and the complications resulting from the interaction of lithium with other drugs.

For the purpose of this presentation side effects have been defined as those drug effects which are not obviously related to lithium's therapeutic action, are likely to impair the patient's level of functioning or well being and can be detected clinically by inspection or routine laboratory tests. Side effects are defined here from the viewpoint of the psychiatrist who uses lithium to stabilize abnormal moods, without influencing other bodily functions, in contrast to the internist or neurologist who may use lithium to treat refractory cases of Grave's disease, Felty's syndrome, or epilepsy.

THE KIDNEY

As the effects of long term lithium treatment on the structure and functions of the kidney have recently attracted a great deal of attention (Hansen, 1982; Jenner, 1979; Mellerup et al., 1978; Vestergaard and Schou, 1981), we focus on them first. The concerns surrounding this issue are quite understandable. Any treatment which would have the long-term potential of endangering a vital function of the body, such as the elimination of waste, would have limited value. As the kidney is the main excretion avenue of lithium, the potential effects of this drug on the kidney have been studied since its introduction into therapy. The classic investigations of Schou (1958) are still relevant today and answer basic questions. However, major concerns arose in the fall of 1977, when Hestbech and co-workers reported structural changes in the kidneys of patients who experienced repeated lithium intoxication and/or polyuria. Although the initial controversy over this report has to some extent settled, the effect of long-term lithium treatment on the kidney remains a very important issue. The following is a summary of our perceptions of the present state of knowledge of the effects of lithium on kidney structure and function.

Changes produced by long-term lithium treatment are functional, and possibly structural. The main effects of lithium on the kidney which the clinician has to keep in mind include polyuria associated with polydipsia, urinary concentrating defect, and possibly structural change of the type of interstitial nephritis. At the functional level, long-term lithium treatment leads to a urinary concentrating defect in many patients. This may manifest as clinically significant polyuria in 10-20% of chronically treated patients, and infrequently as a fully developed, vasopressin-resistant diabetis insipidus-like syndrome. Polydipsia appears to be mainly secondary to renal physiological changes but may also have a central component, due to the effects of lithium on the thirst center. From clinical experience polyuria and polydipsia generally subside with discontinuation of the medication. However, whether this is fully reversible remains uncertain due to lack of data.

Reduced renal concentrating ability is a common, and the most prominent, lithium-induced renal complication with long-term lithium treatment. The impairment of renal concentrating ability is correlated to both the duration of lithium treatment and the serum lithium concentration. Some data suggests that this impairment of renal concentrating ability parallels histological changes in the distal tubules. The reduced primary concentration makes the lithium treated patients probably more susceptible to dehydration due to increased extrarenal water and sodium loss.

The reduction in the maximum urinary osmolality is not of hypothalamic but of renal origin. In these patients the hypothalamic region remains reactive to stimuli such as water loading and water deprivation but hypothalamus is secondarily involved as arginine–vasopressin plasma levels are increased in the afflicted patients.

Glomerular filtration rate, renal albumin and beta-two-microglobulin excretion are normal or almost normal in nearly all patients. These findings are incompatible within the idea of toxic action of lithium on the glomeruli and the proximal tubules. Thus, in patients with no pre-existing renal pathology long-term lithium treatment does not have any demonstrable effects on glomerular filtration (Jenner, 1979; Grof et al., 1980, 1982). The question remains, however, whether lithium facilitates or increases the chances of functional worsening of already impaired glomeruli.

Structural changes in the kidney are common after lithium intoxication. However, there is no good evidence that long-term lithium treatment leads to structural changes in a healthy kidney. Studies have demonstrated that affectively ill patients show more structural renal abnormalities than matched controls even before they ever received lithium, and the observed trends for more structural pathology in patients on lithium have not reached statistical significance.

Lithium-induced renal lesions, if they develop, are probably located in the distal part of the nephron where also the highest lithium concentrations are reached. Lithium-induced nephropathy has been described histologically as tubular lesions, cystic tubular dilation or cysts. However, a causal relationship between the fibrotic changes and long-term lithium treatment is still debatable since the changes have also been reported in affectively ill patients who have not been treated with lithium.

Renal functional changes which may develop during long-term lithium treatment are not a contraindication for the continuation of treatment. However, these changes do underline the need for careful selection of patients for lithium so that only the patients who really need the treatment and are likely to benefit from it receive lithium treatment for an extended period of time. These renal changes also emphasize the importance of careful monitoring of lithium treatment and active prevention of lithium intoxication which may produce structural changes.

ENDOCRINE AND METABOLIC EFFECTS

Long-term lithium treatment influences the endocrine system in a variety of ways (Birch, 1978; Reisberg and Gershon, 1979). The clinically most important effects include its action on the thyroid hormones and insulin-like effects.

Lithium has been found to affect thyroid function in patients and volunteers. However, the effects are transient and without clinical significance in subjects with adequate thyroid reserve. In comparison with pretreatment values, slightly decreased T4 and elevated TSH levels are found in about one third of the patients on long-term lithium maintenance. As a result of lithium's interference with the thyroid function, one may find clinical hypothyroidism, or goiter, or both. Exaggerated response of TSH to TRH has been found by several investigators and suggests altered regulation of thyroid function on lithium. Anecdotally, benign exophthalmos and hyperthyroidism have also been reported. Elevated thyroid function has been seen after a rapid reduction of lithium dosage or when essential hyperthyroidism develops coincidentally during lithium treatment.

Lithium salts have been shown to interfere with thyroid chemistry at several levels, from iodine uptake into the glands, through glandular synthesis of thyroid hormones, to their release and peripheral utilization. Lithium inhibits TSH induced thyroid response by blocking ATP conversion and/or the effects of cyclic AMP on thyroid cells. Lithium also interferes with the effects of TSH at the glandular level (Berens and Wolff, 1975; Glen, 1978; Wolff, 1979).

In most cases, the interference of lithium with thyroid function remains subclinical, and does not require treatment. However, all patients on long-term lithium should have regular clinical and laboratory monitoring of the thyroid functions as clinically significant hypothyroidism requiring thyroid supplementation has been observed in 15–25% of lithium-treated patients (depending probably on the composition of the patient sample). If hypothyroidism or goiter develops, exogenous thyroid supplementation should be prescribed and carefully titrated.

It should be noted that thyroid requirements do change over time and patients who require thyroid supplementation at one point in time may not require it later. However, exogenous thyroid tends to suppress the production of endogenous hormones and after an extended period of supplementation the intrinsic production of thyroid hormones may get suppressed to the point that a need for supplementation becomes permanent. Therefore, the need for supplementation should be reviewed, particularly during the initial stage.

Of interest is the fact that lithium interference with thyroid function has been successfully explored in internal medicine for the treatment of selected cases of thyrotoxicoses.

The metabolic effects of lithium are complex and involve various biochemical processes. Perhaps the most striking is the insulin-like effect of lithium treatment which tends to increase glycogen synthesis and glucose tolerance. Lithium also has a broad effect on many enzymes of carbohydrate metabolism, especially enzymes with inhibitory actions. Occasionally, the effect of lithium on the metabolism of calcium may result in the overactivity of the parathyroid gland, with corresponding clinical manifestations (Mellerup and Rafaelsen, 1975; Mellerup et al., 1978).

No consistent effects of lithium treatment have been found for resting plasma levels of cortisol, prolactin, and growth hormone. However, several recent reports indicate altered neuroendocrine responses to insulin challenge during lithium treatment. Prolactin responses to both hypogylcemia and TRH appear reduced, along with the increased response of TSH and TRH. The altered neuroendocrine responses clearly suggest altered regulation of neuroendocrine function although the clinical relevance of these findings is not yet clear.

Weight gain is a common side effect of long-term lithium treatment but its actual frequency depends on a number of factors: innate predisposition in terms of individual and family history of obesity, ethnic background, the concomitant use of other psychoactive drugs, carbohydrate and caloric intake, the presence or absence of lithium response, and the duration of treatment. The frequency and extent of weight gain reported in the literature varies as those different variables have not been systematically explored (Grof et al., 1973).

Dramatic weight gain is usually observed only during the first year, and takes place mainly in obesity-prone lithium responders. By contrast, at the end of the first year, the average weight of nonresponders to long-term lithium treatment does not appear increased unless, of course, the patient is also regularly receiving antidepressants and neuroleptics.

It is important to bear in mind that the weight gain in patients on lithium is, on the average, less than that observed in patients on maintenance treatment with neuroleptics, or antidepressants, for similar periods of time. Despite this, lithium is associated with weight gain in the clinician's mind, perhaps because lithium responding patients are more compliant and are willing to stay on lithium longer than on other medications.

The increase in body weight is a real increase in tissue mass and is considered independent of fluid retention. As mentioned before, lithium affects significantly a number of enzymes involved in carbohydrate metabolism, and most explanations for the weight gain refer to the insulin-like effect of lithium on body metabolism, gluconeogenesis, and increased glycogen storage.

Weight gain on lithium can be both effectively treated and prevented by substantially reducing carbohydrates or caloric intake. In practice of course a subtantial reduction of caloric intake (for instance below 1,000 calories) takes place mainly at the expense of carbohydrates. In suitable patients a carefully scheduled intermittent treatment with a period of 4-6 weeks off lithium usually produces dramatic weight reduction in lithium-induced obesity. However, this approach should be restricted to setups specializing in the treatment of affective disorders.

CNS AND NEUROMUSCULAR SYSTEMS

In clinical practice the central nervous system effects of lithium can vary from commonly observed mild symptoms to severe and even irreversible toxicity. While mild effects are quite common, serious toxicity develops almost exclusively in various stages of lithium intoxication, and therefore will not be discussed here.

In view of lithium's significant CNS metabolic effects, it is not surprising that even with ordinary therapeutic dosages lithium has a tendency to produce consistent, electrophysiologically documented CNS effects in the majority of patients (Small, Millstein, and Small, 1972; Mayfield and Brown, 1966; Dimitrakoudi and Jenner, 1975). However, the available evidence indicates that these changes are benign.

It is difficult to assess the effects of lithium treatment on such sensitive functions as memory, since depressed patients, even recovered and unmedicated ones, commonly complain of memory difficulties. There is, however, no evidence that routine lithium treatment adversely affects memory or other neuropsychological functions in patients with primary affective disorders. The same cannot be said for healthy volunteers, schizophrenics, or patients with organic impairment, where further studies are needed to clarify complex relationships.

The relationship between lithium and seizure propensity appears complex and vulnerability to seizure probably depends to a considerable extent on the underlying electrophysiological excitability. Some studies have found lithium suppressing desynchronized activity and helpful in epileptics, particularly in some otherwise treatment resistant cases, whereas other investigators have reported seizures in patients with therapeutic lithium levels, and exacerbation of seizure activity in a majority of patients with temporal lobe epilepsy has also been reported.

During the initial stage of lithium treatment, hand tremor is quite frequent and may be observed in more than half of all patients (Vestergaard,

Amdisen, and Schou, 1980). However, the incidence decreases during extended lithium stabilization and only infrequently persists after years of treatment. The tremor is fine and rapid, frequently fluctuates in intensity, and differs in character from Parkinsonian tremor. Clinically, the tremor is influenced by everyday stresses which excite the sympathetic nervous system. It can frequently be relieved by adrenergic beta blockers, such as propranolol.

Muscular weakness is frequently experienced by patients in the initial state of treatment but the complaints are almost invariably transient. After discontinuation of lithium patients occasionally report improvement in muscle strength, which suggests that on lithium there may be a subtle adaptation to muscular weakness unnoticed by the patient except by contrast, once the drug is discontinued.

GASTROINTESTINAL SYSTEM

Gastrointestinal disturbances are relatively frequent during the first weeks of treatment but their persistence in long-term treatment is less common (Jefferson and Greist, 1977). In long-term therapy, a most common problem is an increased tendency for loose stools, which can be triggered off by such upsets as minor dietary mistakes, abortive virus exposure, etc. Epigastric bloating or pressure, diarrhea, anorexia, nausea, abdominal pain, or vomiting may all occasionally occur in long term treatment but are much more common early in therapy. Gastrointestinal distress tends to be associated with steeper rises in serum lithium levels (with a faster change of the concentration gradient between serum and the tissues). The suggested mechanisms of gastrointestinal side effects include lithium substitution for sodium which decreases the intestinal absorption, and lithium's interference with adenylcyclase resulting in inhibition of insulin, glucagon and gastric/pancreatic hormones. The frequency of upper gastrointestinal side effects in both initial and long-term stage can be reduced by the use of good quality, slow-release lithium preparations.

CARDIAC EFFECTS

Benign, reversible EKG changes are quite common among patients on long-term lithium, and are manifested mainly as T wave flattening or inversion (Jefferson and Greist, 1977; Jefferson and Freist, 1979). The frequency of these changes increases with the sensitivity of monitoring, and may be found in the majority of patients, if carefully looked for.

Other cardiac changes are very uncommon and include conduction and/or rhythm abnormalities, and myocarditis. Mechanism of cardiac side effects can be explained by lithium's partial replacement of potassium, which leads to a relative intracellular potassium deficiency; lithium may also affect the heart by interfering with adenylcyclase and inhibiting the response to epinephrine.

In many patients with recurrent depression the treatment choice is between lithium and tricyclic antidepressants. In our experience the heart, even an impaired heart, usually tolerates lithium better than tricyclic antidepressants. In practice, unfortunately, most patients are treated by a combination of these medications and the cardiac abnormalities are attributed to lithium. These abnormalities frequently disappear during lithium treatment when antidepressants are discontinued.

BLOOD

Lithium produces a relative leucocytosis in most patients and, in healthy volunteers given lithium the extent of the leucocytosis varies from minimal to a three fold increase in cell count. Some degree of leucocytosis may be expected in a substantial proportion of patients on lithium therapy. The actual leucocyte count is usually in the neighborhood of $10\text{-}15,000/\text{ml}^3$. The analysis of the observed changes suggests that a lithium-induced leucocytosis is secondary to neutrophilia and is accompanied by lymphocytopenia. These changes in patients on long-term lithium are sometimes episodic, sometimes persistent, and have not been shown to be directly related to lithium plasma levels (Greco and Breton, 1976; Gupta, Robinson and Smyth, 1975).

SKIN AND BONES

As a rule, lithium treatment is not associated with dermatologic complications, with the exception of psoriasis, which is frequently exacerbated by long-term lithium therapy. This effect is so marked that one probably has to consider clear-cut psoriasis as a relative contraindication to long-term lithium treatment. The possible mechanism of action probably includes interference with skin adenylcyclase which may be reduced in psoriasis. Sporadically and temporarily lithium has been reported in association with maculopapular and acne-like dermatological lesions, hair loss, and dermatitis (Reisberg and Gershon, 1979a,b; Schou, 1968; Vestergaard, Amdisen, and Schou, 1980).

Lithium does accumulate in the bone and may decrease bony calcium. There is little evidence to date, however, that for mature bones this effect is of any clinical significance. Caution may be indicated, however, in long-term treatment of younger individuals as there is evidence that immature, growing bone accumulates lithium much more rapidly (Birch, 1978).

TERATOGENIC EFFECTS

For obvious reasons, the effects of lithium on the offspring of mothers receiving lithium treatment cannot be studied experimentally. Our knowledge about this question is based on reports to the Registers of lithium babies. The findings have not documented an overall increase in malformations; however, the reported rate of cardiovascular malformations was greater than expected and one cannot exclude the possibility of a teratogenic potential of lithium for the developing heart. The issue cannot be considered closed as the Registers depend on information which has been voluntarily brought to their attention, and children with problems are more likely to be reported (Weinstein, 1979; Vacaflor, 1975; Vacaflor, Lehmann, and Ban, 1970).

From the clinical point of view this means that the potential benefits and risks of lithium treatment in pregnancy should be weighed very carefully, considering the mother and the fetus. Whenever possible, lithium treatment should be avoided particularly during the formative months of the first trimester. In the case of planned pregnancy, it is frequently possible to select for the mother the time of the least risk and keep her relatively safely off lithium while the couple is attempting impregnation. The safer, low-risk times can be selected on the basis of thorough knowledge of the natural history of affective disorders.

LITHIUM INTOXICATION

Lithium intoxication is the most serious side effect of lithium treatment and can develop at any time during its administration. As the lithium ion is almost exclusively eliminated by the kidneys, a lithium intake which clearly exceeds the renal lithium elimination rate may lead to elevated serum lithium levels and to lithium intoxication. In comparison with other medications, the therapeutic index of lithium is relatively low, and therefore a clear discrepancy between lithium intake and elimination may lead to intoxication in a matter of days or weeks. Lithium intoxication may be complicated by acute renal shutdown or insufficiency, leading to a "vicious circle," in which lithium intoxication delays lithium elimination which results in worsening the intoxication.

Events leading to increased extrarenal loss of water and sodium, and/or decreased fluid intake frequently preceed lithium intoxication. In dealing with the intoxication, one should provide fluid therapy and replenish the deficient sodium. However, one should not administer excess sodium to patients with already severely impaired renal concentrating ability. Hemodialysis remains the most efficient method for treating the lithium intoxication.

Data on lithium intoxication gathered in southern Ontario indicates that it is most likely to occur within the first six months of treatment. Intoxications are frequently iatrogenic in origin, and probably can frequently be avoided. More education of patients and physicians about lithium treatment, a careful screening for pre-existing renal problems, and improved monitoring of lithium treatment would minimize the occurrence of intoxication.

REDUCING AND PREVENTING SIDE EFFECTS

Frequency and severity of side effects can be influenced by a number of factors, some of them related to the type of treatment, others to the characteristics of the patient. The major treatment-related variables are dosage and blood levels of lithium, type of lithium given, length of treatment, and combination with other drugs. Some of the better understood patient variables are age, diet, and clinical response to lithium stabilization. Most of these variables can be to some extent manipulated in order to reduce side effects.

Most side effects can be alleviated by reducing daily dosage and the serum lithium blood levels. Gastrointestinal symptoms and urinary side effects are good examples. Replacing a fast-absorbing preparation by a delayed or slow-release lithium appears to improve particularly the gastrointestinal side effects, such as nausea or diarrhea. The length of lithium treatment is particularly relevant for reduced urinary concentration, nocturia due to lithium, and increased body weight. Side effects related to the duration of treatment can be reduced by treating the patient intermittently, wherever possible: giving lithium during the periods of high relapse risk and keeping the patient drug free for several weeks during safer times. It has been seen many times that a careless combination of lithium with drugs such as certain diuretics or some antirheumatics can increase lithium concentration in the body, elevate blood levels and produce toxicity. The resulting side effects will essentially reflect the increased concentrations of lithium in the tissues. It is important for the prevention and reduction of side effects to keep the dosage of lithium salts at an effective minimum. As the cell membrane transport of lithium changes with age, and older patients tend to achieve higher intracellular concentrations with the same blood lithium levels, it is advisable to treat older patients with relatively lower plasma lithium levels, reducing the dosage correspondingly.

There are interesting differences between responders and nonresponders to lithium not only in terms of benefit but also as far as adverse effects are concerned. Whereas the nonresponders suffer more from the urinary and thyroid side effects, the responders are more prone to weight gain. This differential sensitivity to both benefit and side effects makes it doubly imperative that patients for long-term lithium treatment are carefully selected and that the clinician limits the length of a therapeutic trial on long-term lithium to the minimum necessary to establish a response (Grof et al., 1982).

PRIORITIES FOR RESEARCH ON SIDE EFFECTS OF
LONG-TERM LITHIUM TREATMENT

The priorities for research include new ways of managing, preventing, and systematically documenting side effects and investigation the crucial variables:

1. Optimal methods of reducing the most common side effects (e.g. polyuria, recurrent bouts of diarrhea).
2. Proper tailoring of thyroid supplementation to fluctuating individual needs.
3. Safety of intermittent lithium treatment and its effectiveness in reducing side effects of long-term lithium treatment.
4. The investigation of the relationship between plasma levels and side effects, in quantitative terms.
5. The effects of long-term lithium treatment on kidney function and structure of patients with pre-existing kidney disease.
6. Continuation of the search on the possible structural changes of the kidney on long-term lithium treatment and in affective disorders who have not received lithium.
7. Differences between responders and nonresponders with regards to side effects.
8. Systematic documentation of the frequency of side effects investigated in carefully selected patients (e.g., lithium responders) treated with lithium only and stratified by the length of treatment.
9. Suitable methods for quantification of lithium side effects.

SUMMARY

With more extensive use of lithium, side effects of long-term treatment have gained increasing attention. For most physically healthy lithium responders, long-term lithium treatment is usually free of clinically relevant side effects. However, it does not come as a surprise that a drug with such a wide array of biological effects has the potential for a variety of unwanted effects in man.

Clinically relevant long-term side effects involve particularly the central nervous system, gastrointestinal tract, neuroendocrine function and the kidney (Table 1). Side effects which are frequent during the first few weeks, such as hand tremor and diarrhea, become less common with the passage of time. Subsequently the clinician becomes more concerned about such problems as weight gain or nocturia. Most side effects actually materialize infrequently and when they occur tend to reflect individual susceptibility and idiosyncratic responses.

Table 1. Frequency of Side Effects during Long-Term
Lithium Treatment[a]

	Percent of patients
Thirst	28
Nocturia	26
Excessive weight gain	16
Hypothyroidism	15
Polyuria	12
Gastrointestinal complications	8
Tremor of hands	5
Goiter	3

[a]Established in a sample of 300 consecutive patients treated at
the Affective Disorders Clinic, Hamilton Psychiatric Hospital.
All patients have been on lithium for more than one year but
the sample is otherwise unselected, and it includes responders
and nonresponders, bipolar, unipolar, and schizoaffective
patients.

It is important to bear in mind that most of the long-term side effects of
lithium treatment can be prevented, ameliorated, or treated. Careful selection of
patients, systematic attention to optimum low dosage, choice of suitable lithium
preparation, close monitoring of the patient's progress, and mindfulness of possible side effects are important steps in long-term lithium management and result
in a low frequency of side effects.

REFERENCES

Amdisen, A., and Schou, M. Lithium. *Side Eff. Drug Annu.* 2:17–29, 1978.
Amdisen, A., and Schou, M. Lithium. *Side Eff. Drug Annu.* 3:22–25, 1979.
Amdisen, A., and Schou, M. Lithium. *Side Eff. Drug Annu.* 4:22–25, 1980.
Berens, S.C., and Wolff, J. The endocrine effects of lithium. In F.N. Johnson,
    ed., *Lithium Research and Therapy,* pp. 443–472. New York: Academic
    Press, 1975.
Birch, M.J. Metabolic effects of lithium. In F.M. Johnson and S. Johnson, eds.,
    Lithium in Medical Practice. Baltimore: University Park Press, 1978.
Brown, W.T. Side effects of lithium therapy and their treatment. In A. Ville-
    neuve, ed., *Lithium in Psychiatry,* pp. 125–144. Quebec City: Les Presses
    de l'Université Laval, 1976.
Dimitrakoudi, M., and Jenner, F.A. Electroencephalographic effects of lithium.
    In F.M. Johnson, ed., *Lithium Research and Therapy,* pp. 507–518. New
    York: Academic Press, 1975.
Glen, A.I.M. Lithium regulation of membrane ATPases. In F.M. Johnson and
    S. Johnson, eds., *Lithium in Medical Practice,* pp. 183–192. Baltimore:
    University Park Press, 1978.

Greco, F.A., and Breton, H.D. Lithium carbonate attenuation of neutropenia. *Cancer Chemiotherapy Proc. Am. Soc. Clin. Oncol.* 17:250, 1976.

Grof, P., Loughrey, E., Saxena, L., Daigle, L., and Quesnell, J. Lithium stabilization and weight gain. In *Psychopharmacology, Sexual Disorders and Drug Abuse,* pp. 323–327. Proceedings CIMP, 1973.

Grof, P., MacCrimmon, D., Saxena, B., Daigle, L., and Prior, M. Bioavailability and side-effects of different lithium carbonate products. *Neuropsychobiology* 2:313–323, 1976.

Grof, P., MacCrimmon, D.J., Smith, E.K.M., Daigle, L., Varma, R., Saxena, B., Keitner, G., and Kenny, J. Long-term lithium treatment and the kidney. *Canad. J. Psychiat.* 25:535–543, 1980.

Grof, P., Hux, M., and Dressler, B. Kidney function and response to lithium treatment. Proceedings of the Vth. CCMP Annual Scientific Meeting, Quebec City, 1982.

Gupta, R.C., Robinson, W.A., and Smyth, C.J. Efficacy of lithium in rheumatoid arthritis with granulocytopenia (Felty's Syndrome): A preliminary report. *Arthritis Rheum.* 18:179–184, 1975.

Hansen, H.E. Renal toxicity of lithium. *Drugs* 22:461–476, 1982.

Hestbech, J., Hansen, H.E., Amdisen, A., and Olsen, S. Chronic renal lesions following long-term treatment with lithium. *Kidney Int.* 12:205–213, 1977.

Jefferson, J.W., and Greist, J.H. *Primer of Lithium Therapy.* Baltimore: Williams & Wilkins, 1977.

Jefferson, J.W., and Greist, J.H. Cardiovascular effects and toxicity of lithium. In Davis and Greenblatt, *Psychopharmacology Update,* pp. 81–104. New York: Grune and Stratton, 1979.

Jenner, F.A. Lithium and the kidney. In T.B. Cooper et al., eds., *Lithium– Controversies and Unresolved Issues,* pp. 567–578. New York: Excerpta Medica, 1979.

Jenner, F.A., and Eastwood, P.R. Renal effects of lithium. In F.M. Johnson and S. Johnson, eds., *Lithium in Medical Practice,* pp. 247–263. Baltimore: University Park Press, 1978.

Mayfield, D., and Brown, R.G. The clinical laboratory and electroencephalographic effects of lithium. *J. Psychiatr. Res.* 4:207–219, 1966.

Mellerup, E.T., Vam, H., Wildschidtz, G., and Rafaelson, O.J. Lithium effects of various diurnal rhythms in manic melancholic patients. In F.M. Johnson and S. Johnson, eds., *Lithium in Medical Practice,* pp. 267–270. Baltimore: University Park Press, 1978.

Perez-Cruet, J., Dencey, J.T., and Waite, J. Lithium effects of leucocytosis and lymphopenia. In F.M. and S. Johnson, eds., *Lithium in Medical Practice.* Baltimore: University Park Press, 1978.

Reisberg, B., and Gershon, S. Toxicology and side-effects of lithium therapy. In T.B. Cooper et al., eds., *Lithium–Controversies and Unresolved Issues,* pp. 449–478. New York: Excerpta Medica, 1979a.

Reisberg, B., and Gershon, S. Side effects associated with lithium therapy. *Arch. Gen. Psych.* 36:879–887, 1979b.

Schou, M. Toxicity. *Acta Pharmacol.* 15:70, 1958.

Schou, M. Lithium in psychiatric therapy and prophylaxis. *J. Psychiatr. Res.* 6: 67, 1968.

Shopsin, B., and Gershon, S. Pharmacology-toxicology of the lithium ion. In S. Gershon, and B. Shopsin, eds., *Lithium–Its Role in Psychiatric Research and Treatment,* pp. 107–146. New York: Plenum Press, 1973.

Small, J.G., Milstein, V., and Small, I.F. EEG and neurophysiological studies of lithium in normal volunteers. *Biol. Psychiat.* 5:65–77, 1972.

Vacaflor, L. Lithium side effects and toxicity: The clinical picture. In F.M. Johnson, ed., *Lithium Research and Therapy,* pp. 211–226. New York: Academic Press, 1975.

Vacaflor, L., Lohmann, H.E., and Ran, T.A. Side effects and teratogenicity of lithium carbonate treatment. *J. Clin. Pharmacol.* 10:387–389, 1970.

Vendsborg, P. Lithium and glucose tolerance. In F.M. and S. Johnson, eds., *Lithium in Medical Practice.* Baltimore: University Park Press, 1978.

Vestergaard, P., Amdisen, A., and Schou, M. Clinically significant side-effects of lithium treatment. *Acta Psychiat. Scand.* 62:193–200, 1980.

Vestergaard, P., and Schou, M. Kidney morphology and function in the lithium-treated patient. *Biblthea Psychiat.* 161:104–114, 1981.

Weinstein, M.R. Lithium teratogenesis: The register of lithium babies. In T.B. Cooper et al., eds., *Lithium–Controversies and Unresolved Issues,* pp. 432–448. New York: Excerpta Medica, 1979.

Weinstein, M.R., and Goldfield, M.D. Administration of lithium during pregnancy. In F.M. Johnson, ed., *Lithium Research and Therapy,* pp. 237–266. New York: Academic Press, 1975.

Wolff, J. Lithium interactions with the thyroid gland. In T.B. Cooper et al., eds., *Lithium–Controversies and Unresolved Issues,* pp. 552–566. New York: Excerpta Medica, 1979.

Zerbi, F., Fenoglio, L., and Tosca, P. EEG changes during lithium treatment. In F.M. Johnson and S. Johnson, eds., *Lithium in Medical Practice,* pp. 189–234. Baltimore: University Park Press, 1978.

8

Clinical Pharmacokinetics
of Antidepressants

W. Z. POTTER

Over a decade of research has established the principle that interindividual differences in response to psychotropic drugs can be related to corresponding differences in rates of drug metabolism and hence steady-state concentrations in plasma (Hammer and Sjöqvist, 1967; for review see Potter et al., 1981a). Disagreement remains, however, concerning the frequency with which pharmacokinetic variance contributes to poor response (Burrows et al., 1974; Ziegler et al., 1976; Kragh-Sorensen et al., 1976; Glassman et al., 1977; Coppen et al., 1978). Consequently, the clinical relevance of monitoring plasma concentrations of psychotropic drugs is constantly being evaluated. Numerous reviews have been written during the last five years and many have contributed useful critical assessments instead of simple tabulations of data (Gram, 1977; Asberg and Sjöqvist, 1978; Risch et al., 1979; Amsterdam et al., 1981; Potter et al., 1981a; Linnoila, 1981).

During this same period preclinical psychopharmacologists have been exploring specific receptor-mediated actions of psychotropic drugs thereby providing a basis for better understanding the full range of actions of psychotropic drugs. Many of these actions fall under the general heading of "side effects" and thus have obvious clinical relevance. Moreover, since many of these effects are more easily quantifiable than degree of clinical improvement, it is frequently possible to establish direct relationships between plasma concentration and effect. Thus, the principle that pharmacokinetic variance is critical to *all* effects of psychotropic drugs should be recognized.

The first part of this paper explains those general principles necessary for evaluating the relevance of pharmacokinetics in the clinical use of one class of psychotropic drugs, antidepressants. The second section will discuss how future clinical studies can use pharmacokinetic approaches for investigating the mechanism of drug action and biochemical abnormalities in affective illness as well as for improving treatment.

PHARMACOKINETIC VARIANCE AMONG ANTIDEPRESSANTS

The major determinant of interindividual pharmacokinetic differences is drug metabolism. There are, of course, other processes which affect plasma drug concentration. These include absorption, distribution and renal clearance which are relatively stable in an otherwise healthy population of depressed patients. Certain conditions are associated with systematic changes in one of these processes, such as decreased renal clearance in the aged, and will be identified in what follows. The importance of drug metabolism for most antidepressants is highlighted by the demonstration that only around one percent is usually excreted unchanged in the urine. Lithium is obviously an exception since it is an ion which is excreted unchanged in the urine. The role of pharmacokinetics in its use as an antidepressant is discussed in a separate chapter.

The monoamine oxidase inhibitors are also exceptions, but for a different reason. Little information is available on their metabolism in man and on their renal excretion. Since those in general use can be classed as irreversible inhibitors of monoamine oxidase their effect on the enzyme will be related to total accumulated amount and not their steady-state concentration. Thus, treatment strategies are aimed at giving enough drug to be confident of enzyme inhibition. Of course, differences in metabolism may very well contribute to variations in the amount of drug necessary to achieve MAO inhibition although this has not been conclusively demonstrated. In the absence of extensive pharmacokinetic data, the use of MAOIs is appropriately handled as a special case in another chapter.

The tricyclic antidepressants (TCAs) account for the majority of prescriptions written for non-bipolar depressed patients. Several non-tricyclic antidepressants have recently been introduced (Crow, 1979); these also share the property of extensive metabolism and hence can be expected to show pharmacokinetic variation. Thus, a fixed dose of a standard TCA will typically produce a ten-fold interindividual range of concentrations when administered to a group of patients (Alexanderson et al., 1969; Reisby et al., 1977) and a non-tricyclic such as zimelidine will produce a two- to four-fold range of its predominant active form, norzimelidine (Potter et al., 1979; Brown et al., 1980).

The relevance of this variation to effect is based on the fundamental pharmacological principle that drug action is directly proportional to the *free* concentration at the site of action. And in the treatment of chronic states such as depression or hypertension this can be logically extended to a principle that effect should be proportional to the mean *steady-state free* concentration. Steady-state is, by definition, the condition in which the amount of drug entering the system is equivalent to the amount being eliminated. As shown in Figure 1, it may take considerable time to achieve steady-state depending on the half-life of elimination of a drug. As a rule of thumb 95% of a steady-state concentration is obtained following fixed dosing over five biologic half-lives. More detailed presentations of these basic pharmacokinetics are readily available (Wagner, 1971; Gibaldi and Perrier, 1975).

These well-established basics are worth remembering because of our increased ability to describe concentration/response curves. A sigmoidal relationship can frequently be established between the $\log_{10}$ concentration and some response as shown in Figure 2. Ideally, a drug would have a single therapeutic

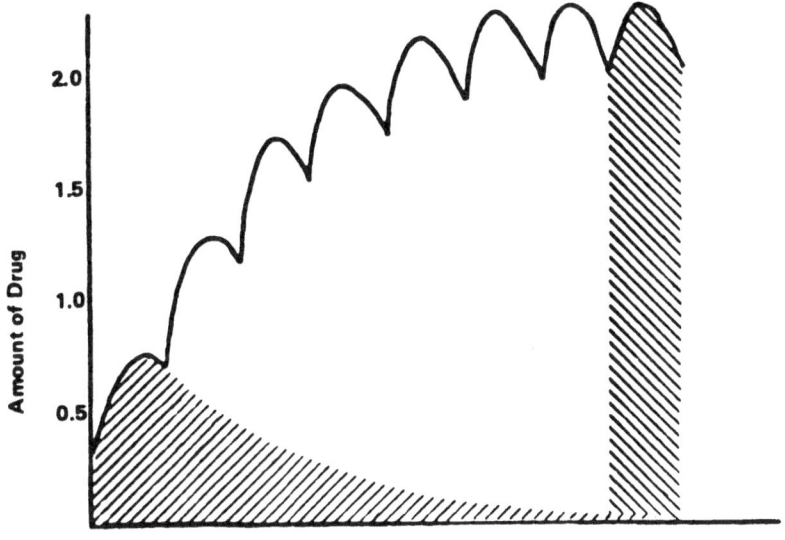

Time (hours)

Figure 1. Accumulation of drug following repeated oral administration with fixed dose and dosing interval 2/3 of the elimination half-life. Thus, a drug with an 18 hour half-life, minimum for most tricyclic antidepressants, administered every 12 hours will require seven dosing intervals (84 hours) or 4.67 half-lives [84 hr/(18 hr/half-life)] to reach steady-state. The area under the plasma concentration-time curve after the first dose is equal to the area under the curve during the dosing interval (see Potter et al., 1981a).

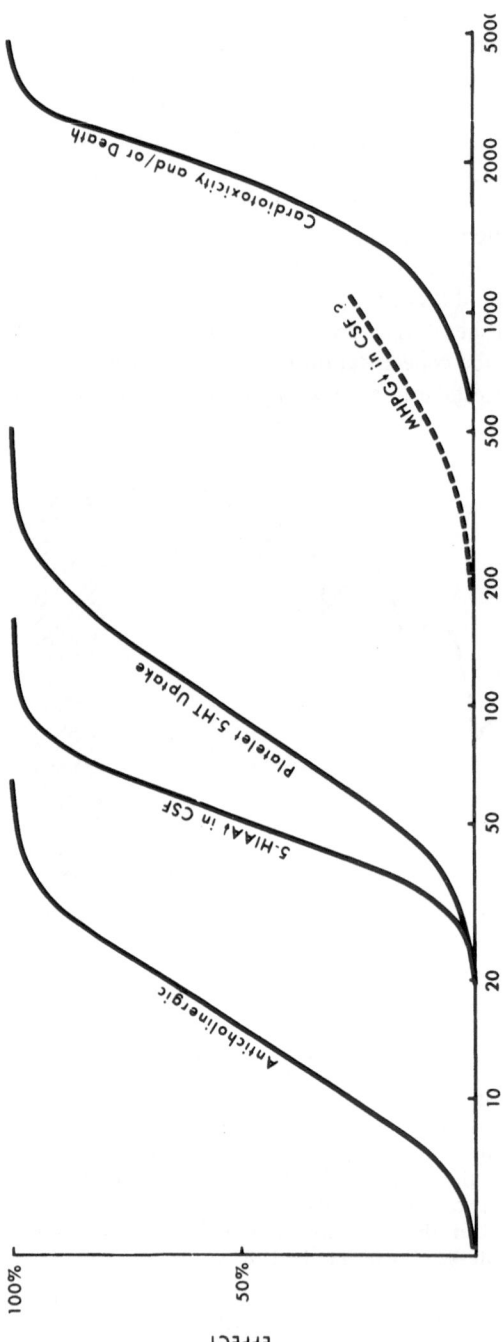

Figure 2. Concentration dependency of amitriptyline effects. See Potter and Linnoila (in press) for details.

action for which a safe concentration producing maximal effect could be identified. Essentially the empirical practice of increasing doses to achieve increased response rate is based on this approach as exemplified in studies which achieve >90% antidepressant response rates simply by using larger doses of such TCAs as desipramine (Stewart et al., 1980). There are two problems with this approach; first, the assumption that the response curve after achieving maximum effect is flat; second, the fact that most antidepressants have multiple effects, many of which are significant within the concentration range usually obtained with therapeutic doses of drugs.

The first problem has been most extensively explored with nortriptyline which clearly is less effective as an antidepressant when higher concentrations are achieved (for review see Asberg and Sjöqvist, 1978). This phenomena of a relatively narrow concentration range being associated with good clinical response has been called a "therapeutic window." Recent demonstrations that chronic treatment with nortriptyline also produces high concentrations of an active hydroxy metabolite (10-OH-nortriptyline) (Kragh-Sorensen et al., 1977; Bertilsson et al., 1979b) have raised the possibility that it is either the hydroxy metabolite or the sum of nortriptyline plus the hydroxy metabolite which truly defines the "therapeutic window." Interestingly, nortriptyline is the only antidepressant for which an upper therapeutic concentration limit has been convincingly demonstrated. We will return to the general principle concerning the importance of active metabolites later.

The second problem is best illustrated by looking at a series of likely concentration response curves for another TCA, desipramine. As shown in Figure 3, within the 50-300 ng/ml range of concentrations likely to be obtained on standard doses there are many complex possibilities concerning the relative extent of different effects. For instance one may have almost maximum effects on noradrenergic parameters as evidenced by 3-methoxy-4-hydroxy phenylglycol (MHPG) decreases in the cerebrospinal fluid (CSF) with minimal effects on serotonergic parameters such as platelet serotonin uptake if one maintains concentrations in the 100 ng/ml range (Potter et al., 1981b; Aberg-Wistedt et al., 1981). Moreover, since it is not possible to assume that effects on one neurotransmitter system are independent of those on another it is conceivable that effects may limit or reverse one another.

Such a possibility is suggested in the findings of Träskman et al., (1979) that clorimipramine induced decreases of the serotonin metabolite, 5-hydroxyindole acetic acid (5HIAA), in cerebrospinal fluid are maximal in the 100 ng/ml range and begin to reverse at higher concentrations which may produce postsynaptic receptor blockade (Ogren et al., 1979). The principle to be extracted here is that with multiple action drugs such as the TCAs there is a high probability of side effects occurring at concentrations close to, overlapping with or even less than therapeutic ones—e.g., for amitriptyline maximum anticholinergic

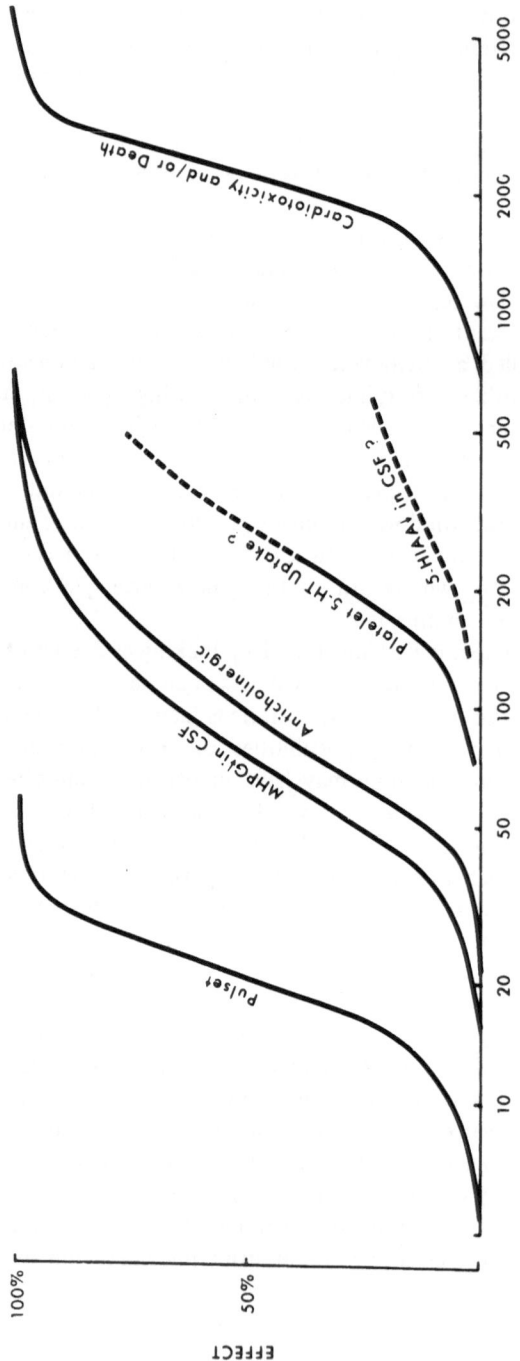

Figure 3. Concentration dependency of desipramine effects. See Potter and Linnoila (in press) for details.

effects may occur at concentrations considerably lower than those required for therapeutic action (Figure 2). Moreover, unless plasma concentrations are obtained, there is a reasonable possibility of falling outside of the therapeutic range while obtaining clear "effects." Again, with amitriptyline, a person may be complaining of a very dry mouth tempting one to reduce the dose, where what is really needed is a dose increase not likely to worsen an already maximal anticholinergic effect.

A final important feature of response curves, referred to in passing, is that effect is related to the *free* or unbound drug concentration (for review see Sellers et al., 1981). Methodological difficulties have prevented the determination of free concentrations in most studies of TCAs; there is considerable disagreement concerning the absolute free concentration even in those reports which do attempt to quantitate unbound drug (for review see Potter et al., 1981a). Although variations in protein binding of TCAs such as increases during inflammatory states which causes elevations of α_1-acid glycoprotein do occur (Piafsky and Borga, 1977), these are rarely great and contribute far less than do variations in metabolism. In populations in which it has been possible to obtain cerebrospinal fluid (CSF), perhaps the best available measure of free drug in the central nervous system (Potter et al., 1979b; Bertilsson et al., 1979a), investigators have found high (>0.90) correlations between total plasma (bound + free) and CSF antidepressant concentrations (Muscettola et al., 1978; Potter et al., 1982) indicating that the plasma concentration is usually an accurate index of relative free concentration and should be appropriate for establishing concentration/response relationships.

Interestingly, large changes in binding are most relevant for the interpretation of unusual plasma concentration data. The simple relationship which best describes the behavior of basic lipophilic drugs which are extensively metabolized is:

$$C_{ss} = \frac{Dose}{pCl_{int}}$$

where

C_{ss} = total steady-state concentration in plasma
p = Fraction "free" (unbound) in plasma
Cl_{int} = intrinsic clearance, which refers to the ability of the liver to remove a drug by all pathways in the absence of any blood flow limitations.

Hence an increase in α_1-acid glycoprotein secondary to an acute inflammatory condition (e.g., pneumonia) would *decrease* the free fraction and produce a

Table 1^a

A correlation between total steady-state plasma concentration of a psychotropic drug and clinical effects in a patient population may be expected when the following criteria are fulfilled:

1. The drug has a reversible action and tolerance at receptor sites does not develop.
2. The total drug concentration in plasma reflects the unbound concentration at receptor sites—binding must be relatively constant within the entire therapeutic range.
3. Factors which modify the relationship between plasma levels and clinical effects are taken into account—e.g., active metabolites, other drugs abnormal plasma protein binding, stage of the disease (e.g., acute vs. chronic).
4. The clinical effects of the drug are indisputable and measured accurately.
5. There *is* variability between individuals both in drug response and drug plasma concentration.
6. The pharmacokinetic properties of the drug are taken into account when sampling plasma (time after dosing, mean C_{ss} or AUC to be measured, etc.)
7. The drug analytical method is sensitive, selective and subject to quality control.

[a]Taken from Potter et al., 1981a.

reciprocal *increase* in the total C_{ss}. The actual free drug concentration ($C_{ss} \times p$), however, would remain the same because of rearrangement of the above: Free drug at steady-state = pC_{ss} = $Dose/Cl_{int}$. Thus free drug concentration is simply a function of the dose and the intrinsic clearance. This demonstrates that it is the interindividual variation in metabolism which is actually responsible for interindividual variation in free drug concentration. Variations in binding would be irrelevant except that one is usually attempting to interpret the total C_{ss} as a measure of free drug. Fortunately, as mentioned above, in most cases this total concentration is a good relative index of the free. The explanation of these perhaps counter-intuitive relationships is beyond the scope of this chapter and are explored in detail elsewhere (Wilkinson and Shand, 1975).

With these principles as background one can use Table 1 to assess whether studies provide convincing evidence of an interpretable concentration/response relationship. The points concerning clinical design and the need to have a quantifiable response variable are elaborated elsewhere (Asberg and Sjöqvist, 1978; Glassman, 1981; Kragh-Sorensen et al., 1981; Potter et al., 1981).

When one considers those investigations which collectively satisfy the clinical prerequisites and pharmacologic criteria for relating concentration to effect the indications for obtaining antidepressant drug levels presented in

Table 2. Indications for Obtaining Plasma TCA Concentrations

I. Compliance	Requires repeated sampling, results from single-dose prediction or urinary measurements to interpret.
II. Failure to Respond	May have very low concentration despite compliance.
III. Exaggerated Responses	High concentrations on low doses, expected in slow hydroxylators ($\sim$5% of population).
IV. High Risk and Polypharmacy	Patients with some type of cardiovascular disease or on drugs which effect TCA metabolism, especially neuroleptics.
V. Maximize Response	Defined for only two TCAs:
Nortriptyline	Aim for 50–150 ng/ml range. Often need to *reduce* dose. Keep *below* 150 ng/ml.
Imipramine	Required combined concentration with metabolite, desipramine, in 200–250 ng/ml range. Usually *increase* dose. No defined upper limit.

Table 2, are currently appropriate. The data and arguments supporting this particular synthesis have been presented elsewhere (Potter et al., 1981a).

Thus, pharmacokinetic variance among antidepressants, principally the TCAs, is of both theoretical and practical concern. Understanding a small number of general principles, however, permits the interpretation of a literature so that specific needs of programs can be met. In other words, a clinical laboratory offering a full range of assays for all antidepressants other than MAOI's might want to issue a caveat that therapeutic ranges are only established for certain drugs and for the remainder concentrations are most useful to assess compliance and whether a person falls far outside of the normal (not therapeutic) range for a given dose. Alternatively, an academic facility might wish to limit itself to the use of antidepressants which appear to have a defined concentration response relationship. Or a researcher might intentionally want to study biochemical changes that occur at concentrations outside of the therapeutic range so as to rule out possible actions as sufficient or necessary for antidepressant effect. Therefore, the utilization of pharmacokinetic information can be counted on to improve both clinical management and research design. The latter point will now be expanded in the following section.

PHARMACOKINETIC APPROACHES TO MECHANISTIC STUDIES OF ANTIDEPRESSANTS

In the more restrictive sense of the term pharmacokinetics is concerned primarily with the movements of substances in and out of various compartments in the body. These can ultimately be described with appropriate mathematical models if given adequate experimental data. There is a large literature devoted to deriving and defending various models, models which frequently involve cumbersome, multi-term equations that discourage the uninitiated and appear to border on art for art's sake. For clinical investigators, this aspect of pharmacokinetics may be best understood as a necessary basic discipline on which can be built more biologically oriented approaches.

One asks how variations in rates of movement; whether absorption, transfer or elimination relate to significant biological effects. Again, using terms in their restrictive sense the study of effects is pharmacodynamics. Under clinical research conditions, however, the study of pharmacokinetics and pharmacodynamics are readily integrated. One cannot fully study drug effects without understanding and taking into account pharmacokinetics. Conversely, simply describing the pharmcokinetics of drugs in man can become an empty exercise.

A pharmacokinetic approach implies that attention is paid to the principles that determine what happens to a drug which, in this broader sense, includes the events involved in its effect(s). Increasing evidence shows that most, if not all, antidepressant drugs have high affinities for specific "receptors" with which the free form combines and may thereby produce selective, not necessarily therapeutic effects (Table 3). The description and assessment of drug-receptor interactions involves the same principles which underly pharmacokinetics including laws of mass action, zero-order, first order, nth order processes, etc. Of equal importance the systematic requirements of obtaining and interpreting data required for pharmacokinetic studies provides a useful framework for clinical pharmacodynamic investigations.

Many empirically developed areas demonstrate important interactions of pharmacokinetics and pharmacodynamics. For instance, if one administers a supramaximal dose of dexamethasone almost everyone will suppress their production of cortisol. By working out the minimal dose (concentration) which produces maximum suppression in the general population it is possible to develop a sensitive test for those who are relatively resistant to this effect of dexamethasone. This is the basis for the 1 mg instead of 2 mg dose currently recommended to identify "non-suppressors" to dexamethasone (Carroll et al., 1981).

Future clinical research can profit by paying close attention to such details. With regard to mechanistic studies of antidepressant activity the greatest focus has centered on a catecholamine "hypothesis" of affective illness (Bunney

Table 3. Interactions of Classic Tricyclic and Newer Nontricyclic
Antidepressants with Various Receptors in Rat Brain[a]

	Serotonergic (^{3}H-d-LSD)	α-Adrenergic (^{3}H-WB-4101)	Muscarinic (^{3}H-QNB)	Histaminergic H$_1$
Tricyclics				
Amitriptyline	++++	++++	+++	++++
Nortriptyline	+++	++	++	++
Imipramine	++	+++	+++	++
Desipramine	++	++	+	+
Chlorimipramine	++	+++	+++	++
Nontricyclics				
Iprindole	+	–	++	+++
Nomifensine	++	+	+	+
Mianserin	+++	+++	++	++++
Zimelidine	–	+	–	+
Norzimelidine	–	+	–	+

[a]Relative potencies (++++ = most potent) are estimates drawn from Richelson, 1978; U'Prichard et al., 1978; Richelson, 1979; Ogren et al., 1979; Hall and Ogren, 1981. A dash means no interaction at concentrations less than 10^{-4} M.

and Davis, 1965; Schildkraut, 1965) and secondarily on an indoleamine "hypothesis" (Coppen, 1967). Investigators have worked with the drugs available to them—usually TCAs with a multitude of biochemical effects such as those discussed above in the examples of amitriptyline and desipramine (Figures 2 and 3). We are therefore handicapped in making interpretations because we have not been able to establish that the TCAs in clinically relevant concentrations produce truly selective biochemical effects on the noradrenergic or serotonergic system. In fact, when close attention is given to pharmacokinetic and pharmacodynamic factors, rather surprising results can emerge. For instance, chlorimipramine, presumed to be a relatively selective inhibitor of serotonin uptake in man, was shown to have predominant effects on the norepinephrine system which correlated best with the substantial steady-state concentrations of its desmethyl metabolite (Träskman et al., 1979).

The problem of active metabolites exemplified in the experience with chlorimipramine is a general one. Since drug metabolism is the crucial determinant of the clearance of TCAs not only is there great variation in parent drug concentrations but also there emerges a wide range of metabolite concentrations. The metabolic scheme for a tertiary amine TCA, imipramine, shown in Figure 4 is typical. Both desmethyl and hydroxy metabolites are biologically active as shown in Table 4. Moreover, as noted in the preceding section for another TCA, nortriptyline (Bertilsson et al., 1979b) these are present in active, unconjugated forms both in plasma and cerebrospinal fluid under steady-state conditions

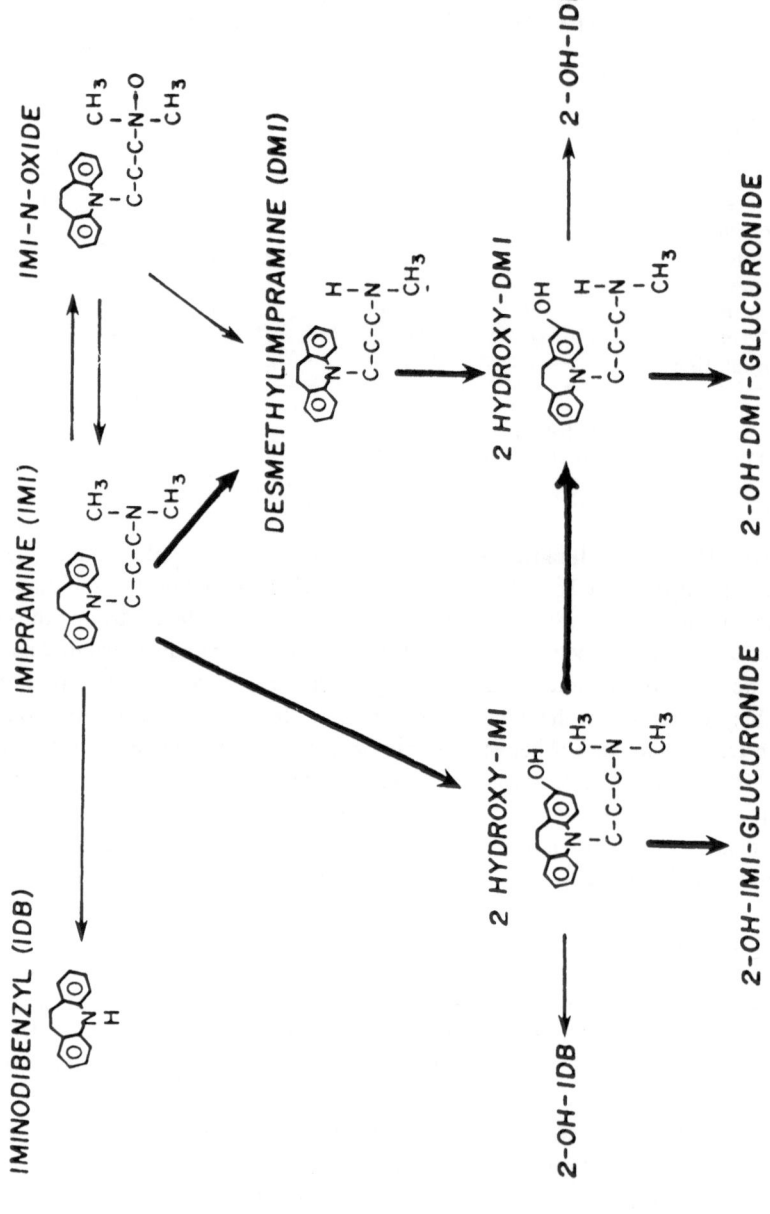

Figure 4. Known metabolic pathways for the major tricyclic antidepressant, imipramine, in man. Similar pathways have been shown for amitriptyline and chlorimipramine.

Table 4. Effect of Metabolites of Tricyclic Antidepressants on the Neuronal Uptake of Norepinephrine (NE) and Serotonin (5HT)

Drug or Metabolite	NE uptake inhibition			5HT uptake inhibition	
	EC_{50} (nmol/liter)	Relative to DMI	Relative to NT	EC_{50} (nmol/liter)	Relative to CLI
Imipramine (IMI)[a]	250	0.22	–	150	0.21
2-OH-IMI	180	0.31	–	320	0.10
Desipramine (DMI)	55	1.00	–	4,230	<0.01
2-OH-DMI	11	0.90	–	4,390	<0.01
Amitriptyline (AT)[b]	380	–	0.2	–	–
Nortriptyline (NT)	75	–	1.0	2,420	0.01
E-10-OH-AT	670	–	0.11	–	–
Z-10-OH-AT	720	–	0.10	–	–
E-10-OH-AT	160	–	0.47	10,120	<0.01
Z-10-OH-NT	160	–	0.47	2,310	0.01
Desmethyl-NT	1,000	–	0.08	–	–
AT-N-Oxide	7,300	–	0.01	–	–
Chlorimipramine (CLI)	–	–	–	31	1.00
8-OH-CLI	–	–	–	52	0.60

[a] Imipramine series, data from Potter et al., (1979).
[b] Amitriptyline series, data from Bertilsson et al., (1979b) NE uptake.
[c] Series on 5HT uptake from Potter et al. (1979).

(Potter et al., 1982). Thus in order to establish specificity of drug action one must rule out the presence of active metabolites or take their concentrations and effects into account.

Given the limitations of in vitro studies for determining drug action it is further necessary to show that antidepressants have selective biochemical effects in man if one is to use them as probes to explore specific biochemical hypotheses. Our experience comparing zimelidine, a selective serotonin uptake inhibitor with active metabolites *not* more potent on other neurotransmitter systems and desipramine, a selective norepinephrine uptake inhibitor at lower concentrations is instructive. We find that these two drugs do produce different biochemical effects in man, generally compatible with their in vitro selectivity, but that important physiological parameters such as the rest-activity pattern are similarly affected (Potter et al., 1981b). Moreover, a single unexpected common biochemical effect also occurs—reduction of urinary 3-methoxy-4-hydroxy-phenylglycol (MHPG), the major metabolite of norepinephrine. Further studies have revealed that the effects on the relationship of norepinephrine to its other major metabolites are quite different after the two drugs leading us to conclude that the mechanisms involved in MHPG reduction must be different (Linnoila et al., 1982). We are currently attempting to establish whether any antidepressant treatment, no matter how selective for other systems in preclinical studies, can be shown *not* to effect the noradrenergic system in actual clinical studies. Thus far, all antidepressant treatments that have been studied—TCA's in clinically relevant concentrations, non-tricyclics such as zimelidine, selective and nonselective MAOI's, ECT, and lithium—show evidence of changes in the noradrenergic system (Potter, Linnoila and Karoum, unpublished data). Our clinical data is consistent with the ability of most, and perhaps all, antidepressants to decrease postsynaptic β-receptor coupled adenylate cyclase stimulation (Vetulani et al., 1976) or β-receptor number (Banerjee et al., 1977) in rat cortex following chronic administration.

It does not necessarily follow that noradrenergic effects are required for antidepressant action. Clearly, such effects are not sufficient since drug-induced changes of norepinephrine or its metabolites can be documented in patients in the absence of concurrent or subsequent clinical improvement (Bertilsson et al., 1974; Muscettola et al., 1978; Potter et al., 1981b). What does follow is that some satisfactory explanation of the effects of norepinephrine must be provided before anyone can convincingly conclude that this neurotransmitter is not directly involved in the etiology and/or treatment of affective illness. Obviously, if an effective antidepressant were developed which could be shown not to effect norepinephrine in man it would have important theoretical implications. Inspection of Table 3 suggests how difficult it may be to find any CNS active drug which does not affect norepinephrine since one or more receptor interactions which may be directly or indirectly related to noradrenergic function is present for all drugs.

Ideally we will find drugs that interact with one receptor at clinically relevant concentrations. Various clinical studies with compounds with putative selective actions based on preclinical work, e.g., clonidine, an α-$_2$ receptor agonist (Checkley et al., 1981a), mianserin, a presynaptic α-receptor blocker (Baumann and Maitre, 1977) salbutamol, a post-synaptic β_2 agonist (Simon et al., 1978), are of greatest value if such biochemical specificites can be shown in man along with other effects being measured. Actual experience with such "specific" drugs as clonidine produce evidence of multiple independently regulated effects, e.g., blood pressure and sympathic function vs. growth hormone (Dollery et al., 1976; Wing et al., 1977; Falkner et al., 1981; Checkley et al., 1981b). In these studies dose and concentration differences contributed greatly to the variable specificity of effects. Other pharmacologic strategies such as pretreatment with an alpha blocker can be used to support the importance of α-stimulation in the mechanism of growth hormone release and may be helpful in clinical studies (Matussek and Laakmann, 1981). Various strategies become obvious once one has numerous selective agonists or antagonists suitable for clinical use and are ultimately only subject to the limitations of quantifying behavioral and biochemical effects in man. Here we emphasize that the successful use of such strategies depends upon a pharmacokinetic approach whereby relationships between concentration, or dose if metabolism is not a problem, and specific effects are established.

A corollary to the above is that altered pharmacodynamics can be a powerful tool to understanding the biochemistry of affective illness. Nonsuppression following dexamethasone in a significant proportion of severely depressed patients (Carroll et al., 1981), as well as patients with other diagnoses (Gerner and Gwirtsman, 1981; Insel et al., 1982), is only a beginning. Blunted response of TSH to TRH may be somewhat more specific (Kierkegaard et al., 1978). Decreased growth hormone release following clonidine (Matussek et al., 1980; Checkley et al., 1981a), and even desipramine may be used to support a derivative hypothesis that post-synaptic α_2 receptors are "down regulated" in affective illness (Matussek and Laakmann, 1981).

These and other challenge paradigms require careful studies to establish whether the concentration/response curve is simply shifted (i.e., greater or lesser sensitivity) or whether the maximum response is altered. In other words, does it simply take a larger dose of agonist to produce growth hormone (GH) release in depressed patients or do these individuals have an absolute reduction in their ability to release GH, no matter how strong the stimulus.

From a practical point of view, understanding mechanisms is not critical to whether or not particular tests in affective illness may be useful. Utility can be prospectively studied by seeing if patients diagnosed and/or treated on the basis of proposed "biological markers" do better than those treated with a traditional clinical approach. Pharmacokinetic control, however, is critical for finding the dose or concentration of a challenging substance which yields the desired combination of sensitivity and selectivity of response.

The ultimate potential of such tests, is moreover, related to their usefulness in understanding mechanisms of antidepressant action and/or the biochemical basis of affective illness. For this to be realized, pharmacokinetic strategies are even more necessary since specificity is critical to mechanistic interpretations. Thus, the clinical pharmacology of antidepressants can be seen as a rapidly growing field of investigation which requires the integration of biochemical and pharmacokinetic studies most promisingly focussing on the evaluation of receptor function.

REFERENCES

Aberg-Wistedt, A., Jostell, K.-G., Ross, S.P., and Westerlund, D. Effects of zimelidine and desipramine on serotonin and noradrenaline uptake mechanisms in relation to plasma concentrations and to therapeutic effects during treatment of depression. *Psychopharmacol.* 74:297–305, 1981.

Alexanderson, B., Price Evans, D.A., and Sjöqvist, F. Steady-state plasma levels of nortriptyline in twins. Influence of genetic factors and drug therapy. *Br. Med. J.* 2:764–768, 1969.

Amsterdam, J., Brunswick, D., and Mendels, J. The clinical application of tricyclic antidepressants and pharmacokinetics and plasma levels. *Am. J. Psychiatry* 137:653–662, 1981.

Asberg, M. and Sjöqvist, F. On the role of plasma level monitoring of tricyclic antidepressants in clinical practice. *Commun. Psychopharmacol.* 2:381–391, 1978.

Banerjee, S.P., Kung, L.S., Riggi, S.J., and Chanda, S.K. Development of β-adrenergic receptor subsensitivity of antidepressants. *Nature* 268:455–456, 1977.

Baumann, P.A., and Maitre, L. Blockade of presynaptic α-receptors and of amine uptake in the rat brain by the antidepressant mianserin. *Naunyn-Schmiedeberg's Arch. Pharmacol.* 300:31–37, 1977.

Bertilsson, L., Asberg, M., and Thoren, P. Differential effect of chlorimipramine and nortriptyline on cerebrospinal fluid metabolites of serotonin and noradrenaline in depression. *Eur. J. Clin. Pharmacol.* 7:365–368, 1974.

Bertilsson, L., Braithwaite, R., Tybring, G., Garle, M., and Borgo, O. Plasma protein binding of desmethylchlorimipramine studied with various techniques. *Clin. Pharmacol. Ther.* 26:265–271, 1979a.

Bertilsson, L., Mellström, B., and Sjöqvist, F. Pronounced inhibition of noradrenaline uptake by 10-hydroxy metabolites of nortriptyline. *Life Sci.* 25:1285–1292, 1979b.

Brown, D., Scott, D.H.T., Scott, D.B., Meyer, M., Westerlund, D., and Lundstrom, J. Pharmacokinetics of zimelidine. *Eur. J. Clin. Pharmacol.* 17:111–116.

Bunney, W.E. and Davis, J.M. Norepinephrine in depressive reactions. A review. *Arch. Gen. Psychiatry* 13:483–494, 1965.

Burrows, G.D., Scoggins, B.A., Turecek, L.R., Davies, B. Plasma nortriptyline and clinical response. *Clin. Pharmacol. Ther.* 16:639–644, 1974.

Carroll, B.J., Feinberg, M. and Greden, J. A specific laboratory test for the diagnosis of melancholia. Standardization validation and clinical utility. *Arch. Gen. Psychiatry* 38:15–22, 1981.

Checkley, S.A., Slade, A.P. and Shur, E. Growth hormone and other responses to clonidine in patients with endogenous depression. *Br. J. Psychiatry* 138: 51–55, 1981a.

Checkley, S.A., Slade, A.P., Shur, E., and Dawling, S. A pilot study of the mechanism of action of desipramine. *Br. J. Psychiatry* 138:248–251, 1981b.

Coppen, A. The biochemistry of affective disorders. *Br. J. Psychiatry* 113:1237–1264, 1967.

Coppen, A., Montgomery, S., Ghose, K., Rama Rao, V.A., Bailey, J., Christiansen, J., Mikkleson, P.L., Van Praag, H.M., Van de Poel, F., Minsker, E.J., Kozulja, V.G., Matussek, N., Kungkunz, G., and Jørgensen, A. Amitriptyline plasma-concentration and clinical effect (A World Health Organization Collaborative Study). *Lancet* 1:63–66, 1978.

Crow, T.J. Biochemical effects of some new antidepressants: Putative mechanisms of antidepressant effect. In: C. Dumont, ed. *Advances in Pharmacology and Therapeutics.* Vol. 5, *Neuropsychopharmacology,* Pergamon Press, Oxford, 1979, pp. 177–185.

Dollery, C.T., Davies, D.S., Draffan, G.H., Dargie, H.J., Dean, C.R., Reid, J.C., Clare, R.A., and Murray, S. Clinical pharmacology and pharmacokinetics of clonidine. *Clin. Pharmacol. Ther.* 19:11–17, 1976.

Falkner, B., Onesti, G., Moskang, T., and Lowenthal, D.T. Growth hormone release in hypertensive adolescents treated with clonidine. *J. Clin. Pharmacol.* 21:31–36, 1981.

Gerner, R.H., and Gwirtsman, H.E. Abnormalities of DST and urinary MHPG in anorexia nervosa. *Am. J. Psychiatry* 138:650–653, 1981.

Gibaldi, M., and Perrier, D. *Pharmacokinetics,* Marcel Dekker, New York, 1975.

Glassman, A.H., Perel, J.M., Shostak, M., Kantor, S.J., and Fleiss, J.L. Clinical implications of imipramine plasma levels for depressive illness. *Arch. Gen. Psychiatry* 34:197–204, 1977.

Glassman, A.H. Plasma levels: pitfalls and power. In: E. Usdin, ed. *Clinical Pharmacology in Psychiatry,* Elsevier, New York, 1981, pp. 277–286.

Gram, L.F. Plasma level monitoring of tricyclic antidepressant therapy. *Clin. Pharmacokinet.* 2:237–251, 1977.

Hall, H., and Ogren, S.-O. Effects of antidepressant drugs on different receptors in the brain. *Eur. J. Pharmacol.* 70:383–407, 1981.

Hammer, W., and Sjöqvist, F. *Life Sci.* 6:1895–1903, 1967.

Insel, T.R., Kalin, N.H., Guttmacher, L.B., Cohen, R.M., and Murphy, D.L. The DST in patients with primary obsessive-compulsive disorder. *Psychiatry Res.* 6:153–160, 1982.

Kierkegaard, C., Nørlem, B., Cohn, D., and Lauridsen, V.B. Thyrotropin-releasing hormone (TRH) stimulation test in manic-depressive illness. *Arch. Gen. Psychiatry* 35:1017–1021, 1978.

Kragh-Sørensen, P., Hansen, C.E., Baastrup, P.C., and Hvidberg, E.G. Self-inhibiting action of nortriptyline's antidepressive effect at high plasma levels: a randomized double-blind study controlled by plasma concentrations in patients with endogenous depression. *Psychopharmacologia* 45: 305–312, 1976.

Kragh-Sørensen, P., Borga, O., Garle, M., Bolvig Hansen, L., Hansen, C.E., Hvidberg, E.F., Larsen, N.E., and Sjöqvist, F.: Effect of simultaneous treatment with low doses of perphenazine on plasma and urine concentrations of nortriptyline and 10-hydroxynortriptyline. *Eur. J. Clin. Pharmacol.* 11:479–483, 1977.

Kragh-Sørenson, P., Gram, L.F., and Larsen, N.-E. Routine use of plasma concentration measurement of tricyclic antidepressant drugs: indications and limitations. In: E. Usdin, ed. *Clinical Pharmacology in Psychiatry*, Elsevier, New York, 1981, pp. 287–300.

Linnoila, M. Relationship between plasma levels of antidepressants and therapeutic response. In: T.A. Ban, R. Gonzales, A.S. Jablensky, N.A. Sartorices, and F.E. Vartanian, eds. *Prevention and Treatment of Depression*. University Park Press, Baltimore, 1981, pp. 219–232.

Linnoila, M., Karoum, F., Calil, H.M., Kopin, I.J., and Potter, W.Z.: Alteration of norepinephrine metabolism with desipramine and zimelidine in depressed patients. *Arch. Gen. Psychiatry* 39:1025–1028, 1982.

Matussek, N., Ackenheil, M., Hippius, H., Müller, F., Schroder, H.Th., Schultes, H., and Wasilewski, B. Effect of clonidine on growth hormone release in psychiatric patients and controls. *Psychiatry Res.* 2:25–36, 1980.

Matussek, N., and Laakmann, G. Growth hormone response in patients with depression. *Acta Psychiatrica Scandinavica*, Suppl. 290, 63:122–126, 1981.

Muscettola, G., Goodwin, F.K., Potter, W.Z., Claeys, M.M., and Markey, S.P. Imipramine and desipramine in plasma and spinal fluid. Relationship to clinical response and serotonin metabolism. *Arch. Gen. Psychiatry* 35:621–625, 1978.

Ogren, S.-O., Fuxe, K., Agnati, L.F., Gustafssonn, J.A., Jonsson, G., and Holm, A.C. Re-evaluation of the indoleamine hypothesis of depression. Evidence for a reduction of functional control 5-HT systems by antidepressant drugs. *J. Neural. Transmission* 46:85–103, 1979.

Piafsky, K.M., and Borga, O. Plasma protein binding of basic drugs. II. Importance of α_1 acid glycoprotein for interindividual variation. *Clin. Pharmacol. Ther.* 22:545–549, 1977.

Potter, W.Z ., Calil, H.M., Extein, I., Zavadil, A.P., III, and Goodwin, F.K. Comparative pharmacokinetics of zimelidine and desipramine in man following acute and chronic administration. *Psychiatry Res.* 1:273–281, 1979a.

Potter, W.Z., Muscettola, G. and Goodwin, F.K. Binding of imipramine to plasma protein and to brain tissue: relationship to CSF tricyclic levels in man. *Psychopharmacology* 63:187–192, 1979b.

Potter, W.Z., Bertilsson, L. and Sjöqvist, F. Clinical pharmacokinetics and psychotropic drugs–fundamental and practical aspects. In: H.M. Van Praag, O. Rafaelseon, M. Lader, and A. Sachar, eds. *The Handbook of Biological Psychiatry*. Part VI, *Practical Applications of Psychotropic Drugs and Other Biological Treatments*. Marcel Dekker, Inc., New York, 1981a, pp. 71–134.

Potter, W.Z., Calil, H.M., Extein, I., Gold, P.W., Wehr, T.A., and Goodwin, F.K. Specific norepinephrine and serotonin uptake inhibitors in man: A crossover study with pharmacokinetic, biochemical, neuroendocrine and behavioral parameters. *Acta Psychi. Scand.*, Suppl. 290, 63:152–165, 1981b.

Potter, W.Z., Calil, H.M., Sutfin, T., Zavadil, A.P., Jusko, W.J., Rapaport, J., and Goodwin, F.K. Active metabolites of imipramine and desipramine in man. *Clin. Pharmacol. Ther.* 31:393–401, 1982.

Potter, W.Z. and Linnoila, M. Tricyclic antidepressant concentrations: Clinical and research implications. In: R.M. Post and J.C. Ballenger, eds. *Neurobiology of Mood Disorders*, Williams and Wilkins, Baltimore, in press.

Reisby, N., Gram, L.F., Beck, P., Nagy, A., Petersen, G.O., Ortmann, J., Ibsen, I., Dincker, S.J., Jocobsen, O., Krautwald, O., Sondergaard, I., and Christiansen, J. Imipramine: clinical effects and pharmacokinetics. *Psychopharmacology* 54:263–272, 1977.

Richelson, E. Tricyclic antidepressants block H, receptors of mense neuroblastoma cells. *Nature* 274:176–177, 1978.

Richelson, E. Tricyclic antidepressants and neurotransmitter receptors. *Psychiatric Annals* 9:186–195, 1979.

Risch, S.C., Huey, L.Y., and Janowsky, D.S. Plasma levels of tricyclic antidepressants and clinical efficacy: Review of the literature, parts I and II. *J. Clin. Psychiatry* 40:4–16, 58–69, 1979.

Simon, P., Lecrubier, Y., Jouvent, R., Puech, A.J., Allilaire, J.F., and Widlöcker, D. Experimental and clinical evidence of the antidepressant effect of a beta-adrenergic stimulant. *Psychological Medicine* 8:335–338, 1978.

Schildkraut, J.J. The catecholamine hypothesis of affective disorders: a review of supporting evidence. *Am. J. Psychiatry* 122:509–522, 1965.

Sellers, E.M., Abel, J.G., Romach, M.K., Khouw, V., and Naranjo, C.A. Sources of variation in binding of psychotherapeutic drugs to plasma proteins. In: E. Usdin, ed. *Clinical Pharmacology in Psychiatry*, Elsevier, New York, 1981, pp. 199–212.

Stewart, J.W., Quitkin, F., Fyer, A., and Klein, D.F. Efficacy of desmethylimipramine in endogenomorphically depressed patients. *Psychopharmacology Bull.* 16(3):52–54, 1980.

Träskman, L., Asberg, M., Bertilsson, L., Cronholm, B., Mellström, B., Neckers, L., Sjöqvist, F., Thoren, P., and Tybring, G. Plasma levels of chlorimipramine and its demethyl metabolite during treatment of depression. *Clin. Pharmacol. Ther.* 26:600–612, 1979.

U'Prichard, D.C., Greenberg, D.A., Sheehan, P.P., and Snyder, S.H. Tricyclic antidepressants: Therapeutic properties and affinity for α-adrenergic receptor binding sites in the brain. *Science* 199:197–198, 1978.

Vetulani, J., Stawarz, R.J., Dingell, J.V., and Sulser, F. A possible carrier mechanism of action of antidepressant treatments. *Naunyn-Schmiedeberg's Arch. Pharmacol.* 293:109–114, 1976.

Wagner, J.G. *Biopharmaceutics and Relevant Pharmacokinetics.* Drug Intelligence Publications, Hamilton, Illinois, 1971.

Wilkinson, G.R. and Shand, D.G. A physiological approach to hepatic drug clearance. *Clin. Pharmacol. Ther.* 18:377–390, 1975.

Wing, L.M.H., Reid, J.L., Davies, D.S., Neill, E.A.M., Tippett, P., and Dollery, C.T. Pharmacokinetic and concentration effect relationships of clonidine in essential hypertension. *Eur. J. Clin. Pharmacol.* 12:463–469, 1977.

Ziegler, V.E., Co, B.T., Taylor, J.R., Clayton, P.J., and Biggs, J.T.: Amitriptyline plasma levels and therapeutic response. *Clin. Pharmacol. Ther.* 19:795–801, 1976.

SECTION II

Schizophrenia

Hints for Clinicians

RATIONALE FOR TREATMENT CHOICE

There is insufficient evidence to favor one antipsychotic agent over another. The striking similarity in the equality and nature of the action of antipsychotics suggests that these drugs share a common and specific mechanism of action. The practical implication of this is that the clinician need only familiarize himself with a few of the numerous neuroleptics available. Choice is then determined empirically by the drug that produced an optimal response with minimum side effects in a given patient.

It is well known that some schizophrenic patients do not appear to respond to neuroleptic drugs. Some of this may be related to non-absorption and can be ameliorated by ensuring absorption of the drug. It has also been suggested that the evidence of brain atropy producing enlarged ventricles and widened sulci may be related to being refractory to neuroleptics. However, the response difference between patients with large and small ventricles is relative, not absolute; the findings have no direct clinical significance. It is suggested that the choice of drug treatment requires a clinical judgment irrespective of enlarged ventricles. In this regard, the relationship of ventricular size and treatment response is more a research than a clinically meaningful finding.

The measurement of variables relating to social functioning indicate that patients receiving both drug and psychotherapy do better than those who receive drug alone. Thus, it appears that while drugs prevent relapse, psychotherapy improves social function. In this sense, then, drugs and psychotherapy complement each other.

MAINTENANCE MEDICATION

Regarding maintenance medication, Davis suggests that for the first episode "reactive" schizophrenic patients or those with hysterical psychosis, it may be reasonable to maintain medication for a short while after symptoms remit to ensure that the patients have a solid recovery from the first episode. Long-term drug maintenance should be avoided. Most patients should be treated with medication for three months to one year after a psychotic episode to be certain that they have recovered from their presenting illness. On the other hand, there is a trend for chronically-ill patients to require lower dosages after a long period of time. This suggests that the schizophrenic process may "burn out" in some very chronic patients. Therefore, all patients should be re-examined periodically to determine whether or not they still need maintenance medication. In fact, efforts should be made to reduce the dose or discontinue medication whenever possible and see if relapse occurs. Medication can be easily reinstituted when necessary, but because tardive dyskinesia is a serious problem, every effort should be made to use the lowest effective dose.

Dr. Davis reviews 35 double blind studies on the effectiveness of antipsychotics in preventing relapse. He points out that in all of the studies, many more patients relapsed on placebo than on drug. Of a total of 3,609 patients studied, 20% relapsed on drug, 53% relapsed on placebo. He suggests that it is very important to note that the risk of relapse remains constant over time. In the studies reviewed by Dr. Davis, the relapse rate varied from 7% to 14% per month in patients not receiving maintenance medication. By comparing to relapse rates on patients maintained on antipsychotic drugs, it can be estimated the neuroleptics reduced the rate of relapse by a factor of from 2.5 to 5.

We do not know which individuals require neuroleptics to stay relatively relapse-free, and which will do equally well, perhaps better, without drugs. High doses of neuroleptics, of course, effectively cut off estrogen secretion in premenopausal women by hormonal feedback mechanisms so that it may be important to keep neuroleptic doses under the amenorrhea threshold; thus, allowing the presumed antipsychotic effect of estrogens to operate and prevent a neuroleptic dose escalation.

For long acting antipsychotics, depot fluphenazine has been shown to be equal or superior to the oral formulation. The depot intramuscular form should be considered for patients who do not show optimal response to oral medication, or who are suspected of poor compliance as evidenced by frequent relapses. The decanoate formulation is often preferred as a long acting depot fluphenazine.

It is suggested that the compliance rate of adhering to a neuroleptic maintenance regime is between 30% and 50%. Unfortunately, there has not been sufficient research into the unpleasant cognitive and emotional effects of neuroleptics, the marked blunting of spontaneity, creativity and affective intensity. These symptoms may, at times, be part of the illness but may also be neuroleptic-induced.

It is known that periodic drug holidays of short duration are possible for some schizophrenic patients, without risk of relapse but that such holidays are hazardous for others. There is evidence that schizophrenia appears to interfere more with left than with right hemisphere learning, suggesting that educational programs would probably be more effective if they addressed the learning potential of the right hemisphere. This would suggest that concrete intuitive, metaphoric, spatial, subjective, wholistic information processing be encouraged.

DOSE

Reported studies consistently fail to show any benefit, from the use of doses of antipsychotics much greater than the equivalent of an average of 300 mg of chlorpromazine per day. More specifically, there is no evidence of additional therapeutic benefit in the use of doses in excess of 600 mg to 1000 mg of chlorpromazine daily. Davis points out that this should lead to a model of therapeutic treatment by considering the dose response curve in the treatment of patients. Thus, the optimal point in the dose response curve is the lowest dose that achieves the maximum clinical effects. In practice, a given dose response curve applies to only one patient at a particular point in time. Different patients may have different dose response curves and a given patient may have different dose response curves at different points in time. Thus, Dr. Davis suggests that one increase the dose as long as the therapeutic effect is noted. When no more therapeutic effect is noted, one has reached the plateau of the curve and further medication should not be added.

TARDIVE DYSKINESIA

A recent study found that prevalence, severity, and distribution of abnormal movements was similar in groups of chronic schizophrenics with a history of extensive neuroleptic treatment and those with no drug treatment. This suggests that further studies must be done to evaluate the role of drug induction of these abnormal movements as compared with those which occur spontaneously to improve the diagnosis and thus treatment. Current investigations report the occurrence of tardive dyskinesia in 20% to 40% of patients maintained on chronic neuroleptic treatment. Casey suggests that a more conservative estimate would be a rate of 10 to 20%, however, the variability in prevalence rates can be accounted for by different criteria of symptoms severity required for identifying "a case" of tardive dyskinesia. Thus, the rates can vary from 5% to 70% depending upon these criteria.

There is a considerable amount of evidence suggesting that there is a steady increase in prevalence of tardive dyskinesia with increasing age. Pooled data from nine studies reported tardive dyskinesia in approximately 10% of patients under 40 years of age and a gradual increase in prevalence to over 50% in patients 60 years of age, or over. There seemed to be no consistent findings to support the association of organic brain disease and neuroleptic induced extrapyramidal symptoms as risk factors in tardive dyskinesia.

Casey confirms Davis's statement that approximately 40% to 60% of patients maintained on neuroleptic medications do not relapse when their medicines are discontinued. This implies that half of the patients may be taking more medicine than is necessary. On the other hand, it also implies that if medicines were discontinued in all patients, half of them would be exposed to potential psychotic exacerbation. Unfortunately, there is no method for predicting which patients may successfully reduce or discontinue their neuroleptic medications. Casey suggests that a periodic reduction of 10 to 20% drug dosage would allow the determination of the lowest effective dose. The data suggest that the most important factor in the risk of developing tardive dyskinesia may be individual vulnerability.

An important step in managing tardive dyskinesia, as well as acute extrapyramidal symptoms, is to control anticholinergic medications properly. Interestingly, the finding that anticholinergic drugs exacerbate tardive dyskinesia has been used to suggest that patients who are potentially susceptible to tardive dyskinesia may be discovered by giving them periodic brief drug trials with anticholinergic agents to uncover the tardive dyskinesia. Such a proposal requires much additional study before it becomes a routine clinical practice. Dr. Casey suggests that the routine prophylactic administration of anticholinergics should be avoided, as this will lead to the prescription of drugs for many patients who do not need them. However, a recent review of the literature found that patients receiving low milligram, high potency neuroleptics and who have well-documented histories of previous extrapyramidal symptoms may need to continue anticholinergic drugs indefinitely.

Patients with tardive dyskinesia and psychosis can be maintained on relatively low neuroleptic doses and have their tardive dyskinesia symptoms gradually improve or resolve over a three or five year period. Thus, discontinuing neuroleptics when tardive dyskinesia is identified is theoretically rational and attractive but often not practical. Some patients may experience a psychotic relapse and must return to drug treatment. In such cases it is important to reconsider the psychiatric diagnosis and evaluate the possibility of treatment with lower doses of antipsychotic medications.

The question of whether drug type and tardive dyskinesia are related has frequently been raised. Although it has been suggested that low milligram, high potency neuroleptics such as depot preparations have higher prevalence rates of tardive dyskinesia, it is very difficult to implicate one drug or one class of drugs as the primary etiological agents of tardive dyskinesia. Further, the biochemical and behavioural differences found in the basic science laboratory have not been translated into important differences in the clinic; drugs which purportedly selectively influence different types of dopamine receptors or brain regions are more similar in the clinic than they are different. Though periodically discontinuing neuroleptic treatment as a "drug holiday" has been recommended in reducing the risk of tardive dyskinesia, the supporting data are conflictive.

Though many drugs have been used to treat tardive dyskinesia, no specific agents have been shown to be both safe and effective over extended treatment periods. These include dopamine antagonists, dopamine agonists, anticholinergics, cholinergic agonists, and drugs which influence GABA.

Blood Levels

The value of monitoring neuroleptic blood levels, currently in the research and development stages, is a promising but uncharted area.

Consent

The question about informed consent is indeed an interesting one. The most practical approach is that the clinician inform the patient, as well as a concerned other person, about the risks and benefits of both treatment and no treatment and that this process by documented in a timely and thoughtful manner, consistent with principles of the doctor-patient relationship.

9

Summary of Guidelines for the Use of Psychotropic Drugs in the Treatment of Schizophrenia

Siu W. Tang

There is overwhelming evidence that neuroleptic drugs provide symptomatic benefits, reduce morbidity and prevent relapses in a large number of schizophrenic patients. As the neuroleptic drugs remain the "drugs of choice" in the treatment of schizophrenia, it is important to establish guidelines for their use. Neuroleptics control and do not cure. Although they are extremely potent in resolving the positive psychotic symptoms, their effects on the negative symptoms are unsatisfactory and many patients remain severely impaired because of these negative symptoms after they have left the hospital. Some patients may not respond to neuroleptics at all. Long-term treatment is inevitable for many patients; the unpleasant side effects of neuroleptics then become a serious problem. Patient drug compliance also becomes a problem for the physician. These and many other problems lead to the necessity to identify areas for future research in psychopharmacology.

GUIDELINES FOR PHARMACOLOGICAL MANAGEMENT OF SCHIZOPHRENIA

1. Neuroleptic drugs are extremely effective in ameliorating the positive symptoms (e.g., hallucinations, delusions, thought disorder) of psychotic patients. Thus, their use is not restricted to schizophrenia alone. They may also be used to treat the psychotic symptoms in affective and organic psychosis.

145

2. Maintenance neuroleptics are indicated for schizophrenic patients at risk for relapse. The relapse rate is constant after medication is discontinued. Most patients should be treated with medication for three months to one year after a psychotic episode. Thereafter, the treatment program should be individualized.

3. In planning for long-term neuroleptic maintenance, the following factors should be taken into consideration:
   − nature and length of the illness
   − previous response to treatment
   − previous relapses
   − social situation
   − occurrence of serious side effects, e.g., tardive dyskinesia.

4. Any of the neuroleptics may be used for maintenance treatment. Aim for an optimal response with a minimum of side effects in a given patient.

5. For most patients, there is no benefit to the use of doses much greater than 300 mg chlorpromazine (CPZ) equivalence per day. Doses above 300 mg CPZ equivalence are equal to or above the optimal dose. Think in terms of minimal therapeutic dose. Administration of high doses over prolonged periods is not recommended. The neuroleptics have serious neurological side effects and also unpleasant effects on the patient's affect and cognitive function.

6. Intramuscular depot neuroleptic drugs should be considered for patients who do not show an optimal response to oral medication, and patients who are suspected of poor compliance.

7. The relationship between clinical response and plasma drug level is still unclear. At present, clinical judgement should guide treatment. Blood levels should be reserved for specific investigation of unusual drug response, e.g., suspected altered absorption or metabolism in a particular patient resulting in too high or too low a drug level.

8. We have no treatment for tardive dyskinesia (TD). Prevention is the main objective. Therefore it is important to recognize involuntary movement disorders early. Consider TD with a differential diagnosis, e.g., other neuroleptic-induced dyskinesia.

9. Presence of TD may necessitate drug discontinuation or re-adjustment of drug to a compromised dosage. Reassess the need for continued drug therapy periodically in patients who developed TD but require neuroleptics for their psychosis.

10. Anticholinergic drugs may aggravate TD once it has developed. Routine prophylactic administration of anticholinergics should be avoided. Many patients can eventually reduce or discontinue their anticholinergic medications. Augmentation of neuroleptics to suppress TD should be avoided.

11. Prevalence and severity of TD increases with advancing age. This, coupled with other complications (e.g., cardiovascular), frequently encountered in this age group suggests cautious use of neuroleptics in geriatric patients.

12. Education about drugs helps patient compliance.

AREAS FOR FUTURE RESEARCH

The areas identified for future research may be grouped under three general headings:

Refinement of the Use of Currently Available Neuroleptic Drugs

Despite all the unpleasant side effects, the neuroleptic drugs, when used appropriately, should benefit a major portion of the schizophrenic population. While the guidelines provided above would apply to most schizophrenic patients, further research should result in the refinement of treatment methods using currently available neuroleptic drugs. An individualized treatment program is emphasized (see in this volume, Chapters by Seeman, Casey, Linden et al., and Chouinard and Steinberg). To reach this goal of individualized treatment, we need research into the factors determining the individual's response to the neuroleptic drugs. At present, we do not know what the optimal blood drug level is for any individual. If there is a therapeutic drug level necessary for response, is this level different at the remission stage from the relapse stage? Our clinical experience suggests that some schizophrenics require less drugs than others. Does this reflect different subtypes of schizophrenia? It is known that differences in metabolism occur between people of different racial background. It has been discovered, for example, that differences exist in the hydroxylation rate of tricyclic antidepressants between Chinese and Caucasians (Dr. W.A. Potter, personal communication). How should one decide on the dosages in patients of different races? We need better ways to separate the neuroleptic non-responders from the responders, to avoid subjecting them to unnecessary neuroleptic treatment. There are many other factors we need to know in order to achieve the ideal goal of treatment individualization (see Seeman, this volume).

New Drugs

Better Neuroleptics. Many patients abandon their neuroleptics because of side effects. Side effects such as sedation, dry mouth, and blurring of vision, commonly complained of by patients, are theoretically avoidable with more specific neuroleptics. Based on the dopamine theory of schizophrenia, an ideal neuroleptic should be a specific potent dopamine D_2 receptor antagonist. It should possess little action (or ideally have no action) on the other neurotransmitter systems. Haloperidol and the other butyrophenones represent a big step towards such a refinement. It is conceivable that further research should result in even more specific D_2 receptor antagonists (Niemegeers and Janssen, 1979) and thus better neuroleptic drugs.

Antipsychotics Devoid of Extrapyramidal and Tardive Dyskinesia Side Effects. Antipsychotics such as clozapine and clozapine-like drugs may relieve psychosis without producing extrapyramidal or tardive dyskinesia side effects. While the mechanism of action of these drugs is still poorly understood, other researchers have attempted to try the dopamine agonists in low doses (e.g., apomorphine, and L-DOPA) in schizophrenics (Calil et al., 1977; Corsini et al., 1977; Smith et al., 1977). Theoretically, low doses of dopamine agonists should stimulate the dopamine autoreceptors, slowing down the activity of the dopamine containing neurons, and thus resulting in a reduction of dopaminergic neurotransmission (Carlson, 1982). The net effect should be compatible with the neuroleptics, which block dopaminergic neurotransmission by acting postsynaptically. However, results from clinical studies are far from conclusive so far. Recently, Carlsson (1982) reported the synthesis of a new compound 3-PPP, an analogue of dopamine, which has a potent agonistic action on the dopamine autoreceptor. From preliminary animal studies, there appears to be great hope that this compound may turn out to be a successful antipsychotic agent without neurological side effects. While much effort in the development of antipsychotic drugs has centered around the dopamine system, there is a need for research into non-dopaminergic mechanisms in psychotic disorders (see chapter by Wyatt and Delisi, this volume; also Barchas et al., this volume). Barchas et al. (1978) cite an example originally described by Marthe Vogt, who noted that the earliest treatments of Parkinson's disease appeared to work by counteracting a hyperactive cholinergic system, yet subsequent studies have shown that the apparent excess of cholinergic activity arises from a severe dopamine deficiency. If dopamine is involved in a potential compensatory system, then treatment should be aimed at the underlying defect. On the other hand, the occurrence of neuroleptic resistant patients raises the possibility that the dopaminergic mechanism may not even be involved in some schizophrenics. The same point is raised by Dr. Weinberger (this volume). The relative ineffectiveness of the neuroleptics in the negative symptoms gives further support for such a possibility.

Subtyping the Schizophrenia Syndrome Biologically

Many believe that the schizophrenia syndrome is more than one single disease. The importance of determining the biological subtypes of schizophrenia cannot be overemphasized. There has been some progress in the subtyping of schizophrenia in the past few years. Weinberger for example, shows that schizoprenics with enlarged cerebral ventricles responded poorly to neuroleptics. They may represent a subgroup for which the dopaminergic mechanism is irrelevant. Other possibilities like slow virus (see Wyatt and Delisi, this volume) or disturbances in other neurotransmitters (Barchas et al., 1978), if proven, should result in better classification and better treatment.

Genetic studies may also help in psychopharmacologic advances. If a certain subtype of schizophrenia is genetically transmittable, then it is important to find out what exactly is the transmittable defect. Identification of the genetic defect or enzymatic defect, for example, has helped in the prevention and management of some genetic metabolic disorders which may result in mental retardation.

So far, the dopamine theory of schizophrenia has provided us with a conceptual basis for psychopharmacologic research in schizophrenia. The next vitally important step now is the biological subtyping of schizophrenia. Once the etiology of the different subtypes of schizophrenia is known, one could visualize that a specific treatment or prevention will follow.

REFERENCES

Barchas, J.D., Elliott, G.R., and Berger, P.A. Biogenic amine hypothesis of schizophrenia. In L.C. Wynne, R.L. Cromwell, and S. Matthysse, *The Nature of Schizophrenia—New Approaches to Research and Treatment*, pp. 126-142. New York: John Wiley & Sons, 1978.

Calil, H.M., Yesavage, J.A., and Hollister, L.E. Low dose levodopa in schizophrenia. *Commun. Psychopharmacol.* 1:593-596, 1977.

Carlsson, A. The search for new monoaminergic receptor agonists. In G. Boysen and O.B. Paulson, Proceedings of the 24th Scandinavian Congress of Neurology. Copenhagen, June 9-12, 1982. Copenhagen: Munksgaard, 1982.

Corsini, G.U., del Zompo, M., Manconi, S., Cinachetti, C., Mangoni, A., and Gessa, G.L. Sedative, hypnotic and antipsychotic effects of low doses of apomorphine in man. *Advan. Biochem. Psychopharmacol.* 16:645-648, 1977.

Niemegeers, C.J.E., and Janssen, P.A.J. A systematic study of the pharmacological activities of dopamine antagonists. *Life Sci.* 24:2201-2216, 1979.

Nowycky, M.C., and Roth, R.H. Dopaminergic neurons: Role of presynaptic receptors in the regulation of transmitter biosynthesis. *Prog. Neuropsychopharm.* 2:139-158, 1978.

Smith, R.C., Tamminga, C., and Davis, J.M. Effect of apomorphine on schizophrenic symptoms. *J. Neurol. Transm.* 40:171-176, 1977.

10

Antipsychotics in the Maintenance Treatment of Schizophrenia

ROBERT LINDEN,
JOHN M. DAVIS, AND JOAN RUBINSTEIN

Shortly following the discovery that chlorpromazine is effective as an antipsychotic agent, it became apparent that patients relapsed after they stopped taking their medication. Therefore clinicians began "maintaining" their patients on medication after their symptoms had resolved in an attempt to reduce the frequency of relapse. In this paper we will review the efficacy of maintenance neuroleptics and discuss the clinical variables which must be evaluated in designing a long-term treatment program.

EFFECTIVENESS OF ANTIPSYCHOTICS IN PREVENTING RELAPSE

The first studies on maintenance medication were initiated early in the era of phenothiazines when sophisticated methodology for controlled investigation of psychotherapeutics had not yet been perfected. These studies performed a pioneering function in the development of quantitative, double-blind research designs, but the methodology used was not as refined as it has become in more recent studies. It is worth noting, however, that both the earlier and the more recent studies yield consistent results. There are presently 35 double-blind studies which compare the relapse rates of patients on placebo vs. on maintenance neuroleptics. Of these studies, 33 present the number of patients who relapsed on placebo vs. antipsychotics and are summarized in Table 1.

Table 1. Antipsychotic Prevention of Relapse

	No. of patients	Percent relapse on placebo	Percent relapse on drug	Percent difference in relapse rate (placebo-drug)
Caffey	250	45	5	40
Prien (1968)	762	42	16	26
Prien (1969a)	325	56	20	36
Schiele	80	60	3	57
Adelson	281	90	49	41
Morton	40	70	25	45
Baro	26	100	0	100
Hershon	62	28	7	21
Rassidakis	84	58	34	24
Melynk	40	50	0	50
Schawver	80	18	5	13
Freeman	94	28	13	16
Whitaker	39	65	8	57
Garfield	27	31	11	20
Diamond	40	70	25	45
Blackburn	53	54	24	30
Gross (1961)	109	58	14	44
Englehardt	294	30	15	15
Leff	30	83	33	50
Hogarty	361	67	31	36
Troshinsky	43	63	4	59
Hirsch	74	66	8	58
Chien	31	87	12	94
Gross (1975)	61	65	34	31
Rifkin	62	68	7	61
Clark	35	78	27	51
Clark	19	70	43	27
Kinross-Wright	40	70	5	65
Andrews	31	35	7	28
Wistedt	38	63	38	25
Cheung	28	62	13	48
Levine (1980) (PO)	33	59	33	26
Levine (1980) (IM)	34	30	18	12

Summary statistics, p less than 1^{-100}

Source: J.M. Davis Overview: Maintenance Therapy in Psychiatry: I. Schizophrenia. *Am. J. Psychiatry* 132:1237–1245, 1975.

In each of the studies included in Table 1, patients were randomly assigned to one of two groups. The first group received antipsychotic medication while the second received an identically appearing placebo. The studies were double-blind in that neither the patients nor the investigators knew which patients belonged to which group. The frequency with which each group relapsed was then measured. These studies were carried out in a variety of settings: in private, state, and Veterans Administration hospitals; in inpatient and outpatient facilities; and in England, Europe, and the United States. While in many of these major studies inpatients were used, there are also adequate data on schizophrenic outpatients.

In all of the studies, many more patients relapsed on placebo than on drug. Of a total of 3,609 patients studied, 20% relapsed on drug, and 53% relapsed on placebo. Taken individually, every one of the studies has shown that more patients relapse on placebo than on maintenance medication. When the studies are combined by the appropriate statistical means (Davis, 1975), this difference is statistically significant with a p-value of less than 10^{-100}. Thus, there is overwhelming statistical evidence that the antipsychotic drugs prevent relapse in schizophrenia.

THE CONCEPT OF RATE OF RELAPSE

In analyzing the data from maintenance studies, Davis (1975) suggested that, rather than thinking in terms of a fixed number of patients who will or will not relapse, it is more appropriate to think in terms of *a rate of relapse*. Specifically, the observation was made that the time course of relapse in a group of patients taken off medication is an exponential function similar to that seen with radioactive half-life ($T^{1/2}$) or the half-life of drugs in plasma. There is a constant rate of relapse, similar to the constant rate of decay seen with radioactive material or the constant rate of disappearance of a drug from plasma.

This can be illustrated by considering a group of 100 patients with a relapse rate of 10% per month. In the first month, 10 patients relapse and 90 remain in the study group. During the second month, 10% of 90 or 9 patients relapse, and 81 patients remain. The next month, 10% of 81 or 8 relapse and so forth, with 10% of the remaining patients relapsing each month. While the actual number of patients relapsing would decrease each month, the 10% rate of relapse remains constant. In this example, the "half-life" is about 6 months. At 12 months, or double the half-life, 25% of the original patients would remain unrelapsed, and at 18 months 12.5% of the original patients would remain unrelapsed.

The literature conveys the impression that there is a substantial group of schizophrenic patients who will not relapse when off medication. It is often

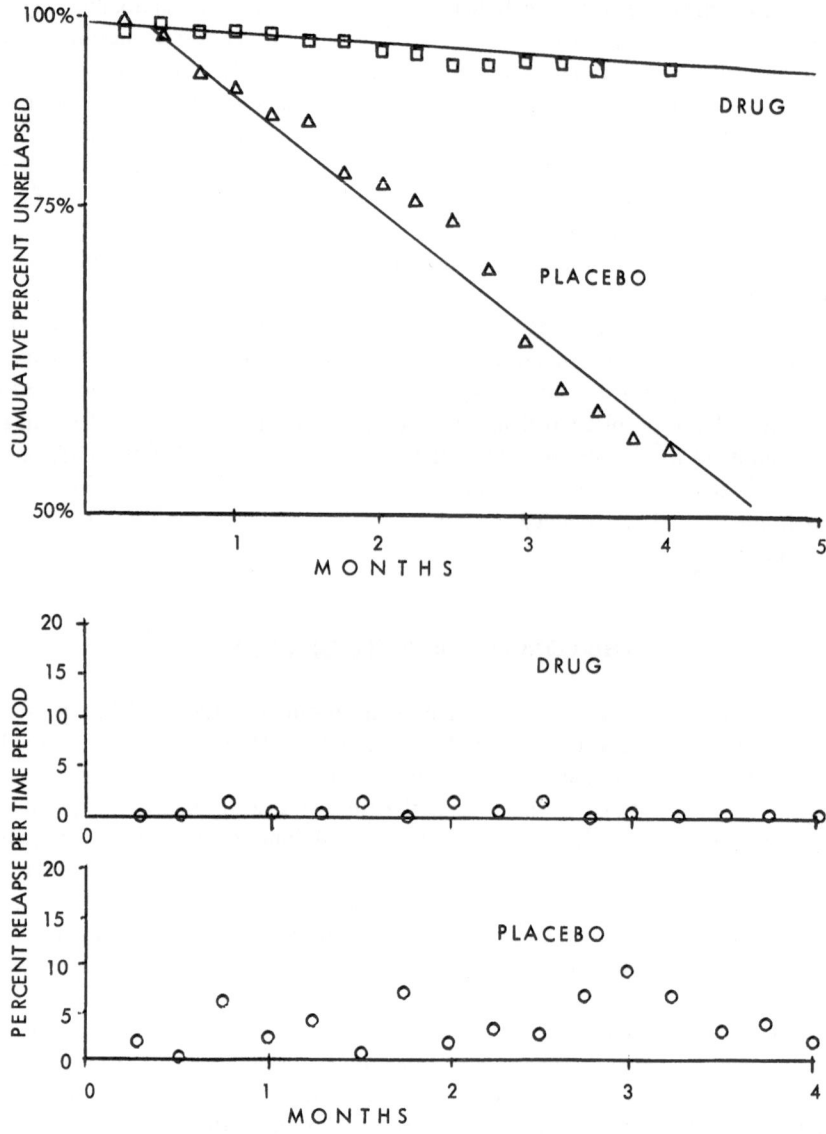

Figure 1. Relapse as a logarithmic function. Relapse over time expressed as the log n_e of percent of patients unrelapsed over time (Data: Caffey et al., 1964). Bottom panel: risk rates, same data. The number of relapses are divided by the number of patients being studied at each time period.

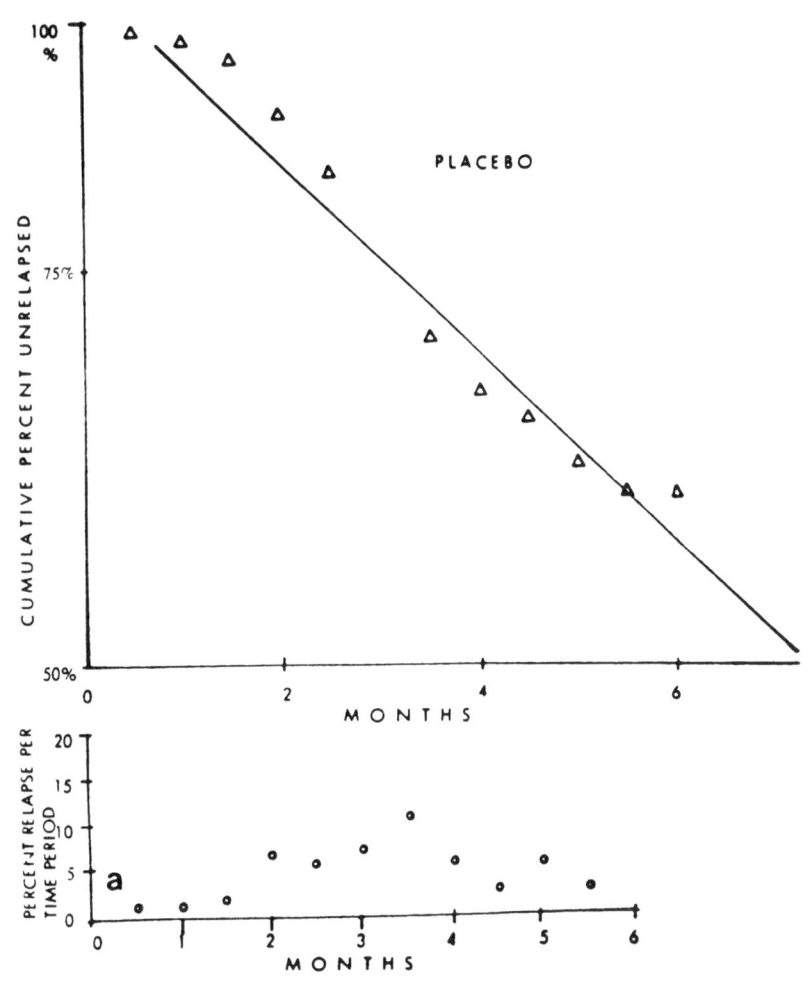

Figure 2.   Relapse as a logarithmic function (Data: Prien & Cole, 1968). See also
Figure 1.

stated that approximately 50% of patients do not relapse when medication is
discontinued and, therefore, maintenance medication is not indicated for a substantial number of patients. It should be noted that several studies from which
the figure of 50% has been culled have a follow-up period limited to 4 to 6
months. This unrelapsed group is not surprising in light of the above discussion;
indeed, data from longer-term studies show that while 50% of patients have not

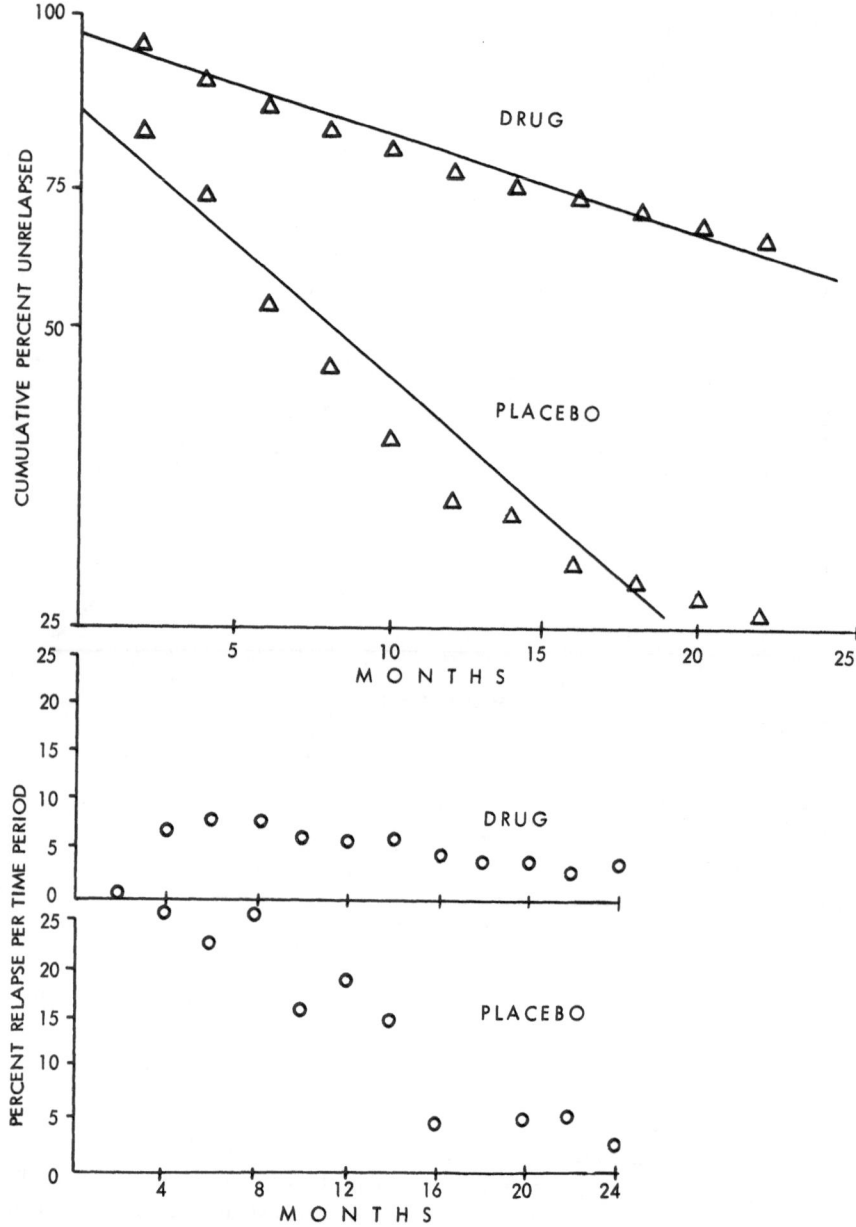

Figure 3. Relapse as a logarithmic function (Data: Hogarty & Goldberg, 1973). See also Figure 1.

relapsed by 4 to 6 months, when followed for 12 to 18 months they continue to relapse at the same constant rate. This shows that patients are not at a relatively greater risk for relapse in the first few months off medication, nor do they become progressively less at risk the longer they have remained without a relapse. Instead, the risk of relapse remains constant over time.

In a statistical analysis of three studies (Hogarty and Goldberg, 1973, Prien and Cole, 1968; Caffey et al., 1964), Davis found that the data was most consistent with a constant relapse rate (Figures 1, 2, 3). The data from these studies fits an exponential curve extremely well, with an r^2 in the neighborhood of 0.96 (Davis, 1980a). In these studies, the relapse rate varied from 7-14% per month in patients not receiving maintenance medication. By comparing to relapse rates in patients maintained on antipsychotic drugs, it can be estimated that neuroleptics reduce the rate of relapse by a factor of from 2.5 to 5.

AN EXTENDED LENGTH STUDY

Of particular interest to the question of maintenance medication and the nature of relapse in schizophrenia is a study by Hogarty and Goldberg (1973). These investigators studied 374 schizophrenic patients after recovery and discharge from the hospital. After an initial outpatient period during which they were stabilized on phenothiazine, the patients were divided into two groups: half were assigned to maintenance chlorpromazine and half were assigned to placebo. Half of each group additionally received outpatient psychotherapy. At the end of one year, 73% of the placebo without psychotherapy group and 63% of the placebo plus psychotherapy group had relapsed. Only 33% of the drug-maintenance group and 26% of the drug-maintenance plus psychotherapy group had relapsed. If those patients in the drug maintenance group who discontinued medication were excluded, the relapse rate for patients on medication for the 12-month period was only 16%. Measurement of variables relating to social functioning indicated that patients who received both drug and psychotherapy did better than those who received drug alone. Thus, it appears that while drugs prevent relapse, psychotherapy improves social functioning. In this sense then drugs and psychotherapy complement each other.

In examining their data in detail it can be seen that the relapse rate is constant up to 18 months, and then appears to decrease. If some patients in the study do not suffer from a recurrent form of illness they would never relapse, and the relapse rate would drop to zero after all the patients with the potential for relapse, do so. To investigate this further, Hogarty (1976) examined the relapse rate of those patients who had not had a relapse for 2 years or longer. As only a few patients in the original placebo group had not experienced a relapse, a statistical study of this group was not possible. However, Hogarty did follow up the larger group of patients who had been on medication and had not relapsed for two years. Antipsychotic medication was discontinued in these patients and relapses occurred in an exponential fashion, with a relapse rate quite similar to that of the initial placebo group. Apparently, while relapse was prevented for a considerable length of time by neuroleptics, when medication was discontinued, the patients repalsed at a rate similar to that of patients initially taken off neuroleptics after only two months of maintenance medication.

WHO NEEDS MAINTENANCE MEDICATION?

So-called reactive schizophrenic patients who may have one florid psychotic episode during adolescence with a fairly quick remission, may constitute a special population from the standpoint of maintenance. There is no firm knowledge based on double blind studies concerning whether maintenance medication is indicated for these patients. Reviews of studies on the natural history of reactive psychosis (brief psychotic disorder, schizophreniform disorder) by such workers as Stephens (1963, 1970) and Astrup (1962, 1966) suggest that the prognosis of these patients may be fairly good, i.e., many of these patients will not relapse even without medication. Therefore, for first episode "reactive" schizophrenic patients or those with hysterical psychosis, it may be reasonable to maintain medication for a short while after symptoms remit to ensure that the patients have a solid recovery from the first episode, but to avoid long-term drug maintenance.

Evidence pertinent to maintenance antipsychotic medication in inpatients was provided by Prien and associates. These investigators combined two NIMH studies of maintenance phenothiazines and found that the patients' history of medication (i.e., the dose levels at which the patients previously had a therapeutic response) presented a reasonably good prediction of relapse (see Table 2).

Table 2. Relapse on Placebo by Prestudy Dose Level
of Chlorpromazine or Equivalent

Prestudy dose level	Total no. of patients	Patients relapsed	
		N	Percent
No medication	30	2	7
Under 300 mg	99	23	23
300 mg to 500 mg	91	47	52
500 mg	81	53	65

The higher the treatment dose, the more likely were the patients to relapse when medication was stopped. This is intuitively sensible because it is reasonable to suppose that patients' dose levels were determined empirically. That is, patients may be maintained on high doses as a consequence of increased symptoms when their physician attempts to lower their dosage.

These studies also revealed a trend for very chronically-ill patients to require lower dosages. This suggests that the schizophrenic process may "burn out" in some very chronically-ill patients. Such patients may have definitely needed drugs years ago but may have changed with time and aging. Therefore, all patients should be reexamined periodically to determine whether or not they still need maintenance medication. On occasion, patients should have their drugs discontinued or their dosage lowered to discover empirically whether the neuroleptic treatment is indeed necessary, or if a lower dose would suffice.

From a common sense perspective, evidence that the patient was initially helped by antipsychotic treatment would be another important indication for maintenance medication, as would the potential consequences to the patient of a relapse. It is important to recognize that relapses for outpatients are a relatively serious event because a wide variety of social variables become involved: the patient's adjustment to his family, job, and social situation may be seriously compromised. A deterioration of the patient's functioning after discontinuance of medication may result in serious work or family problems that place the patient under even greater stress. In addition, the development of psychotic behavior may create serious social repercussions that may harm his later attempt to readjust to his social setting.

Although tardive dyskinesia can occur in outpatients who receive relatively short-term treatment, the incidence of tardive dyskinesia is highest in elderly state hospital patients who have been receiving high doses of medication for many years. In the more controlled situation of the state hospital, relapse can be very quickly treated since the patient is under continuous observation by nursing staff and physicians. Likewise, the social repercussions are minimal compared to those of the outpatient. Therefore, efforts should be made to reduce the dose or to discontinue medication whenever possible and see if relapse occurs. Medication can be easily reinstituted when necessary, but because tardive dyskinesia represents a sufficiently serious problem, every effort should be made to use the lowest effective dose in the hospital. In the outpatient situation much more judgement is required to balance possible benefits against possible risks.

In sum, the patient's psychiatric history (acute vs. chronic, etc.), social situation, and drug history (dose, responsiveness, relapses when decreasing dose), as well as the risks of tardive dyskinesia, must all be evaluated in forming a decision regarding maintenance treatment with neuroleptics.

CHOICE OF DRUG

One of the major treatment decisions facing a psychiatrist is the choice of antipsychotic agent. A widely held, though unconfirmed, belief is that hyper-excitable patients respond best to chlorpromazine (Thorazine) because it is a sedating phenothaizine; and, conversely, withdrawn patients respond best to an alerting phenothiazine, such as fluphenazine (Prolixin) or trifluoperazine (Stela-zine). This relationship has never been proven, and, in fact, the National Insti-tute of Mental Health Collaborative Studies (Goldberg et al., 1967, 1972) indicate that a second-order factor labeled "apthetic and retarded" predicts a differentially good response to chlorpromazine. It should be noted that this finding did not replicate with cross-validation. This underscores the important fact that when studying many predictors, statistical analysis of the data will often yield some statistically significant associations by chance alone. In the past, several systems have been developed to predict which symptom or type of schizophrenic patient would respond optimally to which antipsychotic drug. Subsequent studies to test some of these empirically defined predictions, however, uniformly failed to substantiate them.

An additional property of the antipsychotics that has emerged from clinical studies is their essential equivalency in terms of therapeutic effect. With the exception of promazine and mepazine, all the phenothiazines are clearly superior to placebo, and of equal efficacy to chlorpromazine (for a review, see Davis, 1980b). Inspection of the changes induced by antipsychotics in the various symptoms of schizophrenia further reveal that all of the antipsychotics consistently produce changes in common parameters. The striking similarity in the equality and nature of their action suggest that these drugs share a common and specific mechanism of action. The practical implication of this is that the clinician need only familiarize himself with a few of the numerous neuroleptics available. Choice is then determined empirically by the drug that produces an optimal response with a minimum of side effects in a given patient.

LONG-ACTING ANTIPSYCHOTICS

Of special interest to maintenance therapy of schizophrenia is the avail-ability of a long-acting neuroleptic: fluphenazine. In a number of studies (Hirsch et al., 1973; Hogarty et al., 1979; Levine et al., 1978; Quitkin et al., 1978; Rifkin et al., 1977a, b; Simon et al., 1978; Schooler and Levine, 1978) depot fluphenazine was shown to be equal or superior to the oral formulation. The depot intramuscular form should be considered for patients who do not show an optimal response to oral medication, or who are suspected of poor compli-ance as evidenced by frequent relapses. The different pharmacokinetics of an intramuscular injection, by which the "first-pass effect" of metabolism in the liver is avoided, may be of further benefit to some patients. The two depot formulations of fluphenazine are quite similar and only marginal differences are found, but from the studies which directly compare fluphenazine decanoate to fluphenazine enanthate, it appears that the decanoate form is somewhat more potent, slightly longer acting, and has slightly fewer side effects (Donlon et al., 1978; Kane et al., 1978; Van Praag and Dols, 1973). Thus, the decanoate formulation is probably preferred as a long-acting depot fluphenazine.

Three long-acting antipsychotics which are presently available in Europe are currently undergoing study in the United States: Penfluridol is an orally administered antipsychotic, with a duration of action of about one week. It is equal in efficacy to either oral or depot fluphenazine (Quitkin, 1978). Pipithiazine palmitate is a depot neuroleptic which Simon et al. (1978) found comparable in efficacy to oral antipsychotic and fluphenazine decanoate. Haloperidol decanoate is an injectable depot formulation that can be given monthly. It has been shown to be equivalent in efficacy to bi-weekly injections of fluphenazine decanoate (Roose et al., 1981), and in two open clinical trials it was equal in efficacy to oral haloperidol.

MEDICATION DOSAGE

The most useful way to think about dosage in psychiatry is in terms of a dose–response curve (Figure 4). When a very low dose is given, patients have no clinical response. Then, over a certain dosage range, there is a linear portion of a dose-response curve, in which an increase in dosage produces an increased

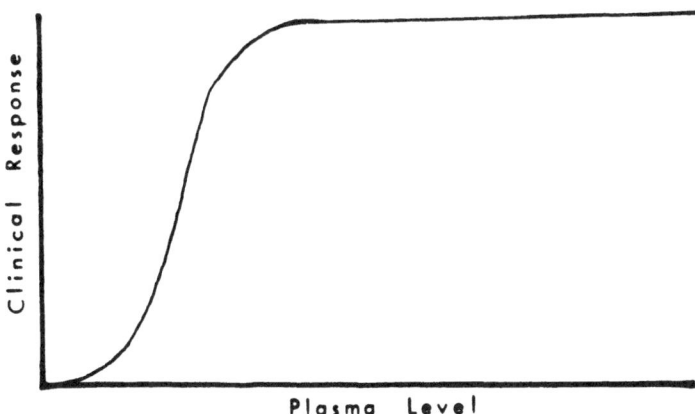

Figure 4. Dose–response curve.

Table 3. Dose Equivalence

Drug	Dose
Chlorpromazine	100
Triflupromazine	28.4 ± 1.8
Thioridazine	95.3 ± 8.2
Prochlorperazine	14.3 ± 1.7
Perphenazine	8.9 ± 0.6
Fluphenazine	1.2 ± 0.1
Trifluoperazine	2.8 ± 0.4
Acetophenazine	23.5 ± 1.5
Carphenazine	24.3 ± 2.7
Butaperazine	8.9 ± 1.1
Mesoridazine	55.3 ± 8.3
Piperacetazine	10.5
Haloperidol	1.6 ± 0.4
Chlorprothixene	43.9 ± 13.9
Thiothixene	5.2 ± 1.3

Source: David, J.M. (1976).

therapeutic response. At some point, a point of diminishing return ensues, when increasing the dose does not increase response, i.e., there is a "ceiling effect." At higher doses, additionally, toxicity may occur. The optimal point on the dose-response curve then is the lowest dose that achieves the maximal clinical effects. In practice, a given dose–response curve applies to only one patient at a particular point in time. Different patients may have different dose-response curves; indeed, a given patient may have different dose-response curves at different points in time.

There is presently a large body of empirical data equating the dose of any given neuroleptic to a standard such as chlorpromazine. This enables the clinician to measure the antipsychotic dose of any neuroleptic and convert it to chlorpromazine equivalents (i.e., the antipsychotic potency of a given neuroleptic needed to produce the same improvement as a 100 mg of chlorpromazine). There are a substantial number of double-blind studies investigating all the neuroleptics, which Davis (1976) reviewed to determine what dose of each neuroleptic is equivalent to the standard of 100 mg of chlorpromazine (Table 3).

Although the pharmacologist often utilizes dose–response curves, this is practically never done in clinical studies. Since the clinician wishes to optimize patients' improvement, virtually all double-blind studies use a flexible dose to achieve an optimal response. Flexible dosage studies, as compared to fixed dosage studies, are more problematic for deriving knowledge of dose-response curves. If a patient, for example, is not clinically responding, the dose is increased. The patient may have had too low a plasma level of drug, or the plasma level

Table 4. Summary of Dose-Response Studies in
Chronic Patients

	Number of studies in which	
Lower dose[a]	Higher dose superior	Both doses equally efficacious
over 300	0	8
300 or less	6	2

[a]Expressed in mg of chlorpromazine equivalence.

may have been adequate but the patient would not have responded at any dosage. Thus, flexible dosage studies give little or no information about the low dose/low response end of the curve and have inflated numbers of high dose/low response results.

In Table 4, we have summarized all studies which used two groups of chronic patients randomly assigned to one of two different fixed dosages, a higher or a lower dosage. Whenever the lower dose was above 300 mg of chlorpromazine equivalence, the higher dose was no more effective than the lower dose. This was true regardless of the particular neuroleptic investigated: two studies used haloperidol (Bjorndal et al., 1980; Rimon et al., 1981), four used fluphenazine (Itil et al., 1970, 1971; Debuck, 1972; MacCreadie and MacDonald, 1977) and two used trifluoperazine (Prien et al., 1969b); Carscallen et al., 1968). Very different results occurred, however, when the lower dose was less than or equal to 300 mg. Three studies showed a higher dose of chlorpromazine to be more effective than a lower dose of 150 or 300 mg (Clark et al., 1970, 1972; Prien and Cole, 1968). Similarly, Dencker et al. (1978) showed that 5300 mg fluphenazine (chlorpromazine equivalent) was superior to 270 mg fluphenazine and Lehmann et al. (1980) found 2600 mg to be superior to 230 mg fluphenazine. However, McClelland et al. (1976) found no differences between 290 and 5850 mg fluphenazine. Additionally, 230 mg thiothixene was just as effective as 910 mg (Gardose et al., 1974), but 440 mg butaperazine was more effective than 56 mg (Simpson et al., 1968).

From these data, it can be inferred that doses above 300 mg chlorpromazine equivalence are equal to or above the optimal dose. Doses at or below 300 mg are on the linear portion of the dose–response curve. In sum, the studies reviewed consistently fail to show any benefit, on the average, to the use of doses of antipsychotics much greater than the equivalence of 300 mg of chlorpromazine per day. While individual patients vary in the amount of neuroleptic they require, for the majority of patients there is no evidence of additional therapeutic benefit to the use of doses in excess of 600 mg to 1000 mg of chlorpromazine.

CONCLUSION

A review of 33 controlled studies on the use of maintenance antipsychotic medication reveals that of 3,609 patients studied, 53% relapsed on placebo, and 20% relapsed on drugs. Maintenance medication clearly prevented relapse in a substantial number of patients and the percent of relapses in the drug-treated groups was less than half that observed in the control groups. Furthermore, when patients previously maintained unrelapsed on medication had their medication withdrawn, they began to relapse at similar rates as the controls. Thus, maintenance antipsychotics are indicated for prophylactic purposes in schizoprenic patients at risk for relapse.

Most patients should be treated with medication for 3 months to 1 year after a psychotic episode to be certain that they have recovered from their present illness. Over longer periods the use of long-term maintenance drugs should be individualized. Such factors as the nature and length of their illness, prior response to drugs, prior relapses and social situation must be taken into consideration. Any of the neuroleptics may be used for maintenance treatment, but in all cases the minimum effective dose should be used.

BIBLIOGRAPHY

Adelson, D., and Epstein, L.A. A study of phenothiazines in male and female chronically-ill schizophrenics. *J. Nerv. Ment. Dis.* 134:543-554, 1962.

Andrews, P., Hall, J.N., and Snaith, R.P. A controlled trial of phenothiazine withdrawal in chronic schizophrenic patients. *Br. J. Psychiatry* 128:451-455, 1976.

Astrup, C., Fossum, A., and Hoomboe, R. *Prognosis in Functional Psychoses.* Springfield, Ill., Charles C Thomas, 1962.

Astrup, C., and Noreik, K. *Functional Psychoses: Diagnosis and Prognostic Models.* Springfield, Ill., Charles C Thomas, 1966.

Baro, F., Brugmans, T., Dom, R., and Lommel, R. Maintenance therapy of chronic psychotic patients with a weekly oral dose of R 16341. *J. Clin. Pharmcol.* 10:330-341, 1970.

Bjorndal, N., Bjerre, M., Gerlach, J., Kristjansen, P., Magelund, G., Oestrich, I.H., and Waehrens, J. High dosage haloperidol therapy in chronic schizophrenic patients: a double-blind study of clinical response, side effects, serum haloperidol, and serum prolactin. *Psychopharm.* 67:17-23, 1980.

Blackburn, H., and Allen, J. Behavioral effects of interrupting and resuming tranquilizing medication among schizophrenics. *J. Nerv. Ment. Dis.* 133:303-307, 1961.

Caffey, E.M., Diamond, L.S., Frank, T.V. et al. Discontinuation or reduction of chemotherapy in chronic schizophrenics. *J. Chronic Dis.* 17:347-358, 1964.

Carscallen, H.B., Rochman, H., and Lovegrove, T.D. High dosage trifluoperazine in schizophrenia. *Canad. Psychiat. Assoc. J.* 13:459-461, 1968.

Cheung, H.K. Schizophrenics fully remitted on neuroleptics for 3-5 years. *Br. J. Psychiatry* 138:490-494, 1981.

Chien, C.P., and Cole, J.O. Drugs and rehabilitation in schizophrenia. In: Greenblatt, M. (ed.), *Drugs in Combination with Other Therapies*, pp. 13-14. Grune & Stratton, Inc., New York, 1975.

Clark, M.L., Huber, W., Hill, D., Wood, F., and Costiloe, J.P. Pimozide in chronic outpatients. *Dis. Nerv. Sys.* 36:137-141, 1975.

Clark, M.L., Huber, W., Serafetinides, E.A., and Colmore, J.P. Pimozide (Oral): A tolerance study. *Clinical Trial Journal Supplement* 2:25-32, 1971.

Clark, M.L., Ramsey, H.R., Ragland, R.E., Rahhal, D., Serafetinides, E., and Costiloe, P. Chlorpromazine in chronic schizophrenia. Behavioral dose-response relationships. *Psychopharm.* 18:260-270, 1970.

Clark, M.L., Ramsey, H.R., Rahhal, D.L., Serafetinides, E., Wood, S., and Costiloe, P. Chlorpromazine in chronic schizophrenia. The effect of age and hospitalization on behavioral dose-response relationships. *Arch. Gen. Psychiatry* 27:479-483, 1972.

Davis, J.M. Maintenance therapy in Psychiatry: I. Schizophrenia. *Am. J. Psychiatry* 132:1237-1245, 1975.

Davis, J.M. Comparative doses and costs of antipsychotic medication. *Arch. Gen. Psychiatry* 33:858-861, 1976.

Davis, J.M., Dysken, M.W., Haberman, S.J., Javaid, J.I., Chang, S.S., and Killian, G.A. Use of survival curves in analysis of antipsychotic relapse studies. In: F. Cattabeni et al., eds., *Long-Term Effects of Neuroleptics* (Adv. Biochem. Psychopharmacol., Vol. 24). Raven Press, New York, 1980a.

Davis, J.M. Antipsychotic Drugs. In: H.I. Kaplan, A.M. Freedman, and B.J. Sadeck, eds., *Comprehensive Textbook of Psychiatry/III* Vol. 3, pp. 2257-2289. Williams and Williams Co., Baltimore, Md., 1980b.

DeBuck, R.P. Relative safety and efficacy of high and low dose administration of fluphenazine HCl to psychotic patients. *Proc. of the 8th International Congress of the C.I.N.P.,* pp. 265-271. North Holland Publishing Co., 1972.

Dencker, S.J., Johansson, R., Lundin, L., and Malm, V. High doses of fluphenazine enanthate in schizophrenia. A controlled study. *Acta Psychiatr. Scand.* 57:405-414, 1978.

Diamond, L.S., and Marks, J.B. Discontinuance of tranquilizers among chronic schizophrenic patients receiving maintenance dosages. *J. Nerv. Ment. Dis.* 131:247-251, 1960.

Donlon, P., Meadow, A., Tupin, J., and Wahby, M. High vs. standard dosage fluphenazine HCl in acute schizophrenia. *J. Clin. Psych.* 39:800, 1978.

Engelhardt, D.M. Rosen, B., Freedman, D., and Margolis, R. Phenothiazines in the prevention of psychiatric hospitalization. *Arch. Gen. Psychiatry* 16:98-99, 1967.

Freeman, L.S., and Alson, E. Prolonged withdrawal of chlorpromazine in chronic patients. *Dis. Nerv. Sys.* 23:321-325, 1966.

Gardose, G., Orzack, H., Finn, G., and Cole, J.O. High and low dose thiothixene treatment in chronic schizophrenia. *Dis. Nerv. Sys.* 35:53-58, 1974.

Garfield, S., Gershon, S., Sletten, L. Newbauer, H., and Fenel, E. Withdrawal of ataractic medication in schizophrenic patients. *Dis. Nerv. Sys.* 27:321-325, 1966.

Goldberg, S.C., Frosch, W.A., Prossman, A.K., Schooler, N.R., and Johnson, G.F.S. Prediction of response to phenothiazines in schizophrenia: A cross-validation study. *Arch. Gen. Psychiatry* 26:367, 1972.

Goldberg, S.C., Mattson, N., Cole, I.O., and Klerman, G.L. Prediction of improvement in schizophrenia under four phenothiazines. *Arch. Gen. Psychiatry* 16:107, 1967.

Gross, H.S. A double-blind study comparison of once-a-day pimozide, trifluoperazine, and placebo in the maintenance care of chronic schizophrenics. *Current Therapeutic Research* 16:696–705, 1975.

Gross, M., and Reeves, W.P. Relapse after withdrawal of ataractic drugs in mental patients in transition. In: M. Greenblatt, ed., *Mental Patients in Transition*, pp. 313–321. Charles C Thomas, Springfield, Ill., 1961.

Hershon, H.I., Kennedy, P.F., and McGuire, R.J. Persistence of extrapyramidal disorders and psychiatric relapse after withdrawal of long-term phenothiazine therapy. *Br. J. Psychiatry* 120:41–50, 1972.

Hirsch, S.R., Gaind, R., Rhode, P.D. et al. Outpatient maintenance of chronic schizophrenic patients with long-acting fluphenazine double-blind placebo trial. *Br. Med. J.* 633–637, 1973.

Hogarty, G.E., and Goldberg, S.C. Drugs and sociotherapy in the aftercare of schizophrenic patients. One-year relapse rates. *Arch. Gen. Psychiatry* 28: 54–62, 1973.

Hogarty, G.E., Schooler, N.R., Ulrich, R., Mussare, F., Ferro, P., and Herron, E. Fluphenazine and social therapy in the aftercare of schizophrenic patients. *Arch. Gen. Psych.* 36:1283, 1979.

Hogarty, G.E., and Ulrich, R.F. Temporal effects of drug and placebo in delaying relapse in schizophrenic outpatients. *Arch. Gen. Psychiatry* 34:297–301, 1977.

Hogarty, G., Ulrich, R., Mussare, F., and Aristigueta, N. Drug discontinuation among long-term successfully maintained schizophrenic outpatients. *Dis. Nerv. Syst.* 37:494, 1976.

Itil, T., Keskiner, A., Heinemann, L., et al. Treatment of resistant schizophrenics with extreme high dosage fluphenazine hydrochloride. *Psychosomatics* 11:456–463, 1970.

Itil, T., Saletu, B., Hsu, W., et al. Clinical and quantitative EEG changes at different dosage levels of fluphenazine treatment. *Acta. Psychiatr. Scand.* 47: 440–451, 1971.

Kane, J., Quitkin, F., Rifkin, A., and Klein, D.F. Comparison of the incidence and severity of extrapyramidal side effects with fluphenazine enanthate and fluphenazine decanoate. *Am. J. Psychiatry* 135:539, 1978.

Kinross-Wright, J., and Charalampous, K.D. A controlled study of a very long acting phenothiazine preparation. *Int. J. Neuropsychiatry* 1:66–70, 1965.

Langfeld, G. The prognosis in schizophrenia. *Acta Psychiat. Neurol. Scand.* (Suppl). 110:7–66, 1956.

Leff, J.P., and Wing, J.K. Trial of maintenance therapy in schizophrenics. *Br. Med. J.* 2:599–604, 1971.

Lehmann, E., Quadbeck, H., Tegeler, J. Fararuni, M., and Heinrich, K. Wirkungsdifferenzen bei Hoch-und Standarddosierung von Fluphenazine-Decanoat in Abhangigkeit von Patienten-Merkmalen. *Pharmakopsychiat.* 13:117–129, 1980.

Levine, J., Schooler, N., and Cassano, G. The role of depot neuroleptics in the treatment of schizophrenic patients. *Psychological Med.* 9:383–386, 1978.

Levine, J., Schooler, N., Serene, F., Escobar, J., Gelenbereg, A., Mandel, H., Somer, R., and Steinbook, R. Discontinuation of oral and depot fluphenazine in schizophrenic patients after one year of continuous medication. In E. Cattabenei, ed., *Long-term Effects of Neuroleptics*, pp. 483–484. Raven Press, New York, 1980.

MacCreadie, R.G., and MacDonald, I.M. High dosage haloperidol in chronic schizophrenia. *Br. J. Psychiatry* 131:310–316, 1977.

McClelland, H.A., Farquharson, R.G., Layburn, P., et al. Very high dose fluphenazine decanoate: A controlled trial in chronic schizophrenia. *Arch. Gen. Psychiatry* 33:1435–1439, 1976.

Melynk, W.T., Worthington, A.G., and Laverty, S.G. Abrupt withdrawal of chlorpromazine and thioridazine from schizophrenic inpatients. *Can. Psych. Ass. J.* 11:410–413, 1966.

Morton, M.R. A study of withdrawal of chlorpromazine or trifluoperazine in chronic schizophrenia. *Am. J. Psychiatry* 124:1585–1588, 1968.

Paredes, A., Baumgold, J., Pugh, L.A. et al. Clinical judgement in the assessment of psychopharmacological effects. *J. Nerv. Ment. Dis.* 142:153–160, 1966.

Prien, R.F., and Cole, J.O.: High dose chlorpromazine therapy in chronic schizophrenia. Report of National Institute of Mental Health Psychopharmacology Research Branch Collaborative Study Group. *Arch. Gen. Psychiatry* 18:482–495, 1968.

Prien, R.F., Cole, J.O., and Belkin, N.F. Relapse in chronic schizophrenics following abrupt withdrawal of tranquilizing drugs. *Br. J. Psychiatry* 115:679–686, 1969a.

Prien, R.F., Levine, J., and Cole, J.O. High dose trifluoperazine therapy in chronic schizophrenia. *Am. J. Psychiatry* 126:305–313, 1969b.

Prien, R.F., Levine, J., and Switalski, R.W. Discontinuation of chemotherapy for chronic schizophrenics. *Hospt. Community Psychiatry* 22:4–7, 1971.

Quitkin, F., Rifkin, A., Kane, J. Ramos-Loren, Jr., and Klein, D.F. Long-acting oral versus injectable antipsychotic drugs in schizophrenics. *Arch. Gen. Psychiatry* 35:889, 1978.

Rassidakis, N.C., Kondakis, X., Papanastassiou, A., and Michalakess, A. Withdrawal of antipsychotic drugs from chronic patients. *Bulletin of the Menninger Clinic* 34:216–222, 1970.

Rifkin, A., Quitkin, F., and Klein, D.F. Fluphenazine decanoate, oral fluphenazine and placebo in treatment of remitted schizophrenics. *Arch. Gen. Psychiat.* 34:1215–1219, 1977a.

Rifkin, A., Quitkin, F., Rabinet, C., and Klein, D.F. Fluphenazine decanoate, oral fluphenazine and placebo in the treatment of remitted schizophrenics: I. Relapse rates after one year. *Arch. Gen. Psychiatry* 34:43–47, 1977b.

Rimon, P., Averbuch, P., Rozick, et al. Serum and CSF levels of haloperidol by radioimmunoassay and radioreceptor assay during high-dose therapy of resistant schizophrenic patients. *Psychopharmacology* 73:197–199, 1981.

Roose, K. Monthly haloperidol decanoate as a replacement for maintenance therapy. *Proc. III World Congress of Biological Psychiatry*, F4 10, 1981.

Schawver, J., Gorham, D.R., Leskin, L.W., Good, W., and Kabnick, D. Comparison of chlorpromazine and reserpine in maintenance drug therapy. *Dis. Nerv. Sys.* 20:452–457, 1959.

Schiele, B.C., Vestre, N.D., and Stein, K.E. A comparison of thioridazine, tri-fluoperazine, chlorpromazine and placebo: A double-blind controlled study on the treatment of chronic, hospitalized, schizophrenic patients. *Journal of Clinical and Experimental Psychopathology* 22:151–162, 1961.

Schooler, N.R., and Levine, J. Fluphenazine and fluphenazine HCl in the treatment of schizophrenic patients. In: *Proc. of the Mtg. of the C.I.N.P.*, Vol. 11, p. 418. Pargamon Press, Oxford, 1978.

Simon, P., Fermanian, J., Ginestet, D., Goujet, M.A., and Peron-Magnan, P. Standard and long-acting depot neuroleptics in chronic schizophrenics: An 18-month open multicentric study. *Arch. Gen. Psychiatry* 35:893, 1978.

Simpson, G.M., Amin, M., Kurz-Bartholini, E., Watts, T., and Laska, E. Problems in the evaluation of the optimal dose of a phenothiazine (butaperazine). *Dis. Nerv. Sys.* 29:478–484, 1968.

Stephens, J.H. Long-term course and prognosis of schizophrenia. *Semin. Psychiatry* 2:464–485, 1970.

Stephens, J.H., and Astrup, C. Prognosis in "process" and "non-process" schizophrenia. *Am. J. Psychiatry* 119:945–953, 1963.

Troshinsky, C.H., Aaronson, H.G., and Stone, R.K. Maintenance phenothiazine in the aftercare of schizophrenic patients. *Pennsylvania Psychiatric Quarterly* 2:11–15, 1962.

Vailant, G.E. Prospective prediction of schizophrenic remission. *Arch. Gen. Psychiatry* 11:509–518, 1964.

Vailant, G.E. The prediction of recovery in schizophrenia. *J. Nerv. Ment. Dis.* 133:534–543, 1962.

Van Praag, H., and Dols, L.C.W. Fluphenazine enanthate and fluphenazine decanoate: A comparison of their duration of action and motor side effects. *Am. J. Psychiatry* 130:801, 1973.

Whitaker, C.B., and Hoy, R.M. Withdrawal of perphenazine in chronic schizophrenia. *Br. J. Psychiatry* 109:422–427, 1963.

Wistedt, B. Withdrawal of long acting neuroleptics in schizophrenic outpatients. *Acta Univ. Upsalinses*: 391–397, 1981.

11

Clinical Applications of Drug Studies

Mary V. Seeman

The efficacy, safety, and optimal use of neuroleptic dopamine blockers in schizophrenia have been studied for thirty years, but many old questions remain unanswered and many new ones continue to arise. Schizophrenia remains a poorly-understood group of disorders with considerable individual variations. Superimposed on these variations are the many complex factors which govern drug response. To complicate matters further, it has recently been hypothesized that long-term drugs may induce brain changes which lead to manifestations perhaps indistinguishable from the symptoms of the original illness.

While researchers sometimes complain that results of their studies are not incorporated into clinical practice more readily and more thoroughly, clinicians maintain that research reports are not relevant to their practice. The captive, drug-compliant long-stay psychiatric inpatient who served as model subject for many of the original neuroleptic efficacy studies is no longer representative of the schizophrenic patient whom clinicians treat. Today's patient is not in hospital and comes to the clinic only when he wishes to or when he is driven there by exasperated families, by poverty and hunger, by behavior perceived as dangerous, or by a militant advocate, insistent that his client have a right to the treatment of his choice in the non-restrictive environment of his choice.

Today's schizophrenic patient lives alone and unsupervised. He is probably unemployed because his relative lack of skills and experience and his considerable interpersonal problems make work unlikely, whether or not residual symptoms of psychosis remain. Mothers, sisters, and female relatives who might have in former times allowed him refuge in their kitchens have deserted the kitchen and now are home to him rarely, probably too exhausted to tolerate his demands and his eccentricity.

The patient is unlikely to be regular in the taking of his prescribed medication or in the taking of his meals. He may spend most of his food allowance on cigarettes, coffee, and beer. He may be popping anticholinergic pills for "kicks" (MacVicar 1977), or under the mistaken impression that they are meant to control his symptoms. He may be exacerbating his symptoms with street drugs (Tsuang et al., 1982) in a vain attempt to feel "normal." If he is on depot neuroleptics, he may have developed severe extrapyramidal symptoms and dyskinetic signs, but no one may have noticed because the changes have been gradual and the doctor may not remember what the patient was like before. Doctors have probably changed periodically and each new one has been afraid to alter the neuroleptic dose or the regimen (Burgoyne, 1976) not knowing what to expect of an unknown, unpredictable, psychosis-prone person.

The relatives and friends of today's patient are suspicious of doctors and of psychiatry. They are no longer quite so naive about psychiatric syndromes as families used to be (Lamb and Oliphant, 1978) and no longer accept blame and responsibility for the patient's illness or for his failure to improve. They expect more from doctors and make demands the doctors cannot meet. They ask embarrassing questions about how the drugs work, and why their relative is receiving a particular drug and not another and why he is having certain side-effects and why he is not being seen more often and why he is getting drugs to chase away his delusions when his delusions are his only pleasure, his only safeguard against despair.

To make it all more confusing for the clinician, today's patient is no longer "schizophrenic." He does not fit the DSM-III or the Catego or the Feighner's or any criteria of schizophrenia. He perhaps has too many emotional upheavals, or drinks too much, or has not been psychotic long enough, or has the wrong kind of symptoms and too few schizophrenic relatives to be classified as schizophrenic. What is he then, and how is he to be treated?

WHAT WE KNOW ABOUT DRUGS AND LENGTHS OF HOSPITAL STAY

We know from the experience of thirty years that neuroleptic drugs alleviate certain symptoms, namely hallucinations, delusions, agitation, and fragmented thinking (Davis et al., 1980). We know that hospital stays for acute schizophrenic psychosis are thereby shortened (Davis et al., 1980).

We do not know how much of the shortening effect is indirect, secondary to the calmer ward atmosphere, improved staff morale, and hence more therapeutic milieu. Given the present attitudinal climate where some believe that psychotic symptoms should not be "unnaturally" interfered with and where patients have a right to refuse treatment, we need to know more about acute treatment without drugs (Carpenter et al., 1977; Mosher and Menn, 1978). How many untreated, acutely-psychotic individuals can be cared for at the same time before the hospital milieu becomes counter-therapeutic? What is the minimum staff/patient ratio required when hospitals become havens for the unfolding and resolution of psychotic illnesses without pharmacologic help? What are the environmental requirements, the personality characteristics, and the therapeutic skills required of the staff? How does the right to refuse treatment affect other patients' length of stay in hospital? If some individuals refuse treatment, what happens to the doses given to other patients on the same ward? Do their doses rise proportionately and, if so, how can this be prevented? Why is it that some inpatient wards use relatively small neuroleptic doses, others relatively high ones? Are the differences related to patient characteristics? Do they influence lengths of stay? In what direction?

WHAT WE KNOW ABOUT THE ADVANTAGES
OF SHORT HOSPITALIZATION

We know that short hospital stays cost less money than long ones.

Are there advantages, other than economic, to shortening a psychotic episode by the intervention of drugs? Are people whose hospitalizations have been short better off one, two, ten years later than those who have had longer admissions (Caffey et al., 1971; Glick et al., 1974; Davis et al., 1980)? What does vigorous treatment of the initial episode accomplish? It probably alleviates suffering and boosts patient, family, and staff morale. But does it give all concerned a realistic perspective on the future course of illness; does it facilitate treatment compliance and long-term planning? Does it prevent suicide and aggressive acts? Does it permit quick return to school, employment, and interpersonal relationships thus ensuring better future outlook in these areas? How does it affect public attitudes toward psychiatry and the psychiatric patient? The answers to these important questions are not yet in.

WHAT WE KNOW ABOUT DRUGS AND SCHIZOPHRENIC RELAPSE

We know that neuroleptics prevent relapse (Davis, 1975; Hogarty and Ulrich, 1977; Davis et al., 1980).

We do not know which individuals require neuroleptics to stay relatively relapse-free, and which will do equally well, perhaps better without drugs (Hogarty et al., 1976; Goldberg et al., 1977; Rappaport et al., 1978; Marder et al., 1979). We do not know which individuals are refractory to the relapse-prevention effect of drugs and therefore do not benefit from maintenance (Davis et al., 1980). We do not know how other factors interact with neuroleptics to reduce or enhance their protectiveness. Dietary factors (Gelenberg, 1980) or hormone levels probably play a role. Estrogens, for instance, are thought to modulate the dopamine receptor and to potentiate neurolepsis in laboratory animals (Labrie et al., 1979; Gordon et al., 1980; DiPaolo et al., 1981).

WHAT WE KNOW ABOUT DRUGS AND GENDER

If estrogens were antidopaminergic in man, one would expect males to be more susceptible than females to the acute dopamine/acetylcholine imbalance induced by neuroleptics—adult females presumably having had the opportunity to adjust gradually to the relative dopamine blockade of cyclic estrogens. Ayd's 1961 study of neurological side-effects of neuroleptics found that men are twice as susceptible as women to the acute dystonias. On the other hand, Ayd found that the akathisia, akinesia, and parkinsonism that occur in the first three months of treatment are more frequent in women. This could be due to higher cumulative dopamine blockade (neuroleptics plus estrogens) or, perhaps, to women's greater compliance in the actual ingestion of prescribed drugs. The probably higher risk of tardive dyskinesia in older women (Smith and Dunn, 1979; Smith et al., 1978) might be due to cumulative effects over years of treatment or, more likely, to estrogen withdrawal at menopause (Bedard et al., 1977).

If estrogens were antidopaminergic in man, one would also expect differential dose requirements in the two sexes. Some studies report higher dose requirements in males (Marriot and Hiip, 1978) as might be expected, but others report higher requirements in women (Goldstein et al., 1978). Our study comparing maintenance dose requirements in chronic schizophrenic men and women from 1978 to 1981 (43 women, 58 men diagnosed by RDC criteria), revealed no difference in the group as a whole. However, when age was taken into account, some interesting differences emerged (Fig. 1).

Younger women (age 20–39) were maintained on lower doses than men. After age 40, women, as a rule, required higher doses than men. This seems to confirm an estrogen effect. In the twenties, schizophrenic men tend to be more aggressive and require higher doses; this gradually diminishes over time. Women require low doses in the twenties and thirties when their estrogen level is high but dose requirements seem to rise in the forties as estrogen levels fall. High doses of neuroleptics, of course, effectively cut off estrogen secretion in premenopausal women via hormonal feedback mechanisms (Beumont et al., 1974) so that it may be important to keep neuroleptic doses in women under the amenorrhea threshold—thus allowing the presumed anti-psychotic effect of estrogens to operate and preventing neuroleptic dose escalation.

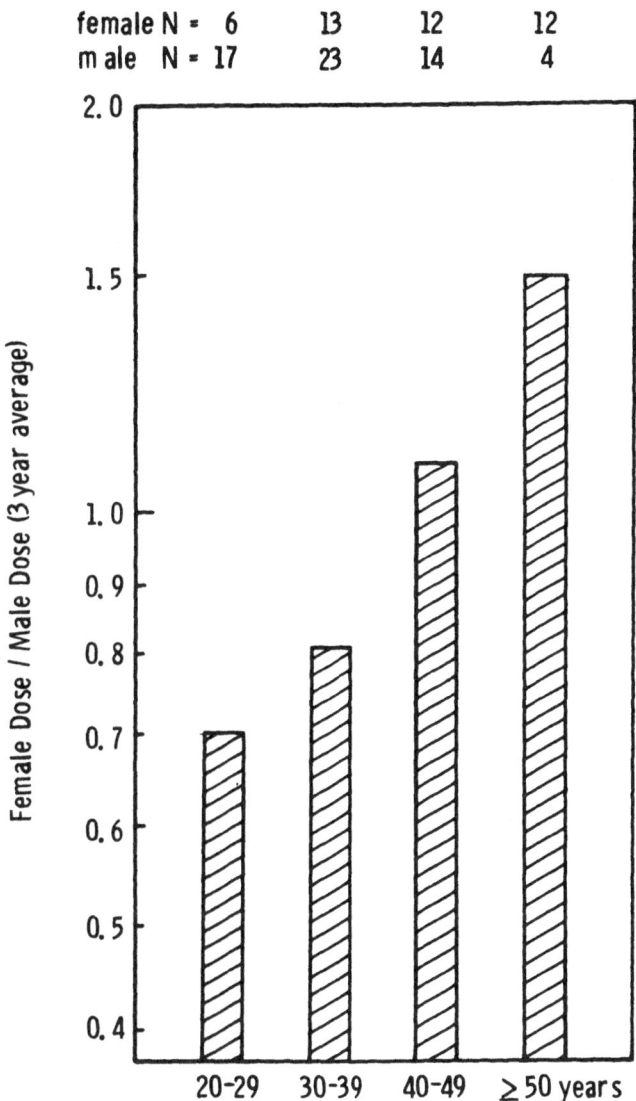

Figure 1. Men require larger neuroleptic doses in youth. Women require larger doses in middle age.

WHAT WE KNOW ABOUT DRUGS AND CHRONICITY

We know that neuroleptics do not alleviate the negative symptoms of schizophrenia (withdrawal, apathy, amotivation) (Pi and Simpson, 1981, Andreasen et al., 1982).

The hope was that energetic treatment of the acute phase would prevent the residual, negative symptoms of schizophrenia, the very symptoms associated with chronicity. Unfortunately this hope has not been met. There is no evidence that neuroleptic treatment affects the development of chronicity.

WHAT WE KNOW ABOUT DRUGS AND DEPRESSION

We known that some patients respond with dysphoria to neuroleptics (Singh and Kay, 1979; Van Putten et al., 1981).

We do not know for certain whether neuroleptics precipitate depression or increase the risk of suicide. Clinical impression is that they may but the bulk of the evidence is negative (Hartmann et al., 1980; Johnson, 1981; Seeman and McGee, 1982; Mandel et al., 1982; Strian et al., 1982).

WHAT WE KNOW ABOUT TOLERANCE

Studies following patients through consecutive admissions for schizophrenic relapse document increasing dose requirements of neuroleptics (Wistedt, 1981). In our three year survey of dose requirements, we found that patients with hospital admissions during the survey period ended up with raised maintenance doses after three years, while those not hospitalized ended the three years with lowered maintenance doses (Fig. 2).

Are these tolerance effects, evidence of supersensitivity psychosis (Chouinard et al., 1978; Davis and Rosenberg, 1979; Chouinard and Jones, 1980) or simply a matter of clinicians prescribing higher doses as they become more familiar with the patient and more anxious, perhaps, to discharge the relapsing patient as quickly as possible? The factors responsible for this phenomenon need to be elucidated. Does the practice lead to ever higher maintenance doses? That it does not need to was shown in our survey where doses, after discharge, could almost always be gradually returned to pre-relapse levels.

WHAT WE KNOW ABOUT COMPLIANCE

We know that the compliance rate of adhering to a neuroleptic maintenance regime is between thirty and fifty percent (Blackwell, 1979; Seltzer and Hoffman, 1980).

We do not know all the factors that contribute to low compliance (Van Putten, 1974; Van Putten et al., 1976). One that has not been sufficiently studied is the unpleasant cognitive and emotional effect of neuroleptics, the marked blunting of spontaneity, creativity and affective intensity which may, at times be part of the illness but which may also be neuroleptic-induced.

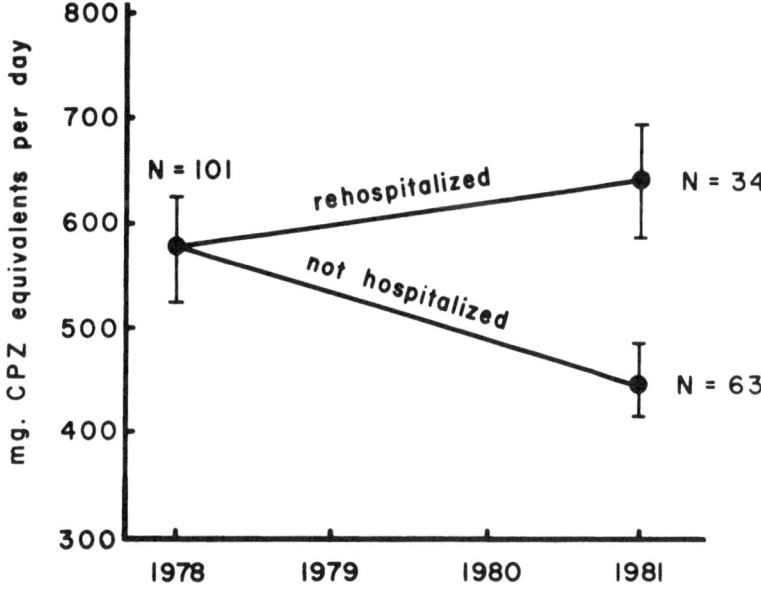

Figure 2. Patients who remain out of hospital over a three-year period can be maintained on a reduced neuroleptic dose.

WHAT WE KNOW ABOUT TARDIVE DYSKINESIA

We know the many factors associated with tardive dyskinesia, we know that the syndrome can be reversible or irreversible, we know that the irreversible dyskinesia is more closely correlated with age than with any other factor, and we know that tardive dyskinesia can be mild and unnoticeable or, more rarely, bothersome, even incapacitating (Alexopoulos, 1979; Berger and Rexroth, 1980; Task Force, 1980; Ezrin-Waters et al., 1981; Seeman, 1981; Rosen et al., 1982).

As clinicians, what we do not know is how to change our clinical practice to accommodate these facts and to plan ahead most effectively for our patients. Do we institute drugs holidays? (Ayd, 1967; Jeste et al., 1979; Carpenter et al., 1980). If we keep neuroleptic doses low in order to prevent tardive dyskinesia, are we achieving optimum function for our patients? Should we attempt to wean our patients off neuroleptics once they reach a certain age and what should that age be? Do we avoid specific neuroleptics for long-term maintenance in favor of others less likely to produce tardive dyskinesia? (Gardos et al., 1977; Csernansky et al., 1981). When does the risk of tardive dyskinesia become equal to the risk of relapse? Do we stay away from anticholinergic drugs for fear of aggravating tardive dyskinesia or does this bring needless suffering to our patients? (Van Putten and May, 1978; Chouinard et al., 1979; Perris et al., 1979; Manos et al., 1981).

WHAT WE KNOW ABOUT DRUG HOLIDAYS

We know that periodic drug holidays of short duration are possible for some schizophrenic patients without risk of relapse but that they are hazardous for others (Marder et al., 1979; Dencker et al., 1980; Sharer and Petit, 1981; Shenoy et al., 1981; Pyke and Seeman, 1981).

As mentioned above, we do not yet know whether drug holidays predispose toward or protect against tardive dyskinesia. We cannot predict who will adhere to the drug holiday regimen and who will take the opportunity to stop treatment altogether and relapse as a consequence. We do not know the duration of drug holiday that is safe for the average person or which factors enter into the decision, although there is some evidence that the safe period off drugs is individual and remains approximately the same for the same person over time (Wistedt, 1981).

WHAT WE KNOW ABOUT LOW MAINTENANCE DOSES

As with drug holidays, we know that some patients can manage with maintenance doses considerably lower than average without sacrificing well-being or increasing the risk of relapse. In fact, functioning may improve when doses are lowered (Gardos and Cole, 1973; Van Putten et al., 1974; Quitkin et al., 1975; Simpson et al., 1976; Marder et al., 1979; Davis et al., 1980).

We do not know enough about timing, frequency of monitoring, patient risk factors, or illness factors. We do not know enough about the specifics of prodromal signs (Docherty et al., 1978; Herz and Melville, 1980) as indicators for the need to increase dose. In our ongoing drug reduction study, we are attempting to elucidate some of these variables. Twenty-five chronic schizophrenic patients on depot neuroleptic maintenance have been selected clinically as "safe" candidates for gradual reduction of their dose. The dose is being decreased by one eighth every two months over a six month total period. Several patient and treatment variables seem to be operating in those able to survive the three reductions without relapse (Table 1) but these findings are still preliminary.

Table 1.   Neuroleptic Maintenance Reduction. Six Month Survival

Patient Factors
Female sex
Older age

Illness Factors
Affective symptoms
Fewer cumulative hospital days

Drug Factors
Higher initial maintenance dose
Longer total time on depot drugs
, Maintained on longer-acting depot drugs
Lesser use of street drugs

WHAT WE KNOW ABOUT DRUG EDUCATION FOR PATIENTS AND FAMILIES

Education about drugs helps patients to adhere to a treatment regimen (Blackwell, 1979; Hansell, 1979; Seltzer et al., 1980). Built into educational programs need to be facts about and probably experiential learning about immediate effects, long-term effects of both neuroleptics and anticholinergics, withdrawal effects (Gardos et al., 1978; Luchins et al., 1980; Lacoursiere, 1980), illness effects (Herz and Melville, 1980), psychological effects (Van Putten et al., 1974), unwanted effects and how to counteract them (Donlon and Stenson, 1976; Marsden and Jenner, 1980; Davis et al., 1980; Simpson et al., 1981).

The principle of titration of dose to stress may need to be taught. This would be easier done with fast-acting drugs of short life rather than with the longer-acting drugs presently available.

Since schizophrenia appears to interfere more with left- than with right-hemisphere learning (Newlin, 1981; Buchsbaum et al., 1982), educational programs would probably be more effective if they addressed the learning potential of the right hemisphere (concrete, intuitive, metaphoric, spatial, subjective, holistic information processing) (Edwards, 1979).

WHAT WE KNOW ABOUT NEUROLEPTIC NON-RESPONSE

We know that there are some schizophrenic patients who do not appear to respond to neuroleptic drugs. There are now some good indications as to who these people are. Some are non-absorbers whose response can be ameliorated by ensuring absorption. These people can now be detected by radioreceptor assay techniques that measure serum neuroleptic levels (Creese and Snyder, 1977; Van Putten et al., 1981; Lascelles, 1981). Some non-responders show evidence of brain atrophy—enlarged ventricles and widened sulci—on CT scans (Weinberger et al., 1980; Andreasen et al., 1982). These same people show negative symptoms of schizophrenia and a predictable pattern of cognitive defect on psychological testing (Andreasen et al., 1982). Hereditary and psychological factors, stress and diet factors may play a role in non-response as may drug interactions (Singh and Kay, 1979; Gelenberg, 1980; Galdi et al., 1981; Kessler and Waletzky, 1981).

We do not know how to treat non-responders although possibilities for treatment regimens have been suggested (Kessler and Waletzky, 1981; Dencker et al., 1981; Pi and Simpson, 1981).

CONCLUSION

Results of large scale controlled studies suggest treatment regimens which must then be tailored to the individual patient. The patient and, ideally, family members, should understand the rationale, benefits and risks of drug treatment and should be encouraged to assist knowledgeably in the treatment process.

REFERENCES

Alexopoulos, G.S. Lack of complaints in schizophrenics with tardive dyskinesia. *J. Nerv. Ment. Dis.* 167:125–127, 1979.
Andreasen, N.C., Olsen, S.A., Dennert, J.W., and Smith, M.R. Ventricular enlargement in schizophrenia: relationship to positive and negative symptoms. *Am. J. Psychiat.* 139:297–302, 1982.
Andreasen, N.C., Smith, M.R., Jacoby, C.G., Dennert, J.W., and Olsen, S.A. Ventricular enlargement in schizophrenia: definition and prevalence. *Am. J. Psychiat.* 139:292–296, 1982.
Ayd, F.J. Jr. Survey of drug-induced extrapyramidal reactions. *J.A.M.A.* 175: 1054–1060, 1961.
Ayd, F.J. Jr. Drug holidays. *Med. Sci.* 59–62, 1967.
Bedard, P., Langelier, P., and Villeneuve, A. Oestrogens and extra-pyramidal system. *Lancet* ii:1367–1368, 1977.
Berger, P.A., and Rexroth, K. Tardive dyskinesia: clinical, biological and pharmacological perspectives. *Schiz. Bull.* 6:102–116, 1980.
Beumont, P.J.V., Gelder, M.G., Friesen, H.G., Harris, G.W., MacKinnon, P.C.B., Mandelbrote, B.M., and Wiles, D.H. The effects of phenothiazines on endocrine function: I. *Br. J. Psychiatry* 124:413–419, 1974.
Blackwell, B. Treatment adherence: A contemporary overview. *Psychosomatics* 20:27–35, 1979.

Burgoyne, R.W. Effect of drug ritual changes on schizophrenic patients. *Am. J. Psychiat.* 133:284–289, 1976.

Buchsbaum, M.S., Ingvar, D.H., Kessler, R., Waters, R.N., Cappelletti, J., van Kammen, D.P., King, A.C., Johnson, J.L., Manning, R.G., Flynn, R.W., Mann, L.S., Bunney, W.E., and Sokoloff, L. Cerebral glucography with positron tomography. *Arch. Gen. Psychiatry* 39:251–259, 1982.

Caffey, E.M., Galbrecht, C.R., and Klett, C.J. Brief hospitalization and aftercare in the treatment of schizophrenia. *Arch. Gen. Psychiat.* 24:81–86, 1971.

Carpenter, T., McGlashan, T.H., and Strauss, J.S. The treatment of acute schizophrenia without drugs: an investigation of some current assumptions. *Am. J. Psychiat.* 134:14–20, 1977.

Carpenter, W.T., Rey, A.C., and Stephens, J.H. Covert dyskinesia in ambulatory schizophrenia. *Lancet* 8187:212–213, 1980.

Chouinard, G., and Jones, B.D. Neuroleptic-induced supersensitivity psychosis: Clinical and pharmacologic characteristics. *Am. J. Psychiat.* 137:16–21, 1980.

Chouinard, G., Jones, B.D., and Annable, L. Neuroleptic-induced supersensitivity psychosis. *Am. J. Psychiat.* 135:1409–1410, 1978.

Chouinard, G., de Montigny, C., and Annable, L. Tardive dyskinesia and antiparkinsonia medication. *Am. J. Psychiat.* 136:228–229, 1979.

Creese, I. and Snyder, S.H. A simple and sensitive radio receptor assay for antischizophrenic drugs in blood. *Nature (London)* 220:180–182, 1977.

Csernansky, J.G., Grabowski, K., Cervantes, J., Kaplan, J., and Yesavage, J.A. Fluphenazine decanoate and tardive dyskinesia: A possible association. *Am. J. Psychiat.* 138:1362–1365, 1981.

Davis, J.M. Overview: Maintenance therapy in psychiatry. I. Schizophrenia. *Am. J. Psychiat.* 132:1237–1245, 1975.

Davis, J.M., Schaffer, C.B., Killian, G.A., Kinard, C., and Chan, C. Important issues in the drug treatment of schizophrenia. *Schiz. Bull.* 6:70–87, 1980.

Davis, K.L., and Rosenberg, G.S. Is there a limbic system equivalent of tardive dyskinesia? *Biol. Psychiat.* 14:699–703, 1979.

Dencker, S.J., Enoksson, P., Johansson, R., Lundin, L., and Malm, U. Late (4–8 years) outcome of treatment with megadoses of fluphenazine enanthate in drug-refractory schizophrenics. *Acta Psychiat. Scand.* 6:1–12, 1981.

Di Paolo, T., Poyet, P., and Labrie, F. Effect of chronic estradiol and haloperidol treatment on striatal dopamine receptors. *European J. Pharmacology* 73:105–106, 1981.

Docherty, J.P., van Kammen, D.P., Siris, S.G., and Marder, S.R. Stages of schizophrenic psychosis. *Am. J. Psychiat.* 135:420–426, 1978.

Donlon, P.T., and Stenson, R.L. Neuroleptic induced extra-pyramidal symptoms. *Dis. Nerv. Syst.* 37:629–635, 1976.

Edwards, B. *Drawing on the Right Side of the Brain.* Los Angeles: J.P. Tarcher Inc., 1979.

Ezrin-Waters, C., Seeman, M.V., and Seeman, P. Tardive dyskinesia in schizophrenic outpatients: Prevalence and significant variables. *J. Clin. Psychiat.* 42:16–22, 1981.

Galdi, J., Rieder, R.O., Silber, D., and Bonato, R.P. Genetic factors in the response to neuroleptics in schizophrenia: a psychopharmacogenetic study. *Psychol. Med.* 11:713–728, 1981.

Gardos, G., and Cole, J.O. The importance of dosage in antipsychotic drug administration: A review of dose response studies. *Psychopharmacologia* 29: 221–230, 1973.

Gardos, G., Cole, J.O., and Labrie, R.A. Drug variables in the etiology of tardive dyskinesia: Application of discriminant function analysis. *Prog. Neuropsychopharmacol.* 1:147–154, 1977.

Gardos, G., Cole, J.O., and Tarsy, D. Withdrawal syndromes associated with antipsychotic drugs. *Am. J. Psychiat.* 135:1321–1324, 1978.

Gelenberg, A.J. Nutrition in psychiatry: we are what we eat? *J. Clin. Psychiat.* 41:328–329, 1980.

Glick, I., Hargreaves, W., and Goldfield, M. Short vs. long hospitalization. *Arch. Gen. Psychiat.* 30:363–369, 1974.

Goldberg, S.C., Schooler, N.R., Hogarty, G.E., and Roper, W. Prediction of relapse in schizophrenic patients treated by drug and sociotherapy. *Arch. Gen. Psychiat.* 34:171–184, 1977.

Goldstein, M.J., Rodnick, E.H., Evans, J.R., May, P.R.A., and Steinberg, M.R. Drug and family therapy in the aftercare of acute schizophrenics. *Arch. Gen. Psychiat.* 35:1169–1177, 1978.

Gordon, J.H., Borison, R.L., and Diamond, B.I. Modulation of dopamine receptor sensitivity by estrogen. *Biol. Psychiat.* 15:389–396, 1980.

Hansell, N. Approaching long-term neuroleptic treatment of schizophrenia. *J.A.M.A.* 242:1293–1294, 1979.

Hartmann, W., Kind, J., Meyer, J.E., Muller, P., and Steuber, H. Neuroleptic drugs and the prevention of relapse in schizophrenia: a workshop report. *Schiz. Bull.* 6:536–543, 1980.

Herz, M.I., and Melville, C. Relapse in schizophrenia. *Am. J. Psychiat.* 137:801–805, 1980.

Hogarty, A.E., and Ulrich, R.F. Temporal effects of drug and placebo in delaying relapse in schizophrenic outpatients. *Arch. Gen. Psych.* 34:297–301, 1977.

Hogarty, G.E., Ulrich, R.F., Mussare, F., and Aristigueta, N. Drug discontinuation among long term, successfully maintained schizophrenic outpatients. *Dis. Nerv. Syst.* 37:494–500, 1976.

Jeste, D.V., Potkin, S.G., Sinha, S., Fedden, S., and Wyatt, R.J. Tardive dyskinesia—reversible and persistent. *Arch. Gen. Psychiat.* 36:585–590, 1979.

Johnson, D.A.W. Studies of depressive symptoms in schizophrenia. *Br. J. Psychiat.* 139:89–101, 1981.

Kessler, K.A., and Waletzky, J.P. Clinical use of the antipsychotics. *Am. J. Psychiat.* 138:202–209, 1981.

Labrie, F., Ferland, L., Veilleux, R., Euvrard, C., and Boissier, J. Influence of estrogens on tuberoinfundibular and striatal dopaminergic systems in the rat. *Acta Psychiat. Belg.* 79:623–637, 1979.

Lacoursiere, R.E. Psychopharmacological precautions in the right to refuse medication. *Am. J. Psychiat.* 137:856–858, 1980.

Lamb, H.R., and Oliphant, E. Schizophrenia through the eyes of families. *Hosp. Comm. Psychiat.* 29:803–806, 1978.

Lascelles, P.T. Drug assays in neuropsychiatry. *Psychol. Med.* 11:661–667, 1981.

Lesser, I.M., and Friedmann, C.T.H. Attitudes toward medication change among chronically impaired psychiatric patients. *Am. J. Psychiat.* 138:801–803, 1981.

Luchins, D.J., Freed, W.J., and Wyatt, R.J. The role of cholinergic supersensitivity in the medical symptoms associated with withdrawal of antipsychotic drugs. *Am. J. Psychiat.* 137:1395–1398, 1980.

MacVicar, K. Abuse of antiparkinsonian drugs by psychiatric patients. *Am. J. Psychiat.* 134:809–811, 1977.

Mandel, M.R., Severe, J.B., Schooler, N.R., Gelenberg, A.J., and Mieske, M. Development and prediction of postpsychotic depression in neuroleptic-treated schizophrenics. *Arch. Gen. Psychiat.* 39:197–203, 1982.

Manos, N., Gkiouzepas, J., and Logothetis, J. The need for continuous use of antiparkinsonian medication with chronic schizophrenic patients receiving long-term neuroleptic therapy. *Am. J. Psychiat.* 138:184–188, 1981.

Marder, S.R., van Kammen, D.P., Docherty, J.P., Payner, J., and Bunney, W.E. Predicting drug-free improvement in schizophrenic psychosis. *Arch. Gen. Psychiat.* 36:1080–1085, 1979.

Marriot, P., and Hiip, A. Drug monitoring at an Australian depot phenothiazine clinic. *J. Clin. Psychiat.* 39:206–207, 1978.

Marsden, C.D., and Jenner, P. The pathophysiology of extrapyramidal side-effects of neuroleptic drugs. *Psychol. Med.* 10:55–72, 1980.

Mosher, L.R., and Menn, A.Z. Community residential treatment for schizophrenia: two year follow-up. *Hosp. Comm. Psychiat.* 29:715–723, 1978.

Newlin, D.B., Carpenter, B., and Golden, C.J. Hemispheric asymmetries in schizophrenia. *Biol. Psychiatry* 16:561–582, 1981.

Perris, C., Dimitrijevic, P., Jacobsson, L., Paulsson, P., Rapp, W., and Froberg, H. Tardive dyskinesia in psychiatric patients treated with neuroleptics. *Br. J. of Psychiat.* 135:509–514, 1979.

Pi, E.J., and Simpson, G.M. The treatment of refractory schizophrenia: pharmacotherapy and clinical implications of blood level measurements of neuroleptics. *Int. Pharmacopsychiat.* 16:154–161, 1981.

Pyke, J., and Seeman, M.V. Neuroleptic-free intervals in the treatment of schizophrenia. *Am. J. Psychiat.* 138:1620–1621, 1981.

Quitkin, F., Rifkin, A., and Klein, D.F. Very high dosage vs. standard dosage fluphenazine in schizophrenia. *Arch. Gen. Psych.* 32:1276–1281, 1975.

Rappoport, M., Hopkins, H.K., Hall, K., Belleza, T., and Silverman, J. Are there schizophrenics for whom drugs may be unnecessary of contraindicated? *Intern. Pharmacopsychiat.* 13:100–111, 1978.

Rosen, A.M., Mukherjee, S., Olarte, S., Varia, V., and Cardenas, C. Perception of tardive dyskinesia in outpatients receiving maintenance neuroleptics. *Am. J. Psychiat.* 139:372–373, 1982.

Rosenblatt, J.E., and Wyatt, R.J. Cerebral ventricular enlargement in chronic schizophrenia. An association with poor response to treatment. *Arch. Gen. Psychiat.* 37:11–13, 1980.

Seeman, M.V. Tardive dyskinesia: two year recovery. *Compr. Psychiatry* 22:187–192, 1981.

Seeman, M.V., and McGee, H. Treatment of depression in schizophrenic patients. *Am. J. Psychotherapy.* 36:14–22, 1982.

Seltzer, A., and Hoffman, B.F. Drug compliance of the psychiatric patient. *Can. Fam. Physician* 26:725–727, 1980.

Seltzer, A., Roncari, I., and Garfinkel, P. Effect of patient education on medication compliance. *Can. J. Psychiat.* 25:638–645, 1980.

Sharer, D.R., and Petit, E. Using drug holidays for chronic outpatients. *Hosp. and Comm. Psychiat.* 32:420–421, 1981.

Shenoy, R.S., Sadler, A.G., Goldberg, S.C., Hamer, R., and Ross, B. Effects of a six-week drug holiday on symptom states, relapse, and tardive dyskinesia in chronic schizophrenics. *J. Clin. Psychopharmacology* 1:141–145, 1981.

Simpson, G.M., Pi, E.H., and Sramek, J.J. Adverse effects of antipsychotic agents. *Drugs* 21:138–151, 1981.

Simpson, G.M., Varga, E., and Haber, E.J. Psychotic exacerbations produced by neuroleptics. *Dis. Nerv. Syst.* 37:367–369, 1976.

Singh, M.M., and Kay, S.R. Dysphoria response to neuroleptic treatment in schizophrenia: its relationship to antonomic arousal and prognosis. *Biol. Psychiat.* 14:277–294, 1979.

Singh. M.M., and Kay, S.R. Therapeutic antagonism between anticholinergic antiparkinsonism agents and neuroleptics in schizophrenia. *Neuropsychobiology* 5:74–86, 1979.

Smith, J.M., and Dunn, D.D. Sex differences in the prevalence of severe tardive dyskinesia. *Am. J. Psychiat.* 136:1080–1082, 1979.

Smith, J.M., Oswald, W.T., Kucharski, T., and Waterman, L.J. Tardive dyskinesia: age and sex differences in hospitalized schizophrenics. *Psychopharm.* 58: 207–211, 1978.

Strian, F., Heger, R., and Klicpera, C. The time structure of depressive mood in schizophrenic patients. *Acta Psychiat. Scand.* 65:66–73, 1982.

Task Force on Late Neurological Effects of Antipsychotic Drugs: Tardive dyskinesia. A summary of a task force report of the APA. *Am. J. Psychiat.* 37:1163–1172, 1980.

Tsuang, M.T., Simpson, J.C., and Kronfol, Z. Subtypes of drug abuse with psychosis. *Arch. Gen. Psychiat.* 39:141–147, 1982.

Van Putten, T. Why do schizophrenic patients refuse to take their drugs? *Arch. Gen. Psychiat.* 31:67–72, 1974.

Van Putten, T., Crumpton, E., and Yale, C. Drug refusal in schizophrenia and the wish to be crazy. *Arch. Gen. Psych.* 33:1443–1446, 1976.

Van Putten, T., and May, P.R.A. Akinetic depression in schizophrenia. *Arch. Gen. Psychiat.* 35:1101–1107, 1978.

Van Putten, T., May, P.R.A., and Jender, D.J. Does a plasma level of chlorpromazine help? *Psychol. Med.* 11:729–734, 1981.

Van Putten, T., May, P.R.A., Marder, S.R., and Wiltmann, L.A. Subjective response to antipsychotic drugs. *Arch. Gen. Psychiat.* 38:187–190, 1981.

Van Putten, T., Mutalipassi, L.R., and Malkin, M.P. Phenothiazine-induced decompensation. *Arch. Gen. Psych.* 30:102–105, 1974.

Weinberger, D.R., Bigelow, L.B., Kleinman, J.E., Klein, S.T., Rosenblatt, J.E., and Wyatt, R.J. Cerebral ventricular enlargement in chronic schizophrenia. An association with poor response to treatment. *Arch. Gen. Psychiat.* 37: 11–13, 1980.

Wistedt, B., A depot neuroleptic withdrawal study. *Acta. Psychiat. Scand.* 64: 65–84, 1981.

12

Tardive Dyskinesia: Management and New Treatment

DANIEL E. CASEY AND JES GERLACH

INTRODUCTION

Tardive dyskinesia (TD) is a neurological syndrome of involuntary, repetitive, purposeless movements in the orofacial, limb, and truncal musculature that occurs during or following prolonged neuroleptic drug treatment (Crane, 1973; Gerlach, 1979; Baldessarini et al., 1980; Casey and Gerlach, 1982). Though first identified in Europe (Schonecker, 1957; Sigwald et al., 1959), it was described in the English literature by Uhrbrand and Faurbye in 1960. This syndrome is of increasing clinical concern because many of the large number of patients receiving neuroleptic drugs may develop irreversible neurological symptoms. Since the neuroleptic medications are clearly efficacious for most psychotic patients, an inescapable dilemma develops: with continued drug treatment, TD may develop or worsen, but without medications the psychosis may exacerbate. This clinical challenge thus requires periodic review of the benefits and risks of extended neuroleptic treatment plans for each individual patient. The aims of this chapter are to present an algorithm for managing TD (Figure 1) based on our current understanding of this syndrome, and to review pharmacological treatment approaches.

CONSIDER TD

Clinical Description

It is important to recognize involuntary movement disorders early in treatment and consider TD with a differential diagnosis. TD is characterized by involuntary, repetitive, irregular, and purposeless hyperkinetic movements comprised

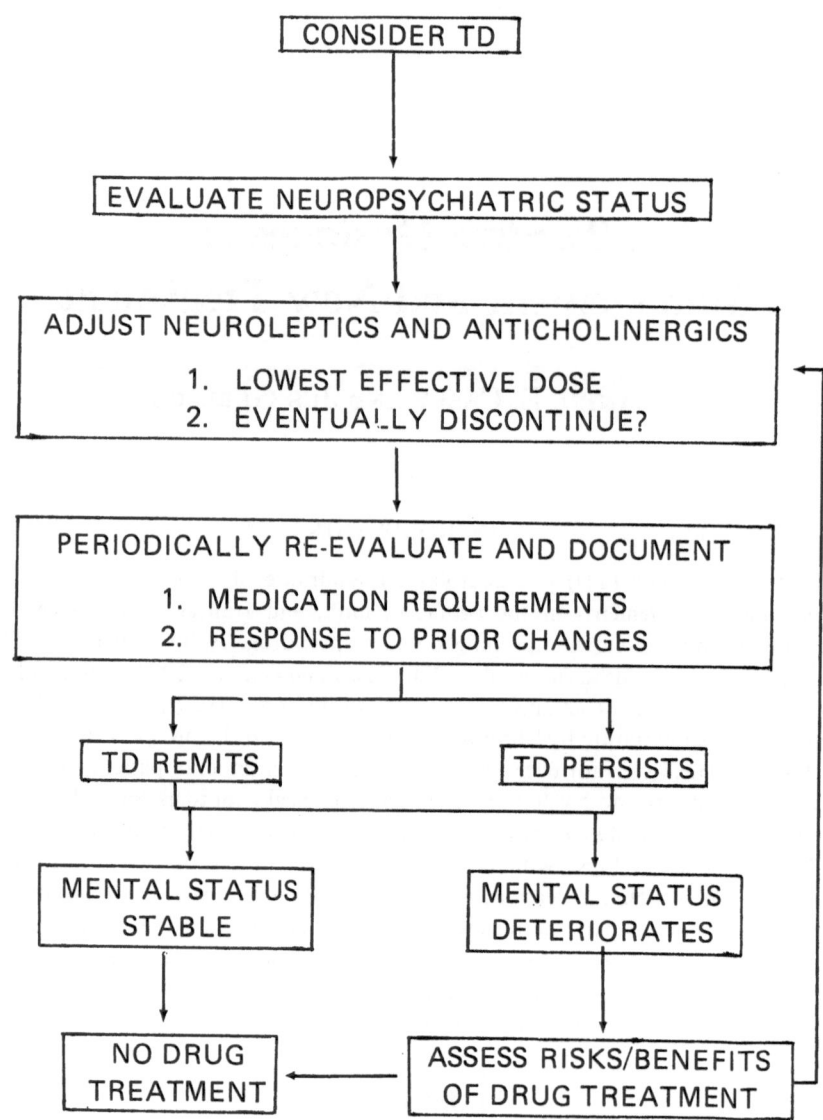

Figure 1. Algorithm for managing tardive dyskinesia.

of an admixture of choreic, athetotic, myoclonic, and dystonic features. Abnormal movements in the mouth, tongue, and facial regions are most commonly found. Usually the symptoms have an insidious onset and slowly progress to more obvious tongue protrusion, puckering, pursing and smacking of the lips, or various combinations of jaw movements that resemble chewing. Other facial muscles can be involved, causing rapid eye blinking, blepharospasm, and brow movements. Axial musculature can also be affected, producing symptoms of forward and backward pelvic thrusting or continuous rotatory hip motions. Both upper and lower extremities can have a combination of irregular choreic and athetotic movements. Occasionally, the hand and fingers move in a repetitive pattern resembling the playing of an invisible piano or guitar. Dystonic symptoms can also be part of the TD syndrome, especially in children and young adults (Polizos et al., 1973; McLean and Casey, 1978). Rarely, TD affects the respiratory pattern so that patients make grunting noises and have irregular rates of breathing (Casey and Rabins, 1978; Weiner et al., 1978).

Differential Diagnosis

Neuroleptic-induced Dyskinesias. TD must be distinguished from the other neuroleptic-induced extrapyramidal symptoms (EPS). Acute dystonia most often occurs in young adult males during the first few days of neuroleptic treatment. Akathisia, a subjective feeling of restlessness that may have motor manifestations of an inability to sit still and continuous motion of the trunk can be misdiagnosed as a psychotic exacerbation or TD (Van Putten, 1975). Neuroleptic-induced parkinsonism (tremor, rigidity, and bradykinesia) is usually easily distinguished from TD. Though the coexistence of TD and other acute neuroleptic-induced EPS is infrequently written about, these dyskinesias may occur in the same patient.

The rabbit syndrome is characterized by twitching in the lips and perioral area (Villeneuve, 1972). It is distinguished from TD by the rapid rhythmical frequency of tremor, localization in the mouth area, and improvement with anticholinergics (Sovner and DiMascio, 1977).

Initial hyperkinesia describes a seldom reported and incompletely understood syndrome that resembles TD. The symptoms are clinically similar, but may be more stereotyped than TD (Gerlach, 1979). Increased cholinergic influences aggravate the symptoms, which are reversed by anticholinergics, or resolve when neuroleptics are discontinued (Gerlach et al., 1974; Casey and Denney, 1977; Moore and Bowers, 1980). This probably occurs more commonly than is recognized, and emphasizes the point that more than one mechanism may be involved in the etiology of hyperkinetic movement disorders.

Other Drug-induced Hyperkinesias. Other drugs can produce hyperkinetic movement disorders that must be differentiated from TD. This distinction can be very difficult, however, if a patient has recently received or is currently taking multiple psychopharmacologically active drugs. Anticholinergic agents have occasionally produced orofacial and limb hyperkinesias after prolonged use (Birket-Smith, 1974) and chronic antihistamine use has also rarely been associated with orofacial hyperkinesias (Thach et al., 1975). Choreic movements, as well as stereotyped behavior called "punding" can occur in conjunction with sustained amphetamine abuse (Rylander, 1972). Tricyclic antidepressants have been implicated as drugs that can both affect pre-existing hyperkinesias and produce movement disorders by themselves. The most common dyskinesia associated with tricyclic antidepressants is a fine tremor, but a few reports have noted orofacial symptoms resembling TD started when tricyclic antidepressants were initiated and resolved when the medications were discontinued (Fann et al., 1976; Dekret et al., 1977). Phenytoin and other anticonvulsants can produce reversible orofacial dyskinesias that are similar to TD (Chadwick et al., 1976). Oral contraceptives are an uncommon cause of hyperkinetic choreic symptoms which also resolve when the medications are discontinued (Nausieda et al., 1979). Chloroquine antimalarial drugs can also produce hyperkinetic dyskinesias (Osifo, 1979).

Dyskinesias Related to Hereditary and Systemic Illnesses. The hereditary neurodegenerative diseases of Huntington's chorea and Wilson's disease (hepatolenticular degeneration) may initially present with signs that resemble TD, but the later presentations of these syndromes are usually distinguishable by clinical signs, laboratory tests, or the family history. Hyperthyroidism, hypoparathyroidism, chorea in pregnancy (chorea gravidarum), systemic lupus erythematosus, Henoch-Schonlein's purpura, and post-encephalitic syndromes can all be associated with hyperkinetic involuntary movements that resemble TD (Casey, 1981).

Idiopathic Dyskinesias. Differing opinions about the association of the psychoses and hyperkinesias can be traced to the original works of Kraepelin and Bleuler. "Athetoid ataxia" was the term used by Kraepelin to describe choreic movements in the face and limbs of chronically institutionalized patients (Kraepelin, 1919). On the other hand, Bleuler believed that chorea was associated with organic, not psychologic disease, and attributed this difference in findings to the problem of varying definitions of terms (Bleuler, 1950). Though it has been suggested that the high incidence of choreoathetoid disorders described in psychiatric patients in earlier articles overinconclusively considered organic neurological diseases (Mettler and Crandall, 1959; Crane, 1973), a recent study found the prevalence, severity, and distribution of abnormal movements was similar in groups of chronic schizophrenics with a history of extensive neuroleptic treatment and those with no drug treatment (Owens et al., 1982).

Idiopathic hyperkinetic movements in the face, limbs, or trunk can occur in older people who have never received medications and who do not have psychiatric disorders. These syndromes have been termed "spontaneous orofacial dyskinesia" (Altrocchi, 1972), "spontaneous buccolinguo-facial dyskinesia" (Delwaide and Desseilles, 1977), and "blepharospasm-oromandibular dystonia syndrome" or "Meige's syndrome" (Marsden, 1976; Casey, 1980). Essential tremor must also be distinguished from TD.

EVALUATE NEUROPSYCHIATRIC STATUS

Since both TD and psychoses can be chronic illnesses, establishing a thorough baseline neurological and psychiatric examination is essential to long-term management. Adjustments to an ongoing treatment plan must take into consideration epidemiological factors of TD to minimize the risks of extended neuroleptic treatment in predisposed patients.

Prevalence

The prevalence of TD varied greatly in past studies, from 0.5% to 56% (A. Jus et al., 1976; Baldessarini et al., 1980; Kane and Smith, 1982). This wide range undoubtedly reflects such variables as criteria for diagnosis and different characteristics of the patients studied. Current investigations report the occurrence of TD in 20% to 40% of patients maintained on chronic neuroleptic treatment (Asnis et al., 1977; J.M. Smith et al., 1979). A more conservative estimate, however, suggests that the rate may be 10% to 20% (Baldessarini et al., 1980; Kane and Smith, 1982). These recent figures apply both to inpatient and outpatient studies, as there are now many chronically psychotic patients maintained on neuroleptics in outpatient clinics.

Some of the variability in prevalence rates can be accounted for by different criteria of symptom severity required for identifying "a case" of TD. When questionable and minimal symptoms are included, prevalence rates may be as high as 60% to 70%, whereas moderate to severe symptoms occur at less than 5% to 10% rates (J.M. Smith et al., 1978; J.M. Smith et al., 1979). Though prevalence estimates are subject to many variables, recent reviews have noted an increase in the prevalence of TD (Jeste and Wyatt, 1981; Kane and Smith, 1982), and thus emphasize the importance of actively managing this syndrome.

Age/Sex

There is a steady increase in prevalence of TD with increasing age. Pooled data from 9 studies reported TD in approximately 10% of patients under 40 years old and a gradual increase in prevalence to over 50% in patients 60 years or older (Smith and Baldessarini, 1980). The severity of TD also increases with advancing age (Smith and Baldessarini, 1980). Early investigations reported TD occurred twice as often in females than in males, but recent reviews question this difference (Baldessarini et al., 1980; Jeste and Wyatt, 1981) or show the sex ratio in TD is influenced by multiple parameters (Kane and Smith, 1982).

Pre-existing Organic Disease/Previous Extrapyramidal Symptoms

Early reports suggested organic brain diseases and neuroleptic-induced EPS as risk factors in TD. A review of these data, however, concluded there are no consistent findings to support the association of these factors with increased risk of TD (Kane and Smith, 1982).

Current Mental Status

Managing patients with TD, as well as patients taking neuroleptics but not showing dyskinetic symptoms, requires periodic reassessment of the current need for continued drug therapy. Acute psychosis is usually responsive to neuroleptic treatment and should be given first priority in defining a treatment plan. When the psychosis is under control, longer-term planning requires a re-evaluation of treatment strategies. Reviews of the practice of maintaining neuroleptic medications in outpatients suffering from chronic schizophrenia concluded that approximately 40% to 60% of the patients maintained on neuroleptic medications do not relapse when their medicines are discontinued (Davis, 1975; Gardos and Cole, 1976; Baldessarini et al., 1980). This implies that half of the patients may be taking more medicine than is necessary. On the other hand, it also implies that if medicines were discontinued in all patients, half of them would be exposed to a potential psychotic exacerbation. Unfortunately, there is no method for predicting which patients may successfully reduce or discontinue their neuroleptic medications, though the patients' responses to previous drug discontinuation may provide useful information.

ADJUST NEUROLEPTICS AND ANTICHOLINERGICS

Neuroleptics

If the available clinical information suggests that a patient may be able to reduce or discontinue neuroleptic medication, this should be done. This step is particularly important if the patient has not clearly benefited from antipsychotic drug treatment. A periodic reduction of 10% to 25% in drug dosage will allow the determination of the lowest effective dose. Many patients can be managed successfully in the extended phase of treatment with lower neuroleptic doses than were required to control the acute psychosis. If psychotic symptoms begin to return, a prompt increase in the dose may quickly control the emerging psychotic symptoms (Branchey et al., 1981). This procedure of gradual dosage reduction may prevent the further development of TD. While some patients develop symptoms during neuroleptic treatment, other patients' symptoms do not become evident until after a few weeks after the medications have been reduced or discontinued. These symptoms have been termed "covert dyskinesias" because they became evident only when a drug dosage reduction unmasked the involuntary movements. If TD symptoms continue, they are called "irreversible" or "persistent" whereas symptoms which gradually resolve when neuroleptics have been withdrawn are termed "reversible" or "withdrawal" dyskinesias (Gardos et al., 1978). Though these clinical distinctions are useful, different underlying pathophysiological processes have not been identified. The most parsimonious explanation of withdrawal and persisting dyskinesias is that a common pathophysiologic process occurs along a continuum of reversible to irreversible, but this must be verified.

Total Dose and Duration of Neuroleptic Drugs. The relationship between total neuroleptic dosage, duration of treatment, and TD is unclear. Though an early report noted this correlation (Crane and Smeets, 1974), later studies failed to find an association between total drug intake and TD (Jus et al., 1976; Simpson et al., 1978; Baldessarini et al., 1980; Kane and Smith, 1982). These data suggest that the most important factor in the risk of developing TD may be individual vulnerability. This predisposition or threshold may be manifested as a sign of TD at any time during the course of extended treatment, and thus be obscured in the data when many years of drug treatment are cumulatively analyzed. In a recent study of patients 55 to 75 years old, the largest increase in TD prevalence rates (up to 70%) occurred within the first 5 years of neuroleptic treatment. Thereafter, there was very little difference in TD prevalence in those patients treated between 5 and 25 years with neuroleptics (Toenniessen and Casey, 1982). These data suggest that future prevalence studies examining total dose and duration of neuroleptic treatment concentrate on the early years of treatment.

The value of monitoring neuroleptic blood levels, currently in the research and development stages, is a promising but uncharted area. Of particular importance is the question of whether TD is related to neuroleptic blood levels, as suggested by one report (Jeste et al., 1979a), but not substantiated in another (Jeste et al., 1981).

Drug Type and TD. The question of drug type and TD has frequently been raised. Low mg, high potency neuroleptics, and in particular depot preparations have been implicated with higher prevalence rates of TD (A. Jus et al.,

1976; Gibson, 1978; R.C. Smith et al., 1978; Csernansky et al., 1981). Contrasting data come from another investigation which reported that chlorpromazine was associated with higher prevalence rates of TD (Gardos et al., 1977). These reports, however, involve mostly retrospective analyses and need to be corroborated by prospective studies. Furthermore, most patients have received a plethora of different neuroleptics over many years, either alone or in combination with other drugs, so that it is very difficult to implicate one drug or one class of drugs as the primary etiological agents of TD.

It has been suggested that "atypical" neuroleptics which preferentially influence the type D-2 dopamine receptors or have "site specificity" may be less likely to produce TD. Though the hypotheses about relationships between the different types of dopamine receptors, pharmacological effects of drugs, and various dyskinesias are intriguing, these suggestions are unsubstantiated and must be tested in comparative clinical trials and with animal models of TD. To date, the biochemical and behavioral differences found in the basic science laboratory have not been translated into important differences in the clinic; drugs which purportedly selectively influence type D-1 or D-2 dopamine receptors or brain regions are more similar in the clinic than they are different.

Trial Periods Without Neuroleptics. Though periodically discontinuing neuroleptic treatment as a "drug holiday" has been recommended for reducing the risk of TD, the supporting data are conflicting. One retrospective study showed a significant correlation between the irreversibility of TD and the number of drug-free intervals (Jeste et al., 1979b), but this finding must be replicated. Other investigations have shown that many patients successfully tolerate periodic drug-free trials and eventually receive lower daily neuroleptic doses, and TD may improve (Levine et al., 1980; Pyke and Seeman, 1981; Casey and Toenniessen, 1982).

Anticholinergic Drugs

Another important step in managing TD, as well as acute EPS, is to properly control anticholinergic medications. There is conflicting correlational evidence both for and against the association of maintenance anticholinergic drugs and the development of TD (A. Jus et al., 1976; Baldessarini et al., 1980; Kane and Smith, 1982), but no conclusive consensus has developed. Anticholinergic drugs, however, may temporarily aggravate TD once it has developed (Gerlach et al., 1974; Casey and Denney, 1977; Klawans and Rubovits, 1974). There are no data to suggest that the temporary aggravation of TD with anticholinergic drugs leads to a permanent increase in symptoms. The ability of anticholinergic drugs to exacerbate TD has been utilized to suggest that patients who are susceptible to TD receive periodic brief drug trials with anticholinergics to uncover

TD (Chouinard and Jones, 1980). Such a proposal requires much additional study before it becomes a routine clinical practice.

Many patients can successfully reduce or discontinue their anticholinergic medications because the acute EPS that initially required these drugs often resolve after a few months (Casey et al., 1982a), though it has frequently been stated that no more than 10% of patients receiving anticholinergic medications will need to continue these drugs beyond 3 months. A recent review of this literature found that patients receiving low mg/high potency neuroleptics and who have well-documented histories of previous EPS may need to continue anticholinergic drugs indefinitely (Casey et al., 1982a). The proper strategy is to decrease the anticholinergic drugs gradually over a few weeks and periodically evaluate the patient for a return of acute EPS. The routine prophylactic administration of anticholinergics should be avoided, as this will lead to the prescription of drugs for many patients who do not need them. On the other hand, there is ample reason to justify anticholinergic drugs when signs of neuroleptic-induced EPS are present and a reduction in the neuroleptic treatment is not feasible due to psychotic symptoms.

PERIODICALLY RE-EVALUATE AND DOCUMENT

The long-term management of TD and chronic mental illnesses requires periodic psychiatric and neurological examinations. At least quarterly re-evaluations should be conducted to augment the initial data base. If possible, more frequent examinations are warranted. Neuroleptic drugs have differential effects in patients diagnosed as schizophrenic. While some patients do very well with modest doses, others require substantial daily doses; some benefit very little from neuroleptics; and still others relapse in spite of stable neuroleptic treatment. Since both schizophrenia and TD can have fluctuating courses, a flexible treatment plan that regularly adjusts to meet the patient's current needs will be most successful.

TD REMITS/PERSISTS

Continued neuroleptic treatment is often necessary in spite of existing TD because of recurring psychosis or rarely disabling dyskinesias. Although it is presumed that continued neuroleptic treatment will contribute to the further development of this syndrome, there is little research to delineate the natural history of TD. Early recognition and subsequent drug reduction or discontinuation are associated with a more favorable prognosis for reversible dyskinesia (Quitkin et al., 1977). Similarly, younger age and shorter durations of treatment are associated with reversible TD (Smith and Baldessarini, 1980; Seeman, 1981). The long-term outcome (2-5 years) for individual patients has been unpredictable; some improved, some were unchanged, and some worsened (Paulson, 1968; A. Jus et al., 1979; Seeman, 1981; J.M. Smith et al., 1981).

Our own clinical experience in a TD and movement disorders clinic where clinical course and drug dosage have been closely monitored has shown that patients with TD and psychosis can be maintained on relatively low neuroleptic doses and have their TD symptoms gradually improve or resolve over a 3-5 year period (Casey and Toenniessen, 1982). Younger patients who were able to discontinue neuroleptics improved the most, followed by older patients who discontinued drugs. Patients who remained on neuroleptic drugs, but at doses lower than their original levels, also had TD improve. Those requiring higher doses had their TD remain stable. These data imply that the neuroleptic drugs can be effectively used to control psychosis without increasing the risk of long-term exacerbation or permanence of TD. If these data are supported by further investigations, it suggests that the undesirable side effects of TD can be avoided in many patients who also benefit from and require extended neuroleptic treatment.

MENTAL STATUS STABLE/DETERIORATES

Discontinuing neuroleptics when TD is identified is theoretically rational and attractive, but often not practical. Some patients can remain off neuroleptics, but many others experience a psychotic relapse and must return to drug treatment (Quitkin et al., 1977; Levine et al., 1980; Jeste et al., 1979b; Pyke and Seeman, 1981). In such cases it is important to reconsider the psychiatric diagnosis and evaluate the possibility of treatment with lower doses of antipyschotic medications or lithium and antidepressants if there are symptoms of an affective disorder. When neuroleptics are to be reinstituted, it is essential to verify that the psychosis is responsive to these drugs. A broadly based treatment program that emphasizes the active management of both pharmacological and nondrug approaches is the most effective strategy for treating schizophrenia and reducing the vulnerability to TD (Gardos and Cole, 1976).

INFORMATION ABOUT RISKS AND BENEFITS OF TREATMENT

The medical-legal dictum of informed consent is readily finding a place in the recommendations for managing schizophrenia and TD. In theory, this concept says that the patient will be adequately informed about the potential risks of receiving neuroleptic medications, whereas in practice this concept is extremely difficult to implement. There are varied recommendations in the psychiatric literature suggesting that TD be discussed with patients at different phases of treatment, or that different informed consent documents be prepared for different situations (Casey and Gerlach, 1982). A more general and practical approach suggests that the clinician inform the patient, as well as a concerned other person, about the risks and benefits of both treatment and no treatment, and that this process be documented in a timely and thoughtful manner consistent with the principles of the doctor-patient relationship (Casey, 1978; Baldessarini et al., 1980).

DRUG TREATMENT

Though many drugs have been used to treat TD, no specific agents have been shown to be both safe and effective over extended treatment periods. The drugs mentioned in the next section include agents aimed at manipulating the dopaminergic, acetylcholinergic, GABAergic, and neuropeptide influences of the basal ganglia, as well as some compounds with unknown mechanisms of action. This list will require periodic revision as new developments occur. Although some compounds are restricted to research use only, they are mentioned because of their theoretical interest.

TD is hypothesized to develop, at least in part, from dopamine receptor hypersensitivity, perhaps of specific receptor subtypes (Klawans, 1973). This may lead to an imbalance between reciprocal dopamine and acetylcholine influences in the nigrostriatal systems. Neurochemical interrelations in the basal ganglia which are mediated by GABA and the endorphins may also play a role in TD (Casey et al., 1981a).

Dopamine

Dopamine Antagonists. The most effective method for suppressing the hyperkinetic symptoms of TD is to reinstitute a reduction of dopaminergic influences with receptor blockers, amine depleters, or drugs with related effects. However, it is essential to raise the caution that treating a syndrome with a group of drugs thought to be pathophysiological agents causing the syndrome may, by temporarily suppressing symptoms, lead to an eventual further aggravation.

Theoretically, all the neuroleptics commercially available are capable of both temporarily masking TD and producing this syndrome (Baldessarini et al., 1980). However, whether one particular drug is more capable than another of producing or suppressing TD is unclear and a subject of ongoing research. Many retrospective epidemiological studies have attempted to clarify the relationship between drug type, dosage, and duration of treatment, but the results have been inconsistent. This may not be surprising, however, if the predisposing vulnerability of the individual to develop TD is of greater importance than varying drug parameters. Though long-term studies of suppressing TD with neuroleptics are limited, we have been able to maintain patients on low doses of neuroleptics for up to 5 years without aggravating TD (Casey and Toenniessen, 1982). Perhaps the most important approach is to *not* suppress TD because the degree of suppression may be related to the degree of eventual aggravation.

Recent interest has been shown in reducing dopaminergic influences via presynaptic amine depletion. Reserpine has produced variable effects ranging from nearly complete suppression of TD to only modest symptomatic improvement (Crane, 1973; A. Jus et al., 1979; Huang et al., 1981). If reserpine is used, doses must be started in the antihypertensive range of approximately 0.25 mg/day and gradually increased. Potential side effects of depression, hypotension, diarrhea, and nasal congestion may be encountered as the doses are gradually increased. Other research strategies with the amine depletor have included tetrabenazine (Kazamatsuri et al., 1972; Asher and Aminoff, 1981), the synthesis inhibitor alpha-methyl-para-tyrosine (Magelund et al., 1979), and the false transmitter alpha-methyl-dopa (Huang et al., 1981). Although reserpine has only rarely been associated with causing TD, it should be cautiously considered as a treatment because the caveat holds that it may be reproducing similar neurochemical alterations which are implicated in animal models of this syndrome (Tarsy and Baldessarini, 1974).

Dopamine Agonists. Altering the purported dopamine receptor hypersensitivity underlying TD has been attempted with drugs that increase available dopamine. This approach reasons that if dopamine receptors have developed increased sensitivity due to receptor blockade, stimulating the receptors with dopamine agonists might "reset" receptor sensitivity to a normal range of function. The initial trial reported encouraging results in TD (Alpert and Friedhoff, 1980). In a subsequent study, TD was treated for 4 to 8 weeks with levodopa + benserazide, a peripheral decarboxylase inhibitor, over a wide dose range, corresponding to 3.0-9.0 grams/day of levodopa. TD scores moderately increased during levodopa. After the drug was discontinued, TD scores returned to pretreatment baseline levels without further improvement in the 9 patients receiving concurrent neuroleptic medications, but in the neuroleptic-free patients TD scores decreased 25% in 3 patients and resolved in one younger patient. Psychological effects of depression or increased psychotic symptoms occurred at higher drug doses (Casey et al., 1982b). These results do not support the proposal that receptor sensitivity modification with levodopa is an effective therapeutic approach to TD, though selected patient and drug treatment variables, including other DA agonists, are considerations for further investigation.

Direct receptor stimulation with dopamine agonists has also been used in experimental trials for TD. Apomorphine, a partial dopamine agonist, usually decreased TD, perhaps through presynaptic mechanisms (R.C. Smith et al., 1977). The ergot dopamine agonists bromocriptine and CF 25-397 failed to affect TD (Tamminga and Chase, 1980). These inconsistent findings with dopamine agonists will require further study to provide additional information about the mechanisms of actions and the clinical effects of dopamine agonists in TD.

Acetylcholine

Anticholinergics. Cholinergic hypofunction is a purported pathophysiological factor underlying TD, possibly interacting with dopamine receptor hypersensitivity. As discussed above, anticholinergic drugs can aggravate or uncover existing TD. Anticholinergics, when given in combination with neuroleptics, may markedly reduce the antihyperkinetic effect of neuroleptics on TD (Gerlach and Simmelsgaard, 1978). In a few reports, anticholinergics have reduced rather than aggravated TD (Gerlach et al., 1974; Granacher et al., 1975; Casey and Denney, 1977; Moore and Bowers, 1980). It is not yet clear if there is a subgroup of patients with TD that may benefit from anticholinergics, or if these infrequently reported cases of improvement with anticholinergics actually represent patients with the seldom recognized syndrome of initial hyperkinesia (described above).

Cholinergic Agonists. Augmenting a relatively underfunctioning cholinergic system has been a logical experimental approach to TD. Physostigmine, an acetylcholine esterase inhibitor, usually decreased TD, but may have variable effects (Casey et al., 1981a) that are complicated by undesirable effects of sedation, dizziness, nausea, and vomiting. Treating TD via cholinergic precursor loading with deanol produced inconsistent results (Casey, 1977). Choline moderately reduced TD symptoms (Growdon et al., 1977), though side effects limit the widespread use of this compound. Lecithin also moderately suppressed TD (Gelenberg et al., 1979). Though the idea that the cholinergic system could be modified by precursor loading is theoretically attractive, further research is needed to develop practical, effective, and safe compounds.

GABA

Recent investigations of striato-nigral mechanisms suggest that increased GABAergic influences may have an inhibitory effect on dopaminergic function. The GABA agonist muscimol decreased TD, but this experimental compound has untoward psychotomimetic effects (Tamminga et al., 1979). Another experimental GABA agonist, THIP, had no significant effect in TD, however (Korsgaard et al., 1982). Gamma-acetylenic GABA, an irreversible catalytic inhibitor of the degradative enzyme GABA-transaminase, also significantly reduced TD (Casey et al., 1980). Interestingly, this experimental GABA agonist had significantly greater antihyperkinetic effects in older patients taking neuroleptic drugs, suggesting that increased GABA influences may reduce TD by indirect effects on dopaminergic mechanisms.

Sodium valproate (Depakene) may increase brain GABA via GABA-trans-aminase inhibition, though there is some question whether doses used in the clinic are large enough to affect brain GABA. After the initial positive report of sodium valproate in TD (Linnoila et al., 1976), less encouraging reports appeared. As with gamma-acetylenic GABA, sodium valproate was more effective in suppressing TD when it was combined with a neuroleptic (Nair et al., 1980). Baclofen (Lioresal), a structural analog of GABA, with unclear effects on GABA mechanisms, moderately suppressed TD, potentiated the neuroleptic antihyperkinetic effects, and was substantially less effective in suppressing TD when not used in combination with neuroleptics (Korsgaard, 1976; Gerlach et al., 1978; Nair et al., 1980).

Benzodiazepines may also act as GABA agonists. Diazepam (Valium) has both reduced (K. Jus et al., 1974; Singh et al., 1980) and aggravated TD (Rosenbaum and de la Fuente, 1979), but further controlled trials are needed to corroborate these reports. Clonazepam (Clonopin), a benzodiazepine that may also affect serotonin, was as effective as phenobarbital in reducing TD (Bobruff et al., 1981), and again raises the question of whether the antihyperkinetic effects of benzodiazepines in TD occur primarily through GABAergic mechanisms, via nonspecific sedative effects, or through other processes.

Neuropeptides

The recent identification of endogenous opiate receptors in the central nervous system has stimulated much research into the effects of these neurochemical systems in psychiatric and neurological syndromes. The β-lipotropin hormone, $_{61-91}(\beta\text{-LPH}_{61-91})$ compound and its peptide fragments have been found to affect dopamine-mediated mechanisms, and thus may be involved in the pathophysiology of schizophrenia and TD.

The met-enkephalin ($\beta\text{-LPH}_{61-65}$) synthetic analog FK 33-824 was compared with the naturally occurring agonist morphine, and the antagonist naloxone (Narcan). FK 33-824 produced only a modest suppression of TD; even less effect was produced by morphine. Naloxone, an opiate antagonist, had no consistent effect on TD. The most pronounced decrease in TD was seen in patients who were concurrently receiving a high neuroleptic dose (Bjørndal et al., 1980). Recent reports have shown that the non-opiate $\beta\text{-LPH}_{62-77}$ fragment, des-tyrosine-γ-endorphin (DTγE), also had no effect on TD (Casey et al., 1981b). The initial results do not suggest a primary role for these specific peptide fragments in the pathophysiology or treatment of TD, though new molecular subdivisions of the β-lipotropin hormone will undoubtedly be considered in future research.

Other Drug Trials

Many other medications for TD have been investigated, varying from controlled trials to individual case reports. Although the initial reports with lithium carbonate were encouraging, later double-blind studies showed no benefit or improvement only in selected patients (Yassa and Ananth, 1980). Lithium offers little promise as a primary treatment for TD, but if patients with diagnoses of schizophrenia and TD also have affective symptoms, an adequate clinical trial with lithium may be able to reduce or replace the neuroleptic medication and thus reduce the long-term TD risks. Papaverine, a derivtive of opium, moderately decreased TD, perhaps through its weak dopamine antagonist properties (Gardos et al., 1976). Estrogen has also produced inconsistent results in TD (Villeneuve et al., 1978; Koller et al., 1982); Hydergine, an ergot alkaloid, may reduce TD (Gomez, 1977). Tryptophan has not been generally effective in TD (Prange et al., 1973; K. Jus et al., 1974). Amantadine and methylphenidate also have inconsistently affected TD (Janowsky et al., 1972; Fann et al., 1973). Clonidine (Freedman et al., 1980) and propranolol (Bacher and Lewis, 1980) are also under investigation as potential treatments for TD.

SUMMARY

During the past two and a half decades, neuroleptic medications have provided a practical and efficacious treatment of acute and chronic psychoses. It is clear, however, that this advancement in clinical psychopharmacology has been at the unanticipated cost of producing the potentially irreversible neurological syndrome of TD. This tradeoff between risks and benefits now leads to a timely reassessment of the clinical use of neuroleptic medications. The overall ineffectiveness or troublesome side effects of the currently available clinical and research drugs to treat TD supports the contention that it will be far better to direct efforts toward preventing the syndrome than trying to control TD once it develops. The ultimate goal of psychopharmacological research is to develop an effective antipsychotic drug which is free of neurological and other troublesome side effects. Until that time, if we minimize the risks and maximize the benefits of appropriate neuroleptic treatment, TD will become a less frequent and less disabling consequence of psychopharmacological treatment of psychoses.

ACKNOWLEDGMENTS

This work was supported in part by the Veterans Administration Research Career Development program and The Grass Foundation.

BIBLIOGRAPHY

Alpert, M., and Friedhoff, A. Clinical application of receptor modification treatment. In W.E. Fann, R.C. Smith, J.M. Davis, and E.F. Domino, eds., *Tardive Dyskinesia: Research and Treatment*. New York: Spectrum Books, 1980, pp. 471-473.

Altrocchi, P.H. (1972). Spontaneous oral-facial dyskinesia. *Arch. Neurol.* 26: 505-512, 1972.

Asher, S.W., and Aminoff, M.J. Tetrabenazine and movement disorders. *Neurology* 31:1051-1054, 1981.

Asnis, G.M., Leopold, M.A., Duvoisin, R.C., and Schwartz, A. A survey of tardive dyskinesia in psychiatric outpatients. *Am. J. Psychiatry* 134:1367-1370, 1977.

Bacher, N.N., and Lewis, H.A. Low-dose propranolol in tardive dyskinesia. *Am. J. Psychiatry* 137:495-497, 1980.

Baldessarini, R.J., Cole, J.O., Davis, J.J., Gardos, G., Preskorn, S., Simpson, G., and Tarsy, D. *Tardive Dyskinesia: A Task Force Report*. Washington, D.C.: American Psychiatric Association, 1980.

Birket-Smith, E. Abnormal involuntary movements induced by anticholinergic therapy. *Acta Neurol. Scand.* 50:801-811, 1974.

Bjørndal, N., Casey, D.E., and Gerlach, J. Enkephalin, morphine, and naloxone in tardive dyskinesia. *Psychopharmacol.* 69(2):133-136, 1980.

Bleuler, E.E. *Dementia Praecox or the Group of Schizophrenias*. New York: International Universities Press, 1950.

Bobruff, A.A., Gardos, G., Tarsy, D., Rapkin, R.M., Cole, J., and Moore, P. Clonazepam and phenobarbital in tardive dyskinesia. *Am. J. Psychiatry* 138: 189-193, 1981.

Branchey, M.H., Branchey, L.B., and Richardson, M. Effects of neuroleptic adjustment on clinical conditions and tardive dyskinesia in schizophrenic patients. *Am. J. Psychiatry* 138:608-612, 1981.

Casey, D.E. Deanol in the management of involuntary movement disorders: a review. *Dis. Nerv. Syst.* 38 (Sect. 2):7-15, 1977.

Casey, D.E. Managing tardive dyskinesia. *J. Clin. Psychiatry* 39:748-753, 1978.

Casey, D.E. Pharmacology of blepharospasm-oromandibular dystonia syndrome. *Neurology* 30:690-695, 1980.

Casey, D.E. The differential diagnosis of tardive dyskinesia. *Acta Psychiat. Scand.* (Suppl. 291) 63:71-87, 1981.

Casey, D.E., and Denney, D. Pharmacological characterization of tardive dyskinesia. *Psychopharmacol.* 54:1-8, 1977.

Casey, D.E., and Gerlach, J. Clinical management of tardive dyskinesia. In J. DeVeaugh-Geiss, ed., *Tardive Dyskinesia and Related Involuntary Movement Disorders: The Long-Term Effects of Antipsychotic Drugs*. Boston: John Wright PSG, 1982, pp. 85-107.

Casey, D.E., and Rabins, P. Tardive dyskinesia as a life-threatening illness. *Am. J. Psychiatry* 135:486-488, 1978.

Casey, D.E., and Toenniessen, L.M. Tardive dyskinesia: changes during five years. *Proc. Amer. Psychiat. Assoc.*, 68E:171-172, 1982.

Casey, D.E., Gerlach, J., Magelund, G. and Christensen, T.-R. Gamma-acetylenic GABA in tardive dyskinesia. *Arch. Gen. Psychiatry* 37:1376-1379, 1980.

Casey, D.E., Gerlach, J., and Korsgaard, S. Clinical pharmacological approaches to evaluating tardive dyskinesia. In E. Usdin, S.G. Dahl, L.F. Gram, and O. Lingjaerde, eds., *Clin. Pharmacol. in Psychiatry: Neuroleptic and Antidepressant Research*. London: MacMillan, pp. 369-383, 1981a.

Casey, D.E., Korsgaard, S., Gerlach, J., Jørgensen, A., Simmelsgaard, H. Effect of des-tyrosine-γ-endorphin in tardive dyskinesia. *Arch. Gen. Psychiatry* 38:158-160, 1981b.

Casey, D.E., Clappison, V., and Keepers, G. Anticholinergic drugs in neuroleptic-induced extrapyramidal symptoms. *Psychopharmacology*, in press.

Casey, D.E., Gerlach, J., and Bjørndal, N. Levodopa and receptor sensitivity modification in tardive dyskinesia. *Psychopharmacol.* 78:89-92, 1982.

Chadwick, D., Reynolds, E.H., and Marsden, C.D. Anticonvulsant-induced dyskinesias: a comparison with dyskinesias induced by neuroleptics. *J. Neurol. Neurosurg. Psychiatry* 39:1210-1218, 1976.

Chouinard, G., and Jones, B.D. Anticholinergics and tardive dyskinesia. *Am. J. Psychiatry* 137:1470-1471, 1980.

Crane, G.E. Persistent dyskinesia. *Br. J. Psychiatry* 122:395-405, 1973.

Crane, G.E., and Smeets, R.A. Tardive dyskinesia and drug therapy in geriatric patients. *Arch. Gen. Psychiatry* 30:341-343, 1974.

Csernansky, J.G., Grabowski, K., Cervantes, J., Kaplan, J., and Yesavage, J. Fluphenazine decanoate and tardive dyskinesia: a possible association. *Am. J. Psychiatry* 138:1362-1365, 1981.

Davis, J.M. Overview: Maintenance therapy in psychiatry: I. Schizophrenia. *Am. J. Psychiatry* 132:1237-1245, 1975.

Dekret, J.J., Maany, I., Ramsey, A., and Mendels, J. A case of oral dyskinesia associated with imipramine treatment. *Am. J. Psychiatry* 134:1297, 1977.

Delwaide, P.J., and Desseilles, M. Spontaneous buccolinguofacial dyskinesia in the elderly. *Acta Neurol. Scand.* 56:256-262, 1977.

Fann, W.E., Davis, J.M., and Wilson, I.C. Methylphenidate in tardive dyskinesia. *Am. J. Psychiatry* 130:922-924, 1973.

Fann, W.E., Sullivan, J.L., and Richman, B.W. Dyskinesias associated with tricyclic antidepressants. *Br. J. Psychiatry* 128:490-493, 1976.

Freedman, R., Bell, J., and Kirch, D. Clonidine therapy for coexisting psychosis and tardive dyskinesia. *Am. J. Psychiatry* 137:629-630, 1980.

Gardos, G., and Cole, J.O. Maintenance antipsychotic therapy: is the cure worse than the disease? *Am. J. Psychiatry* 133:32-36, 1976.

Gardos, G., Cole, J.O., and Sniffen, C. An evaluation of papaverine in tardive dyskinesia. *J. Clin. Pharmacol.* 16:304-310, 1976.

Gardos, G., Cole, J.O., and LaBrie, R.A. Drug variables in the etiology of tardive dyskinesia. Application of discriminant function analysis. *Prog. Neuro-Psychopharmacology* 1:147-154, 1977.

Gardos, G., Cole, J.O., and Tarsy, D. Withdrawal syndromes associated with antipsychotic drugs. *Am. J. Psychiatry* 135:1321-1324, 1978.

Gelenberg, A., Doller-Wojcik, J.C., and Growdon, J. Choline and lecithin in the treatment of tardive dyskinesia: preliminary results from a pilot study. *Am. J. Psychiatry* 136:772-776, 1979.

Gerlach, J. Tardive dyskinesia. *Dan. Med. Bull.* 26:209-245, 1979.

Gerlach, J., and Simmelsgaard, H. Tardive dyskinesia during and following treatment with haloperidol, haloperidol + biperiden, thioridazine, and clozapine. *Psychopharmacol.* 59:105-112, 1978.

Gerlach, J., Reisby, N., and Randrup, A. Dopaminergic hypersensitivity and cholinergic hypofunction in the pathophysiology of tardive dyskinesia. *Psychopharmacologia* 34:21-35, 1974.

Gerlach, J., Rye, T., and Kristjansen, P. Effect of baclofen on tardive dyskinesia. *Psychopharmacol.* 56:145-151, 1978.

Gibson, A.C. Depot injections and tardive dyskinesia. *Br. J. Psychiatry* 132:361-365, 1978.

Gomez, E. Clinical observations in the treatment of tardive dyskinesia with dihydrogenated ergot alklaoids (Hydergine); preliminary findings. *Psychiatry J. Univ. Ottawa* 2:67-71, 1977.

Granacher, R.P., Baldessarini, Ross, J., and Cole, J.O. Deanol for tardive dyskinesia. *N. Engl. J. Med.* 292:926-927, 1975.

Growdon, J.H., Hirsch, M.J., Wurtman, R.J., and Wiener, W. Oral choline administration to patients with tardive dyskinesia. *N. Engl. J. Med.* 297:524-527, 1977.

Huang, C.C., Wang, R.I., Hasegawa, A., and Alverno, L. Reserpine and alpha-methyldopa in the treatment of tardive dyskinesia. *Psychopharmacol.* 73: 359-362, 1981.

Janowsky, D.S., El-Yousef, M.K., Davis, J.M., Sekerke, H.J., Morris, D.R., and Decker, B. Effects of amantadine on tardive dyskinesia and pseudoparkinsonism. *N. Engl. J. Med.* 286:785, 1972.

Jeste, D.V., and Wyatt, R. Changing epidemiology of tardive dyskinesia: an overview. *Am. J. Psychiatry* 138:297-309, 1981.

Jeste, D.V., Rosenblatt, J.E., Wagner, R.L., Wyatt, R. High serum neuroleptic levels in tardive dyskinesia? *N. Engl. J. Med.* 21:1184, 1979a.

Jeste, D.V., Potkin, S.G., Sinha, S., Feder, S., and Wyatt, R. Tardive dyskinesia—reversible and persistent. *Arch. Gen. Psychiatry* 36:585-590, 1979b.

Jeste, D.V., DeLisi, L.E., Zalcman, S., Wise, D., Phelps, B., Rosenblatt, J., Potkin, S., Bridge, P., and Wyatt, R. A biochemical study of tardive dyskinesia in young male patients. *Psychiatry Res.* 4:327-334, 1981.

Jus, A., Pineau, R., Lachance, R., Pelchat, C., Jus, K., Pires, P., and Villeneuve, R. Epidemiology of tardive dyskinesia. *Dis. Nerv. Syst.* 37:210-214; 257-261, 1976.

Jus, A., Jus, K., and Fontaine, P. Long-term treatment of tardive dyskinesia. *J. Clin. Psychiatry* 40:72-77, 1979.

Jus, K., Jus, A., Gautier, J., Villeneuve, A., Pires, P., Pineau, R., and Villeneuve, R. Studies on the action of certain pharmacological agents on tardive dyskinesia and on the rabbit syndrome. *Int. J. Clin. Pharmacol.* 9:138-145, 1974.

Kane, J.M., and Smith, J.M. Tardive dyskinesia. *Arch. Gen. Psychiatry* 39:473-481, 1982.

Kazamatsuri, H., Chien, C.-P., and Cole, J.O. The treatment of tardive dyskinesia. I. Clinical efficacy of a dopamine-depleting agent, tetrabenazine. *Arch. Gen. Psychiatry* 27:95-99, 1972.

Klawans, H.L. The pharmacology of tardive dyskinesia. *Am. J. Psychiatry* 130: 82-86, 1973.

Klawans, H.L., and Rubovits, R. Effect of cholinergic and anticholinergic agents on tardive dyskinesia. *J. Neurol. Neurosurg. Psychiatry* 37:941-947, 1974.

Koller, W.C., Barr, A., and Biary, N. Estrogen treatment of dyskinetic disorders. *Neurology* 32:547-549, 1982.

Korsgaard, S. Baclofen (Lioresal) in the treatment of neuroleptic induced tardive dyskinesia. *Acta Psychiat. Scand.* 54:17-24, 1976.

Korsgaard, S., Casey, D.E., Gerlach, J., Hetmar, O., Kaldan, B., and Mikkelsen, L. The effect of THIP, a new GABA agonist, in tardive dyskinesia. *Arch. Gen. Psychiatry* 39:1017-1031, 1982.

Kraepelin, E. *Dementia Praecox and Paraphrenia.* Edinburgh: E&S Livingstone, 1919, pp. 43-83.

Levine, J., Schooler, N., Severe, J., Escobar, J., Gelenberg, A., Mandel, M., Sovner, R., and Steinbook, R. Discontinuation of oral and depot fluphenazine in schizophrenic patients after one year of continuous medication: a controlled study. In F. Cattabeni, G. Racagni, P.F. Spano, and E. Costa, eds., *Long-Term Effects of Neuroleptics.* New York: Raven Press, 1980, pp. 483-493.

Linnoila, M., Viukari, M., and Hietala, O. Effect of sodium valproate on tardive dyskinesia. *Br. J. Psychiatry* 129:114-119, 1976.

Magelund, G., Gerlach, J., and Casey, D.E. Neuroleptic-potentiating effect of α-methyl-p-tyrosine compared with haloperidol and placebo in a double-blind crossover trial. *Acta Psychiat. Scand.* 60:185-189, 1979.

Marsden, C.D. Blepharospasm-oromandibular dystonia syndrome (Breughel's syndrome). *J. Neurol. Neurosurg. Psychiatry* 39:1204-1209, 1976.

McLean, P., and Casey, D.E. Tardive dyskinesia in an adolescent. *Am. J. Psychiatry* 135:969-971, 1978.

Mettler, F.A., and Crandall, A. Neurologic disorders in psychiatric institutions. *J. Nerv. Ment. Dis.* 128:148, 1959.

Moore, D.C., and Bowers, M.B. Identification of a subgroup of tardive dyskinesia patients by pharmacologic probes. *Am. J. Psychiatry* 137:1202-1205, 1980.

Nair, N.P.V., Lal, S., Schwartz, G., and Thavundayil, J.X. Effect of sodium valproate and baclofen in tardive dyskinesia: clinical and neuroendocrine studies. In F. Cattabeni, G. Racagni, P.F. Spano, and E. Costa, eds., *Long-Term Effects of Neuroleptics.* New York: Raven Press, 1980, pp. 437-441.

Nausieda, P., Koller, W.C., Weiner, W.J., and Klawans, H. Chorea induced by oral contraceptives. *Neurology* 29:1605-1609, 1979.

Osifo, N.G. Drug-related transient dyskinesias. *Clin. Pharmacol. Ther.* 25:767-771, 1979.

Owens, D.G.C., Johnstone, E., and Frith, C.D. Spontaneous involuntary disorders of movement. *Arch. Gen. Psychiatry* 39:452-461, 1982.

Paulson, G.W. An evaluation of the permanence of the "tardive dyskinesias." *Dis. Nerv. Syst.* 29:692-694, 1968.

Polizos, P., Engelhardt, D.M., Hoffman, S.P., and Waizer, J. CNS consequences of psychotropic drug withdrawal in schizophrenic children. *Psychopharmacol. Bull.* 9:34, 1973.

Prange, A.J., Wilson, I.C., Morris, C.E., and Hall, C.D. Preliminary experience with tryptophan and lithium in the treatment of tardive dyskinesia. *Psychopharmacol. Bull.* 9:36-37, 1973.

Pyke, J., and Seeman, M.V. Neuroleptic-free intervals in the treatment of schizophrenia. *Am. J. Psychiatry* 138:1620-1621, 1981.

Quitkin, F., Rifkin, A., Gochfeld, L., and Klein, D. Tardive dyskinesia: are first signs reversible? *Am. J. Psychiatry* 134:84-87, 1977.

Rosenbaum, A.H., de la Fuente, J.R. Benzodiazepines and tardive dyskinesia. *Lancet* 2(8148):900, 1979.

Rylander, G. Psychoses and punding and choreiform syndromes in addiction to central stimulant drugs. *Psychiat. Neurol. Neurochirg.* 75:203–212, 1972.

Schonecker, M. Ein eigentumliches syndrom im oralen bereich bei megaphen applikation. *Nervenarzt* 28:35, 1957.

Seeman, M. Tardive dyskinesia: two-year recovery. *Compr. Psychiatry* 22:189–192, 1981.

Sigwald, J., Bouttier, D., Raymondeaud, C. Quatre cas de dyskinesie facio-bucco-linguo-masticatrice a l'evolution prolongee secondaire a un traitement par les neuroleptiques. *Rev. Neurol.* 100:751–755, 1959.

Simpson, G.M., Varga, E.E., Lee, H.J., and Zoubok, B. Tardive dyskinesia and psychotropic drug history. *Psychopharmacology* 58:117–124, 1978.

Singh, M.M., Nasrallah, H.A., Lal, H., Pitman, R., Becker, R., Kucharski, T., Karkalas, J., and Fox, R. Treatment of tardive dyskinesia with diazepam: indirect evidence for the involvement of limbic, possibly GABAergic mechanisms. *Brain Res. Bull.* (Suppl. 2) 5:673–680, 1980.

Smith, J.M., Oswald, W.T., Kucharski, L.T., and Waterman, L.J. Tardive dyskinesia: age and sex differences in hospitalized schizophrenics. *Psychopharmacology* 58:207–211, 1978.

Smith, J.M., Kucharski, L.T., Eblen, C., Knutsen, E., and Linn, C. An assessment of tardive dyskinesia in schizophrenic outpatients. *Psychopharmacology* 64:99–104, 1979.

Smith, J.M., and Baldessarini, R.J. Changes in prevalence, severity, and recovery in tardive dyskinesia with age. *Arch. Gen. Psychiatry* 37:1368–1373, 1980.

Smith, J.M., Burke, M.P., and Moon, C.O. Long-term changes in AIMS ratings and their relation to medication history. *Psychopharmacol. Bull.* 17:120–121, 1981.

Smith, R.C., Tamminga, C., Haraszti, J., Pandey, G., and Davis, J. Effects of dopamine agonists in tardive dyskinesia. *Am. J. Psychiatry* 134:763–768, 1977.

Smith, R.C., Strizich, M., and Klass, D. Drug history and tardive dyskinesia. *Am. J. Psychiatry* 135:1402–1403, 1978.

Sovner, R., and DiMascio, A. The effect of benztropine mesylate in the rabbit syndome and tardive dyskinesia. *Am. J. Psychiatry* 134:1301–1302, 1977.

Tamminga, C., and Chase, T.N. Bromocriptine and CF 25-397 in the treatment of tardive dyskinesia. *Arch. Neurol.* 37:204–205, 1980.

Tamminga, C., Crayton, J.W., and Chase, T.N. (1979). Improvement in tardive dyskinesia after muscimol therapy. *Arch. Gen. Psychiatry* 36:595–598, 1979.

Tarsy, D.J., and Baldessarini, R.J. Behavioral supersensitivity to apomorphine following chronic treatment with drugs which interfere with synaptic function of catecholamines. *Neuropharmacol.* 13:927–940, 1974.

Thach, B.T., Chase, T.N., and Bosma, J.F. Oral facial dyskinesia associated with prolonged use of antihistaminic decongestants. *N. Engl. J. Med.* 293:486–487, 1975.

Toenniessen, L.M., and Casey, D.E. Duration of neuroleptic exposure and risk of tardive dyskinesia. *Proc. Soc. Biol. Psychiatry*, 69:100, 1982.

Uhrbrand, L., and Faurbye, A. Reversible and irreversible dyskinesia after treatment with perphenazine, chlorpromazine, reserpine, and electroconvulsive therapy. *Psychopharmacologia* 1:408–418, 1960.

Van Putten, T. The many faces of akathisia. *Compr. Psychiatry* 16:43–47, 1975.

Villeneuve, A. The rabbit syndrome: a peculiar extrapyramidal reaction. *Canad. Psychiatric Assoc. J.* 17:69–72, 1972.

Villeneuve, A., Langelier, P., and Bedard, P. Estrogens, dopamine and dyskinesias. *Canad. Psychiatric Assoc. J.* 23:68–70, 1978.

Weiner, W.J., Goetz, C.G., Nausieda, P.A., and Klawans, H. Respiratory dyskinesias, extrapyramidal dysfunction and dyspnea. *Ann. Intern. Med.* 88:327–331, 1978.

Yassa, R., and Ananth, J. Lithium carbonate in the treatment of movement disorders. *Int. Pharmacopsychiat.* 15:301–308, 1980.

13

New Clinical Concepts on Neuroleptic-Induced Supersensitivity Disorders: Tardive Dyskinesia and Supersensitivity Psychosis

GUY CHOUINARD AND SUSANNE STEINBERG

INTRODUCTION

The use of antipsychotic drugs in the management of schizophrenia became widespread as no other equally effective treatment existed. Although these drugs appeared safe at the beginning, it was soon discovered that their long-term side effects were associated with the central nervous system. First, tardive dyskinesia (Shonecker, 1957; Faurbye et al., 1964) and then supersensitivity psychosis (Chouinard, Jones and Annable, 1978; Chouinard and Jones, 1980) were recognized following prolonged neuroleptic administration. Several theories have been proposed for these long-term side effects. The dopamine theory, which attributes them to postsynaptic dopamine receptor supersensitivity (Klawans, 1980) best explains clinical findings. Withdrawal of neuroleptics after prolonged blockade results in a release of dopamine with manifest supersensitivity symptoms, while neuroleptic reinstitution has a masking effect.

We propose the concept of type I and type II risk factors of neuroleptic-induced supersensitivity disorders and in particular of tardive dyskinesia. Type I factor is defined as a risk leading primarily to a reversible form of tardive

Table 1.   Risk Factors for Tardive Dyskinesia

Type I factors: Factors which lead to reversible and withdrawal dyskinesia.

Type II factors: Factors which lead to masked and irreversible overt dysinesia.

A) *Drug Factor:*

   1) Central anticholinergic drugs (antiparkinsonian, antihistamine, antidepressant)

   2) Dopamine agonists or precursors

   3) Type I neuroleptics

     a) Endogenous neuroleptic (weak neuroleptic activity): estrogens. High ratio of postsynaptic to presynaptic receptor blockade.

     b) Diphenylbutylpiperidines: pimozide, fluspirilene, penfluridol. High specificity for postsynaptic receptor and relatively high ratio of postsynaptic/presynaptic activity.

B) *Patient Factor (Host Factor):*

   1) Age under 40.

   2) Good prognosis schizophrenia (good response or fewer days in hospital).

   3) Akathisia and tremor

A) *Drug Factor:* Type II Neuroleptics:

   1) Neuroleptics which block equally both pre- and postsynaptic dopamine receptors (low ratio of post-synaptic to presynaptic activity): high potency neurolpetics (haloperidol, fluphenazine).

   2) Low specificity for a particular neurotransmitter receptor site and for pre- or postsynaptic: low potency (chlorpromazine).

B) *Patient Factor (Host Factor):*

   1) Age (over 40)

   2) Poor prognosis schizophrenia (little drug response or more days in hospital)

   3) Hypokinetic parkinsonian features

   4) Brain injury or damage, or previous history of brain disease, mental retardation.

   5) Female over 65.

dyskinesia, while type II factors to irreversible forms of the disorder. The greater the number of type I factors the milder, less frequent and more reversible the syndrome. The more numerous the type II factors, the higher the incidence, the greater the severity and the more likely the disorder will be irreversible. Drug and host (patient) profiles are defined for each category of risk factors (Table 1). The following drug activities are associated with reversible or type I tardive dyskinesia: 1) central anticholinergic agents unmask or exacerbate tardive dyskinesia but do not increase its incidence or its severity;   2) dopamine agonists tend to initially cause a reversible exacerbation of these involuntary movements by stimulation of sensitized postsynaptic dopamine receptors; and 3) the neuroleptics involved have a relatively high postsynaptic to presynaptic ratio blockade activity. Type I host factors have the following patient characteristics: 1) age under 40; 2) good prognosis schizophrenia and/or brief hospital admission; and 3) akathisia and tremor.

The type II tardive dyskinesia is overt, which makes the challenge with anticholinergics unnecessary. Significant increases in dosages of neuroleptics are needed to mask the dyskinesia, with only moderate effect. The drug profile for type II tardive dyskinesia consists of the following characteristics: 1) the neuroleptics involved block both pre- and post-synaptic dopamine receptors and are considered to have a low postsynaptic to presynaptic receptor ratio; 2) some of them are of low specificity for a particular neurotransmittor receptor site; and 3) they are especially efficacious in the acute treatment. The patient's profile consists of: 1) age over 40; 2) poor prognosis schizophrenia, as manifested by poor response to drug treatment or long periods in hospital; 3) hypokinetic parkinsonian features; 4) history of brain injury or disease; and 5) female over 65.

Type I and II factors are associated with differences in pathophysiology. The presence of type I factors suggests that only postsynaptic dopaminergic receptors are affected. In contrast, for irreversible tardive dyskinesia, presynaptic changes occur which may consist of neuronal sprouting, in response to dopamine blockade in the brain. In this chapter, we present clinical evidence from which this concept of tardive dyskinesia was derived. Drug trials will be discussed in regard to their contribution to this theory. An epidemiological survey will be described which explains our choice of host criteria. Then, supersensitivity psychosis will be defined and compared to tardive dyskinesia.

TARDIVE DYSKINESIA

Drug Factors

Anticholinergic Agents. Central anticholinergic drugs best represent the drug profile leading to reversible dyskinesia. We present three clinical trials documenting the reversible effect of anticholinergic drugs on dyskinesia. In a study designed to investigate antiparkinsonian drugs and tardive dyskinesia, we examined the effects of administration and subsequent withdrawal of procyclidine HCL (Chouinard, DeMontigny and Annable, 1979). All patients were without antiparkinsonian agents for three weeks before the onset of the study. Then, the neuroleptic dosages were kept constant and the subjects completed a two-week trial, one week with 30 mg of procyclidine daily and one week without it. The presence of procyclidine significantly decreased parkinsonism and increased

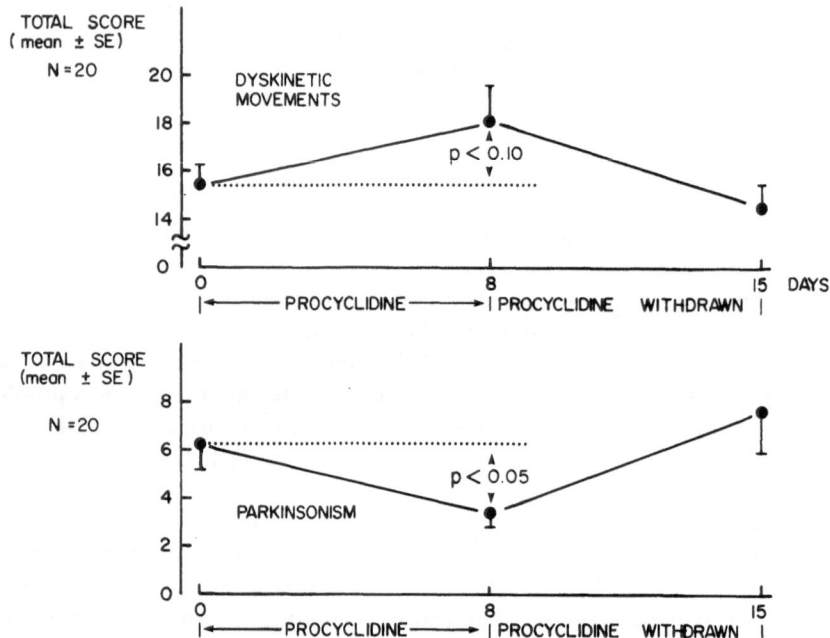

Figure 1. Weekly mean total score for tardive dyskinesia and parkinsonism of the Extrapyramidal Symptom Rating Scale in patients treated with procyclidine and withdrawn from procyclidine.

tardive dyskinesia. When procyclidine was withdrawn, the parkinsonism reverted to its original state and the dyskinesia diminished. Figure 1 illustrates the parallel but inverse relationship between the dyskinesia and the parkinsonism. These findings are consistent with the dopamine supersensitivity hypothesis of tardive dyskinesia. The exacerbation of dyskinesia by procyclidine may be accounted for by its dopamine reuptake blocking property and/or its central anticholinergic activity, which exaggerates the dopaminergic-cholinergic imbalance. The study also shows the reversibility of this effect after short-term administration. As there is evidence that early signs of tardive dyskinesia may be reversible (Chouinard and Bradwejn, 1982; Quitkin et al., 1977), uncovering the syndrome with central anticholinergic drugs may aid in its detection and prevention at its onset.

In another study, 24 patients were placed on neuroleptics plus bupropion, a weak dopamine re-uptake inhibitor, or placebo. Bupropion was found to be equivalent to placebo in its effect upon extrapyramidal symptoms. Patients remained on this drug regimen for 37 to 65 days and the procyclidine was

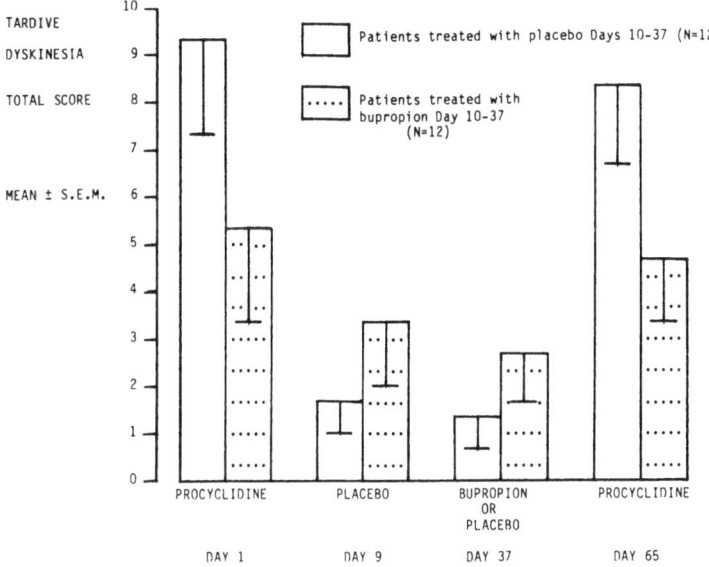

Figure 2. Course of tardive dyskinesia during bupropion trial for patients treated with bupropion or placebo as measured by weekly mean total scores. Patients were treated before and after with procyclidine.

restarted for two weeks at previous levels. During the placebo washout, and the later bupropion or placebo period, the masking effect of neuroleptics acted to diminish dyskinetic movements. The exacerbation of dyskinesia by anticholinergics was found to be completely reversible, and did not exceed the severity manifested during previous antiparkinsonian treatment (Figure 2). Ratings for bucco-lingual-masticatory (BLM) syndrome and choreoathetoid movements of extremities were examined separately. There was a similar pattern of exacerbation and reversibility regardless of the region of the body involved. However, the masking effect of the neuroleptics or the uncovering effect of the antiparkinsonian agents appeared more important for the abnormal movements of the extremities. This suggests that reversibility is more likely to occur in the dyskinetic movements of the limbs than those involving the mouth, tongue and jaw.

In a third study of 12 weeks duration, ethopropazine was compared to benztropine in the treatment of neuroleptic-induced parkinsonism (Chouinard, Annable and Ross-Chouinard, 1979a). While ethopropazine and benztropine were equally effective in controlling these symptoms, only benztropine-treated patients had a significant increase in tardive dyskinesia. The magnitude of exacerbation by benztropine is related to its greater anticholinergic potency, a fact confirmed by greater atropinic peripheral side effects, such as dry mouth, constipation and blurred vision, in benztropine-treated patients. Overall, neither drug increased the incidence of tardive dyskinesia, which is in agreement with our previous epidemiological study (Chouinard, Annable and Ross-Chouinard, 1979b). In animal studies, prolonged administration of anticholinergics did not increase the incidence of tardive dyskinesia (Christensen and Nielsen, 1979). Thus, central anticholinergic drugs appear as a prototype of type I drug factor which increases the clinical manifestation of the disorder but not its overall incidence.

Dopamine Agonist and Precursor. L-dopa is known to induce reversible dyskinesia in idiopathic parkinsonian patients. However, its effect on neuroleptic induced extrapyramidal symptoms is not as well documented. L-dopa was at first discarded following uncontrolled studies which reported that it was ineffective and exacerbated psychotic symptoms (Yaryura-Tobias, Wolpert, Dana, and Merlis, 1970) Several controlled studies (Gerlach and Luhdorf, 1975; Inanaga et al., 1972) have found a therapeutic effect for L-dopa given in association with neuroleptics in the treatment of schizophrenia. Alpert and Friedhoff suggested the use of L-dopa in the prevention of tardive dyskinesia through a possible desensitization effect, and published encouraging results (Alpert and Friedhoff, 1976).

In order to reassess the effect of L-dopa, we undertook a study including twenty schizophrenic inpatients, who were first gradually withdrawn from their antiparkinsonian medication and then stabilized on fluphenazine HCl (Chouinard, Annable and Jones, 1980). Ten patients were allocated randomly to each of two treatments: placebo or prolopa (L-dopa 100 mg and benserazide 25 mg), for a period of three weeks and then given the standard anticholinergic drug, procyclidine. L-dopa significantly reduced both parkinsonism and the positive symptoms of schizophrenia in comparison with placebo but aggravated tardive dyskinesia. When procyclidine was substituted, there was a return to previous psychopathology in L-dopa patients. The procyclidine also increased the dyskinetic movements in both groups but caused an earlier and more intense response in the prolopa-treated patients. It appears that L-dopa has a differential effect on dopamine receptors in the neostriatal and mesolimbic systems after short-term administration. In the neostriatum, L-dopa failed to desensitize the dopamine receptors. Further research would be needed to clarify whether more prolonged use of L-dopa treats tardive dyskinesia (we have undertaken a long-term study to this effect). In the mesolimbic region of the brain, where positive symptoms of schizophrenia originate, L-dopa appears to alter dopamine receptor responses. L-dopa, in association with neuroleptics, may represent a form of prevention if not treatment for supersensitivity psychosis. The exacerbation of psychosis by L-dopa described previously has two possible explanations. First, in studies where neuroleptics were replaced by L-dopa the symptoms produced may be due to the action of L-dopa on already sensitized dopamine receptors (Chouinard et al., 1978; Chouinard and Jones, 1980). Second, L-dopa may induce a toxic psychosis superimposed on the schizophrenic illness rather than cause a relapse of the original illness (Alpert and Friedhoff, 1976).

Animal studies provide further information concerning dopamine agonists. These drugs increase the stereotyped behavior in rats, possibly due to stimulation of the sensitized postsynaptic receptor (Veith, 1977; Carey and DeVeaugh-Geiss, 1982; Waddington and Gamble, 1980). In addition, dopamine agonists might prevent the development of dopamine receptors supersensitivity associated with neuroleptic use (Christensen and Nielsen, 1979) and reverse this disorder when induced by reserpine (Ezrin-Waters and Seeman, 1978). Investigations of dopamine agonists suggest an important role for them in clinical management and in understanding the biology of schizophrenia and of neuroleptic-induced supersensitivity disorders.

Neuroleptic Drugs. We propose a new classification of neuroleptic drugs. This concept was derived from three double-blind controlled studies comparing chlorpromazine with diphenylbutylpiperidine neuroleptics in the treatment of 113 acute schizophrenic patients and from an epidemiological survey including 261 patients on long-term maintenance treatment. In accordance with our previous model of risk factors for tardive dyskinesia, we divide neuroleptics into two types. Type I neuroleptics are associated with milder and more reversible tardive dyskinesia, while type II are associated with severe and irreversible forms.

At this stage, we consider estrogens and diphenylbutylpiperidines, both relatively specific postsynaptic receptor blocking agents, to be type I neuroleptics. Furthermore, we hypothesize that estrogen acts as an endogenous weak neuroleptic and that its dopamine antagonist activity accounts for the differences in male and female schizophrenics regarding therapeutic response, onset, severity of illness and prevalence of tardive dyskinesia. Such a theoretical explanation seemed indicated in view of the reports of two major epidemiological studies of a greater prevalence of severe forms of tardive dyskinesia among men from 20 to 67 and among women beyond that age range. The premenopausal woman benefits from the potentiation of neuroleptic activity by hormones with a better response to treatment, but suffers from more complete masking of tardive dyskinesia. As estrogen levels decline, the true extent of denervation supersensitivity manifests itself. An anticholinergic challenge or an abrupt decrease of dopamine blocking agents is not as effective in women in an early recognition of this disorder. Since reversibility is dependent upon immediate diagnosis and management, women are at risk for a more persistent form of this condition. In fact, the symptoms of tardive dyskinesia were masked in 80% of one population administered estrogens (Villeneuve, Czaejust and Cote, 1980).

In an animal study, Raymond et al. (1978) demonstrated the potent nature of this estrogen activity. Prior incubation of pituitary cells with estradiol resulted in a 35 to 45% increase in basal prolactin release and almost completely reversed dopamine agonist inhibition. Fields and Gordon (1982) reported that estradiol, administered to rats after neuroleptic withdrawal, was associated with a decrease in the number of dopamine receptors toward control levels. The increase in receptor density induced by chronic haloperidol administration was substantially prevented. In addition, when a course of estradiol was administered to the rats and then withdrawn, an initial suppression was followed by an augmentation in stereotypy. This receptor supersensitivity is similar to the one observed during neuroleptic withdrawal.

We suggest that estrogens have a high ratio of postsynaptic/presynaptic dopamine receptor blockade that permits a compensatory presynaptic effect. With increasing age, this compensatory phenomenon loses its intensity, permitting overt expression of tardive dyskinesia, particularly in those women receiving neuroleptics but also in the elderly female population in general. Consequently, the drug of choice for women of childbearing age is one which specifically blocks postsynaptic dopamine receptors and allows presynaptic activity to occur, such as pimozide or fluspirilene. In our opinion, standard neuroleptics with a low post to presynaptic ratio are not particularly suitable for female patients. Prescribing neuroleptics to women over 40 may be contraindicated due to their susceptibility to develop severe tardive dyskinesia.

The other type I neuroleptics included in our model are the diphenylbutylpiperidines which have been consistently found to differ from the classical neuroleptics. We examined the effect of pimozide and chlorpromazine in 40 newly admitted schizophrenic patients (Chouinard and Annable, 1982) and found pimozide had less of an effect on the acute symptoms of schizophrenia, even at high doses (70 mg/day). This may be explained by a strong dopamine blockade at postsynaptic receptors and weak effect upon presynaptic receptors in comparison with other neuroleptics (Walters and Roth, 1976). The ability of the classical neuroleptics, such as chlorpromazine, to block both pre- and post-synaptic receptors is thought to lead to a temporary increase in dopamine turnover followed by a decrease due to an apparent depolarization inhibition. The eventual decrease in dopamine in the synaptic cleft brought about by these drugs is considered to be responsible for their delayed onset of action and for the development of supersensitivity phenomena such as a decline in parkinsonian symptoms with time and the emergence of tardive dyskinesia. If pimozide has only a weak effect on presynaptic receptors, it may not deplete dopamine to as great an extent as neuroleptics which block both pre- and postsynaptic receptors. Pimozide may therefore be less efficacious in the treatment of the acute phase of the illness during which positive symptoms such as hallucinations and thought disturbance predominate, but in the long run may induce less postsynaptic receptor supersensitivity and consequently less tardive dyskinesia than the classical neuroleptics. A weak effect upon presynaptic dopamine blockade may protect against the development of tardive dyskinesia by a mechanism similar to estrogens. Women, in fact, required less pimozide to achieve a therapeutic response than men. In regard to tardive dyskinesia, pimozide patients demonstrated levels equivalent to chlorpromazine despite higher amounts of anticholinergic agents. These findings support the view that pimozide administration leads to less of a supersensitivity phenomenon.

In another double-blind controlled study (Chouinard, Annable and Denis, 1980) including 40 newly admitted schizophrenic patients, similar findings were obtained with another diphenylbutylpiperidine, fluspirilene: 1) a higher proportion of females with a favorable response to the drug; 2) more parkinsonian side effects in the acute treatment; 3) greater need for anticholinergic antiparkinsonian drug without a significant effect on the manifestation of tardive dyskinesia. In an earlier study comparing penfluridol to chlorpromazine, we also found penfluridol to be less efficacious for the most acutely ill patients (Chouinard and Annable, 1976). In conclusion, the diphenylbutylpiperidines differ from classical neuroleptics in their limited effect upon receptors other than dopamine, in their specificity for postsynaptic receptors, in their greater effectiveness in women than men and in a diminished tendency to induce supersensitivity suggested by less tardive dyskinesia despite more anticholinergic agents. However, they are not specific in any region of the brain.

Type II neuroleptics have been divided into two classes. The first class includes high potency neuroleptics, such as haloperidol or fluphenazine, which are more specific for dopamine receptors and are the ideal treatment during the acute stage of the illness. The second class includes low potency neuroleptics, such as chlorpromazine or thioridazine, which block numerous receptors (cholinergic, muscarinic, alpha-adrenergic, H_1 histaminic, H_2 histaminic and serotoninergic) as well as dopamine. We conducted a study to further investigate the differences between these two classes, in which 26 chronic schizophrenic outpatients receiving low potency antipsychotic agents gradually converted to equivalent doses of high potency neuroleptics (Chouinard et al., unpublished). The incidence of tardive dyskinesia in the population (N = 17) treated with low potency neuroleptics was 76%, compared with 54% for those (N = 48) on high potency neuroleptics and 67% for those receiving both. The trend in favor of a higher incidence of tardive dyskinesia in those managed with low potency neuroleptics may be due to a simultaneous blockade of both cholinergic and dopaminergic receptors. The effect seems similar to a challenge with antiparkinsonian agents in the neuroleptic-treated patients. Another explanation for the increased incidence is the relatively stronger presynaptic blocking activity of these low potency neuroleptics in contrast with high potency drugs. This may result in the formation of greater numbers of new synapses, permanent structural changes in the brain and a type II irreversible tardive dyskinesia. In addition, the low potency neuroleptics, having strong anticholinergic properties, were associated with a high incidence of withdrawal symptoms (85%) that makes patients reluctant to discontinue their use. Complete withdrawal of low potency medication was achieved in only nine patients over a period of two years. They may consequently be open to abuse in a way similar to that reported for the anticholinergic antiparkinsonian drugs (Smith, 1980). These rebound phenomena may also make it difficult for the minimum therapeutic dosage to be achieved, thus exposing the patient to an unnecessary risk of long-term side effects, such as tardive dyskinesia.

Patient (Host) Factors: Epidemiological Studies

Although various groups of investigators have carried out epidemiological studies of tardive dyskinesia (Fann et al., 1972; Jus et al., 1976; Asnis et al., 1977; Gardos et al., 1977; Bell and Smith, 1978; Smith et al., 1978; Jeste et al., 1978; Gardos et al., 1980; Ezrin-Waters and Seeman, 1981; Mukherjee et al., 1982), there is little consensus as to the prevalence and etiology of the disorder. Most of the recent studies report an incidence of 30 to 40% in patients undergoing long-term neuroleptic therapy, though estimates have varied by as much as 0.5 to 56%. Factors that obviously need to be considered when assessing this wide variation in the reported prevalence rate are differences in study populations, the lack of uniformity of diagnostic definition and the varying skills of raters in identifying the disorder. We think that differences in neuroleptic regimens and in the times of evaluations may also be critical factors responsible for these discrepancies. Unfortunately, none of the previously mentioned studies took into account the time of the last dose of neuroleptics and antiparkinsonian medication. For instance, patients on a QID neuroleptic regimen may show less tardive dyskinesia than those on a once-a-day regimen (Jeste, Olgiati and Chali,

Table 2.   Variables Significantly Related to Presence of Tardive Dyskinesia According to Stepwise Logistic Regression Analysis.

Variable	Significance
Age	$p < .001$
Days in hospital	$p = .03$
CGI therapeutic effect	$p = .05$
Fluphenazine treatment	$p = .03$
Parkinsonism total score (negatively related)	$p = .06*$

*$p = .03$ when score for tremors is excluded from parkinsonism total score; $p = .02$ when scores for tremors and akathisia are excluded from parkinsonism total score. (From Chouinard et al., *Am. J. Psychiatry* 136(1):79–83, 1979.)

Table 3. Variables Contributing Significantly to Multiple Regression
Relationship with Total Score for Tardive Dyskinesia,*
As Entered by Stepwise Inclusion.

	Significance	Multiple Correlation Coefficient	Partial Correlation Coefficient
All patients included (n=261)			
Age	p<.001	.29	.29
CGI therapeutic effect	p = .003	.34	.19
Parkinsonism total score			
(negatively related)	p = .026	.37	-.14
Fluphenazine treatment	p = .013	.39	.15
Days in hospital	p = .050	.41	.12
Sex (male)	p = .049	.43	.12
Only tardive dyskinesia patients (n=80)			
Brain damage	p = .003	.33	.33
CGI therapeutic effect	p = .045	.39	.23
Age	p = .089	.43	.19
Parkinsonism total score			
(negatively related)	p = .079	.47	-.20
Sex (male)	p = .077	.50	.20

*Scores for tremors and akathisia are excluded from total score for parkinsonian symptoms.
(From Chouinard, Annable, Ross-Chouinard et al., *Am. J. Psychiatry* 136(1):79–83, 1979.

1977) if the latter are evaluated when the drug concentrations are declining. Similarly, there may be a tendency for patients treated with long-acting neuroleptics to show more dyskinetic movements toward the end of their injection interval (Chouinard et al., 1979b).

Age. Many of the studies attempting to identify the factors contributing to the development of the disorder are flawed by univariate statistical analyses which do not consider the possible interrelationships between the explanatory variables (Chouinard and Annable, unpublished). However, most investigators (using a variety of statistical techniques) confirm that the risk of tardive dyskinesia increases with age. This may be related to changes in dopamine receptor sensitivity that occur in elderly patients. In our own survey of tardive dyskinesia in 261 schizophrenic outpatients whose neuroleptic maintenance therapy was under rigorous control, stepwise multiple logistic regression analysis determined age to be the variable most closely linked to the occurrence of the disorder (Tables 2 and 3) (Chouinard et al., 1979b). It has also been proposed that the older the patients when first started on neuroleptics, the more likely they are to develop tardive dyskinesia (Chouinard et al., 1979b). Furthermore, the elderly display an increased sensitivity to regular doses of neuroleptics and a greater tendency toward toxicity. Animal studies, in which neuroleptics were administered to various age groups, found significantly greater behavioral stereotypy in the elderly than the younger population on the same regimen (Smith and Lucavathi, 1980). It appears valid to include advancing age among factors which lead to an irreversible form of the disorder. Smith and Baldessarini reviewed the subject and concluded also that age was the most significant factor in the development of tardive dyskinesia (Smith and Baldessarini, 1980).

Poor Drug Responders. Other factors found to be associated with a higher incidence of the disorder were longer records of hospitalization and poor therapeutic response (Tables 2 and 3) (Chouinard et al., 1979b). Kucharski et al. (1980) reported less tardive dyskinesia in discharged schizophrenia patients than in the non-discharged group, which supports our finding that therapeutic response may be an important variable. Thus, patients with poor prognosis, defined as having poor therapeutic response or longer stays in hospital, are more likely to develop tardive dyskinesia independent of their age. These same patients may have an abnormal CAT scan and more severe dopamine deficiency in the mesolimbic, and to a lesser extent in the neostriatal, regions of the brain (Chouinard and Jones, 1978). The administration of high doses over prolonged periods is not recommended for patients with poor prognosis schizophrenia.

Parkinsonian Symptoms. The inverse relationship between tardive dyskinesia and parkinsonian symptoms has been discussed by other authors, but not studied in epidemiological surveys. Crane (1968, 1973) has reported that severe tardive dyskinesia is seldom observed in patients with severe parkinsonism and vice versa. In our clinical experience, the patient with tremors or akathisia may manifest tardive dyskinesia, whereas a patient with akinesia and rigidity does to a lesser extent. It is possible that the hyperkinetic parkinsonian symptoms of tremor and akathisia are precursors of tardive dyskinesia and may be used as early predictors of risk. In contrast, the hypokinetic parkinsonian symptoms of rigidity and akinesia could mask this disorder. Thus, tardive dyskinesia will be more difficult to diagnose in the early phases in this group of patients and will be more likely to progress to the irreversible type II form.

History of Brain Damage. In earlier surveys, tardive dyskinesia was found to be more prevalent in patients with a history of brain damage (Crane, 1973). In our study, previous brain damage tended to be present in the more severe cases of tardive dyskinesia but was not implicated in the appearance of the disorder, thus suggesting that initially only the most severe forms were reported. Since these forms are incapacitating, a history of brain damage would be a relative contraindication for neuroleptic treatment.

Gender. Previous investigations reported a higher incidence of tardive dyskinesia in female patients, but there is some evidence that this may be age-related. In our study of patients aged 19 to 67 years, we found a higher mean incidence of the disorder (Chouinard et al., 1979b). When Smith and Dunn (1979) initially examined their data it appeared that there was an overall higher prevalence in female patients between 20 and 91 years, but on reanalysis severe forms were more prevalent in men up to age 67, after which they were more common in women. We have suggested that these age and sex differences in the prevalence of tardive dyskinesia may be related to the hormonal status of women (Chouinard, Annable, Jones and Ross-Chouinard, 1980). It has been shown that estradiols have dopamine antagonist activity. Until menopause, estrogen may "coat" the dopamine receptors, potentiating the effect of the neuroleptic in the neostriatum and resulting in less tardive dyskinesia than in male patients. However, after menopause such protection would disappear and this might lead to a greater degree of dopaminergic supersensitivity and greater vulnerability to tardive dyskinesia than in men of a comparable age.

Type of Neuroleptics. Fluphenazine in both depot and oral preparations has also been associated with a high prevalence of tardive dyskinesia (Gardos et al., 1977; Smith et al., 1978). Although a higher incidence of tardive dyskinesia among patients treated with depot neuroleptics has been found, this is probably related to length of the interval between injections and the timing of evaluations. In our study all patients were rated at the end of the injection period, when neuroleptic concentrations are expected to be low (Chouinard et al., 1979b). Unfortunately, other studies do not mention the time between the injection and the day of evaluation. There is some evidence suggesting that diphenylbutylpiperidines would tend to induce less tardive dyskinesia (Gardos et al., 1980; Gibson, 1978).

Drug Holidays. Another important issue is the effect of drug holidays. It has been suggested that drug holidays reduce the incidence of tardive dyskinesia. However, Jeste et al. (1979) presented evidence disputing this belief. In any case, complete drug holidays are clinically impossible for most patients and we prefer to think in terms of minimal therapeutic dose.

SUPERSENSITIVITY PSYCHOSIS

The adverse behavioral reactions associated with neuroleptics have been divided recently by Hollister (1982) into the following four categories: toxic confusional state, akinetic depression, akathisic agitation and supersensitivity psychosis. Only the latter will be discussed here since the first one is related to

anticholinergic effects, the akinesia-depression and akathisia agitation to dopamine receptor blockade, while only the last one is due to supersensitivity
receptor phenomenon. One way to help to understand supersensitivity psychosis
is to compare it with tardive dyskinesia.

Description

Tardive dyskinesia and supersensitivity psychosis share a common history.
In both instances, there has been a reluctance to believe in their existence and a
tendency to underestimate the incidence. In fact, supersensitivity psychosis is
presently in this phase, whereas a 30 to 40% incidence of tardive dyskinesia has
been generally accepted. There are difficulties associated with the diagnosis of
supersensitivity psychosis (Chouinard, 1982). Psychotic symptoms are nearly the
same as the disease process itself: the distinctions being that only positive symptoms of schizophrenia are exhibited, that the symptoms parallel neuroleptic drug
administration, and that the relapses occur more rapidly than would be expected
from the normal course of the illness. Similarly, symptoms of tardive dyskinesia
could be mistaken for mannerisms of schizophrenia, hyperkinetic parkinsonian
side effects (akathisia or tremors), and normally occurring senile choreid
movements.

As with tardive dyskinesia, clinical symptoms are masked by neuroleptics.
Since all the neuroleptics presently available have prolonged half-lives, the recognition of the disorder is difficult (Chouinard and Jones, 1982). One would
predict that metaclopramide, a short-acting dopamine receptor blocking agent,
when given in doses effective in treating schizophrenia, would give clear evidence
of supersensitivity relapse upon abrupt withdrawal. Swedish investigators have
reported several cases of supersensitivity psychosis following withdrawal of
clozapine (Ekholm, Eriksson and Lindstrom, 1981), a drug with a short half-life
and a greater affinity for mesolimbic than striatal dopamine receptors.

The nature of the neuroleptic profile may obscure the diagnosis. The low
potency neuroleptic, known to block alpha-adrenergic, cholinergic, serotonergic
and histaminergic receptors, produces rebound cholinergic activity upon its
cessation which interferes with the expression of psychotic symptoms. This may
explain the higher incidence of supersensitivity psychosis reported in the literature among patients treated with the more potent neuroleptics. We observed
supersensitivity psychosis in approximately 30% of 300 schizophrenic outpatients administered high potency neuroleptics without attempts at abrupt drug
withdrawal.

Finally, both disorders are identified most readily when the patients are
under stress. In regard to tardive dyskinesia, increased concentration, motor
activity or anxiety augments the involuntary movements. In regard to supersensitivity psychosis, the most potent stressors are the activities of the patients'
normal lives, difficult to recreate in hospital settings.

Diagnosis

The criteria required for diagnosis of this syndrome are listed in Table 4. The inclusion criteria consist of: 1) a history of relatively prolonged exposure to neuroleptic drugs; 2) a close association of the symptoms with changes in neuroleptic dosages; 3) tolerance to the antipsychotic effect of medication; 4) an exacerbation of the disorder by stress or alcohol intake; and 5) rapid improvement with treatment unless severe tolerance has occurred. The exclusion criteria consist of patients in the acute phase of the illness or suffering continuous psychosis.

Mechanism

The two supersensitivity disorders are thought to be caused by alteration of dopamine receptors secondary to prolonged neuroleptic antagonist activity at these sites. Tardive dyskinesia appears to result from changes occurring in the neostriatum, whereas supersensitivity psychosis is more likely to be a consequence of receptors alterations in the mesolimbic system. In animal studies, there is evidence of induction of receptor supersensitivity in the mesolimbic system by long-term neuroleptic treatment (Seeger and Gardner, 1979). In postmortem brain studies, dopamine receptor binding sites have been found to be increased in these regions and to correlate with length of previous neuroleptic treatment (Owen et al., 1979).

Both syndromes may be explained by a common mechanism. Initially, chemical denervation of the postsynaptic membranes produces postsynaptic receptor proliferation. This is followed by "sprouting," that is, new synaptic bouton appearance, in the presynaptic receptor. Sprouting leads to the formation of new synaptic structures. The increased numbers of new synapses may induce permanent postsynaptic neuronal overactivity. Staton and Brumback (1980) explained the stages of reversibility in terms of this conceptual model. Stage I refers to the early period of dopamine neurotransmission blockade, when the supersensitivity disorder disappears completely following cessation of neuroleptic therapy. In this phase, neuronal overactivity is due to excessive receptor numbers without reinnervation sprout connections and is reversible. Stage II neuronal overactivity would be present once sufficient reinnervation synapses have developed to produce irreversible alteration of brain structure and function. Stage IIA refers to covert irreversible neuronal overactivity in which the supersensitivity disorder appears and improves after cessation of drug therapy but leaves residual symptoms. The amelioration is explained by the disappearance of receptors not in contact with new synaptic boutons. Stage IIB refers to overt irreversible neuronal activity in which the dyskinesia or psychosis appears during treatment and results in permanent impairment despite cessation. In this

Table 4. Criteria for Supersensitivity Psychosis

I.   History of receiving neuroleptics or antipsychotics for at *least 6 months*

II. A) Patient has had a *decrease or discontinuation* of medication

    1) has shown appearance of psychotic symptoms within *6 weeks for oral* medication
       or
    2) *3 months for i.m. medication*

  or

  B) Has had *no decrease or discontinuation* of medication during treatment

    1) has shown *greater frequency of relapse* with time
       and/or
    2) *tolerance* to the antipsychotic effect of the neuroleptic

III. At least 2 of the following criteria for definite and 1 for probable

  A) *Those who had a decrease of medication*

    1) psychotic symptoms upon decrease of medication were:
       i) *not previously seen*
         or
       ii) are of *greater severity*
    2) patient has shown *greater frequency* of relapse with time
    3) *tolerance* to the antipsychotic effect
    4) *tardive dyskinesia* is present (a standard examination must be used)
    5) *rapid improvement* of psychotic symptoms when the effective neuroleptic dose is increased after a decrease or discontinuation of medication
    6) patient has shown clear exacerbation of psychotic symptoms by *stress*
    7) if patient is treated *only with i.m. long-acting*, has shown appearance of psychotic symptoms at *the end of the injection interval*

  or

  B) Those who had no decrease of medication (only one required if II.B)i) + II.B)ii)

    1) *tardive dyskinesia* is present (a standard examination is required)
    2) patient has shown clear exacerbation of psychotic symptoms by *stress*
    3) if patient is treated *only with i.m. long-acting*, has shown appearance of psychotic symptoms at *the end of the injection interval*

IV. *Exclusion* Criteria:

    1) Patients in the *acute phase* of the illness.
    2) Patients with *continued psychotic* illness which did not respond to neuroleptic treatment.

case, sufficient numbers of new synapses have developed and cause moderate to severe clinical disability which responds to neuroleptics. However, such management only perpetuates the process of new synapse formation and should be avoided.

Supersensitivity psychosis appears more readily reversible than tardive dyskinesia through desensitization by a gradual decrease of 5% of the neuroleptic dosage every three to four weeks. Thus, supersensitivity psychosis tends to remain at Stage I in which proliferation of receptors but no synapse formation has occurred. This may be a function of high dopamine turnover in cell bodies of the mesolimbic system (Agnati et al., 1980).

Prognosis

We surveyed the incidence of supersensitivity psychosis in 261 schizophrenic outpatients treated with neuroleptics and found it more frequently among good prognosis than poor prognosis patients. In contrast, when we studied the incidence of tardive dyskinesia in the same population, we found that patients less responsive to neuroleptics (presumably poor prognosis) were more likely to develop tardive dyskinesia (Chouinard et al., 1979b). Overlap of the two syndromes also occurs. In the poor prognosis patient who manifests severe tardive dyskinesia without supersensitivity psychosis, there may no longer be sufficient dopamine available in those regions of the brain involved in the production of positive symptoms of schizophrenia. In cases where the two syndromes overlap, such a dopamine depletion may not exist. Thus, such coexistence may indicate a milder or more reversible form of tardive dyskinesia.

Tolerance

Supersensitivity disorders may be associated with CNS tolerance to the therapeutic effect of neuroleptics. The tolerance is reflected in increasing requirements of medications to maintain the same state of wellbeing. Relapses occur at levels previously sufficient to obtain stability. In a double-blind controlled study (Chouinard, Annable and Ross-Chouinard, 1982) of seven months duration, we compared fluphenazine enanthate with fluphenazine decanoate in the maintenance treatment of 48 schizophrenic outpatients. Before entering the trial, patients underwent a one-month period of stabilization. Twenty-four patients were assigned to each treatment at random and the dosages of either drug were adjusted according to therapeutic response. Twelve patients (50%) treated with decanoate and nine (37.5%) treated with enanthate required gradual increases in dosage. By week 8, there had been significant increases in geometric mean doses of decanoate (range: 2.5 to 250 mg; mean 32.1 mg) and enanthate (range 2.5 to 325 mg; mean: 40.2 mg). Thus, substantial increases in dosage were required to maintain the mean therapeutic effect. Our investigation demonstrates the capacity of humans to develop tolerance to the therapeutic effect of neuro-leptics. Animals, after prolonged exposure to neuroleptics, require increased dosages to block the behavioral effects of apomorphine (Asper et al., 1973; Moller Neilson et al., 1974).

Another study (Capstick, 1980) on neuroleptic withdrawal with fluphena-zine decanoate reports that 80% of their 47 patients relapsed on withdrawal of neuroleptics (half during withdrawal itself and half after withdrawal). The authors report that patients relapsing during withdrawal exhibited significantly more symptoms, different from those of their original illness, than those re-lapsing after withdrawal. In regard to supersensitivity psychosis, an indica-tion of tolerance could be the repeated appearance of symptoms at the end of the injection period, despite the prescription of larger dosages of neuro-leptics.

Other Features for Comparison

Another area for research is the influence of varying hormonal levels during the menstrual cycle upon the supersensitivity disorders. Reports exist of premenstrual exacerbation of schizophrenic symptoms (Glick and Steward, 1980). It could be postulated that the physiological decline in estrogens dimin-ishes dopamine blockade and unmasks a supersensitivity psychosis. If this proves to be the case, avoidance of increasing medications at these times would prevent further structural change in the brain.

Alcohol like estrogen has been found in recent animal studies to serve as a dopamine antagonist and to cause supersensitivity in both the mesolimbic (Engel and Liljequest, 1976) and nigrostriatal systems (Lai et al., 1979). We would like to suggest that patients who are abusers of alcohol are at an increased risk for supersensitivity disorders.

CONCLUSION

Two neuroleptic-induced supersensitivity disorders, tardive dyskinesia and supersensitivity psychosis, have been described, and type I and type II risk factors discussed for tardive dyskinesia. Since tardive dyskinesia can be a severe, disabling, irreversible disorder for which we have no treatment, prevention must be the main objective. Even though supersensitivity psychosis appears more reversible than tardive dyskinesia, if not recognized it may lead to unnecessary neuroleptic drug treatment. Clinical findings, as reported in this paper, lead us to make the following recommendations.

First, it is mandatory to establish the need for maintenance treatment and the minimum therapeutic doses for each patient. This cannot be assessed without recognizing that some symptoms during neuroleptic withdrawal may be related to supersensitivity psychosis. The second recommendation regards the choice of neuroleptic. It is preferable to use drugs that act primarily on post-synaptic dopamine receptor sites (type I neuroleptic), especially in young women with good prognoses. Pimozide and fluspirilene at present most closely satisfy these requirements. Clearly, the characteristics of the host alter the strategy of drug prescription. The patient with a poor prognosis may require high potency neuroleptics (type II) at dosages beyond the recommended therapeutic range, which should be administered only for short periods of time. The elderly and brain damaged patients require minimum therapeutic doses with indications for treatment clearly defined.

Third, careful history and standard neurological examination should be completed at each visit. Special efforts to uncover tardive dyskinesia should be made either with tasks that require concentration or produce stress, or by manipulations of neuroleptics and anticholinergic agents. Augmentation of neuroleptics in an attempt to treat the disorder should be avoided as it perpetuates the denervation process, unless the dyskinesia or illness become life-threatening.

Fourth, it is essential to identify patients with supersensitivity psychosis in order to avoid treating patients for symptoms related to rebound phenomenon. The supersensitivity psychosis is similar in many respects to tardive dyskinesia, especially the type I variety. However, it differs in that it is observed more frequently in good prognosis patients, and appears more reversible. The recognition of this disorder has implications in the clinical management of the patient. The appearance of positive symptoms of psychosis in this context does not require an increase in the dosage of neuroleptics. Injectable long-acting forms of neuroleptics are preferable as they allow early recognition of the syndrome. Reversibility through desensitization requires gradual reduction of the drugs. Should this approach fail, patients should be given antipsychotic agents with other profiles such as the diphenylbutylpiperidines. For those patients who have developed tolerance, we recommend an abrupt switch to the diphenylbutyl-piperidines.

Fifth, the classification of neuroleptics into two types leads to a different approach in the acute treatment of schizophrenia versus the maintenance treatment. Although type II neuroleptics, such as haloperidol or fluphenazine, appear to be the ideal treatment for the acute episode, their long-term use may have to be restricted to subgroups of patients with poor response to type I neuroleptics. Further investigation is needed to document the more irreversible form of supersensitivity psychosis and identify the risk factors involved. Meanwhile, tardive dyskinesia could serve as a model.

REFERENCES

Agnati, L.F., Fuxe, K., Andersson, F., Benfenati, P., Cortelli, D'Alessandro, R. The mesolimbic dopamine system: evidence for high amine turnover and for a heterogeneity of the dopamine neuron population. *Neurosci. Lett.* 18:45–51, 1980.

Alpert, M., and Friedhoff, A.J. Receptor sensitivity modification in the treatment of tardive dyskinesia. *Clin. Pharmacol. Ther.* 19:103, 1976.

Asnis, G.M., Leopold, M.A., Duvoisin, R.C. Schwartz, A.H. A survey of tardive dyskinesia in psychiatric outpatients. *Am. J. Psychiatry* 134:1367–1370, 1977.

Asper, H., Baggraline, M., Burki, H.R. et al. Tolerance phenomena with neuroleptics: catalepsy, apomorphine stereotypes and striatal dopamine metabolism in the rat after single and repeated administration of loxapine and haloperidol. *Eur. J. Pharmacol.* 22:287–294, 1973.

Bell, R.C.H., and Smith, R.C. Tardive dyskinesia: characterization and prevalence in a statewide system. *J. Clin. Psychiatry* 39:39–42, 46–47, 1978.

Capstick, N. Long-term fluphenazine decanoate maintenance dosage requirements of chronic schizophrenic patient. *Acta. Psychiat. Scand.* 61:256–262, 1980.

Carey, R., and DeVeaugh-Geiss, J. Chronic benztropine and haloperidol administration induce behaviorably equivalent pharmacological hypersensitivities separately but not in combination. *Psychopharmacology* 76:341–345, 1982.

Chouinard, G. Neuroleptic-induced supersensitivity psychosis. In: DeVeaugh-Geiss, J., Ed. *Tardive Dyskinesia and Related Involuntary Movement Disorders.* John Wright PSG of Boston, Massachusetts, 1982, pp. 109–115.

Chouinard, G., and Annable, L. Penfluridol in the treatment of newly admitted schizophrenic patients in a brief therapy unit. *Am. J. Psychiatry* 133:820–823, 1976.

Chouinard, G., and Annable, L. Pimozide in the treatment of newly admitted schizophrenic patients. *Psychopharmacology* 76:13–19, 1982.

Chouinard, G., Annable, L., and Denis, J.F. Fluspirilene in the treatment of acute schizophrenia. Scientific Proceedings of the 30th Annual Meeting of the Canadian Psychiatric Association, Toronto, Ontario, No. 86, pp. 77–78, 1980.

Chouinard, G., Annable, L., Jones, B.D. L-dopa in drug-induced extrapyramidal symptoms. Synopsis, 12th C.I.N.P. Congress (Collegium Internationale Neuropsychopharmacologicum), Goteborg, Sweden, p. 106, 1980.

Chouinard, G., Annable, L., Jones, B.D., Ross-Chouinard, A. Sex differences and tardive dyskinesia. *Am. J. Psychiatry* 137:507, 1980.

Chouinard, G., Annable, L., Ross-Chouinard, A. Comparison of fluphenazine esters in the treatment of schizophrenic outpatients: extrapyramidal symptoms and therapeutic effect. *Am. J. Psychiatry* 139:312–318, 1982.

Chouinard, G., Annable, L., Ross-Chouinard, A., Kropsky, M. Ethopropazine and benztropine in neuroleptic-induced parkinsonism. *J. Clin. Psychiatry* 40:147–152, 1979a.

Chouinard, G., Annable, L., Ross-Chouinard, A. Nestoros, J. Factors related to tardive dyskinesia. *Am. J. Psychiatry* 136:79–83, 1979b.

Chouinard, G., Bradwejn, J. Reversible and irreversible tardive dyskinesia. *Am. J. Psychiatry* 139:360-362, 1982.

Chouinard, G., De Montigny, C., and Annable, L. Tardive dyskinesia and anti-parkinsonian medications. *Am. J. Psychiatry* 136:228-229, 1979.

Chouinard, G., and Jones, B.D. Schizophrenia as dopamine-deficiency disease. *Lancet* 2:99-100, 1978.

Chouinard, G., and Jones, B.D. Neuroleptic-induced supersensitivity psychosis: clinical and pharmacologic characteristics. *Am. J. Psychiatry* 137:16-21, 1980.

Chouinard, G., and Jones, B.D. Neuroleptic-induced supersensitivity psychosis, the hump course and tardive dyskinesia. *J. Clin. Psychopharmacol.* 2:143-144, 1982.

Chouinard, G., Jones, B.D., and Annable, L. Neuroleptic-induced supersensitivity psychosis. *Am. J. Psychiatry* 135:1409-1410, 1978.

Christensen, A.V., and Nielsen, I.M. Dopaminergic supersensitivity: influence of dopamine agonists, cholinergics, anticholinergics, and drugs used for the treatment of tardive dyskinesia. *Psychopharmacology* 62:111-116, 1979.

Crane, G.E. Dyskinesia and neuroleptics. *Arch. Gen. Psychiatry* 19:700-703, 1968.

Crane, G.E. Persistent dyskinesia. *Br. J. Psychiatry* 122:395-405, 1973.

Ekholm, B., Eriksson, H., and Lindstrom, L. Tardive psychosis: hypothesis or reality. *Lakartidninger* 78:1-5, 1981.

Engel, J., and Liljequest, S. The effect of long-term ethanol treatment on the sensitivity of dopamine receptors in the nucleus accumbus. *Psychopharmacology* 49:247-253, 1976.

Ezrin-Waters, C., and Seeman, P. L-dopa reversal of hyperdopaminergic behavior. *Life Sci.* 22:1027-1032, 1978.

Ezrin-Waters, C., Seeman, M.V., and Seeman, P. Tardive dyskinesia in schizophrenic outpatients: prevalence and significant variables. *J. Clin. Psychiatry* 42:16-22, 1981.

Fann, W.E., Davis, J.M., and Janowsky, D.S. The prevalence of tardive dyskinesias in mental hospital patients. *Dis. Nerv. Syst.* 33:182-186, 1972.

Faurbye, A., Rasch, P.J., Petersen, P.B. Brandborg, G., and Pakkenberg, H. Neurological symptoms in pharmacotherapy of psychoses. *Acta. Psychiatr. Scand.* 40:10-27, 1964.

Fields, J., and Gordon, J. Estrogen inhibits supersensitivity induced by neuroleptics. *Life Sci.* 3:229-234, 1982.

Gardos, G., Cole, J.O., and La Brie, R.A. Drug variables in the etiology of tardive dyskinesia application of discriminant function analysis. *Prog. Neuropsychopharmacol.* 1:147-154, 1977.

Gardos, G., Samu, I., Kallos, M., and Cole, J.O. Absence of severe tardive dyskinesia in Hungarian schizophrenic out-patients. *Psychopharmacology* 71:29-34, 1980.

Gerlach, J., and Luhdorf, K. The effect of L-dopa on young patients with simple schizophrenia, treated with neuroleptic drugs. *Psychopharmacology* 44:105-110, 1975.

Gibson, A.C. Depot injections and tardive dyskinesia. *Br. J. Psychiatry* 132:361-365, 1978.

Glick, I., and Steward, D. A new drug treatment for premenstrual exacerbation of schizophrenia. *Compr. Psychiatry* 21:281-287, 1980.

Hollister, L.E. Drugs for schizophrenia. *Rational Drug Therapy* 16(8):1–6, 1982.
Inanaga, K., Inoue, K., Tachibana, H., Oshima, M., and Kotorii, T. Effect of L-dopa in schizophrenia. *Folia Psychiatr. Neurol. Jpn.* 26:145–157, 1972.
Jeste, D.V., Olgiati, S.G., and Chali, A.Y. Masking of tardive dyskinesia with four times-a-day administration of chlorpromazine. *Dis. Nerv. Syst.* 38: 755–758, 1977.
Jeste, D.V., Potkim, S.G., Sinha, S., Feder, S., and Wyatt, R.J. Tardive dyskinesia—reversible and persistent. *Arch. Gen. Psychiatry* 36:1080–1082, 1979.
Jus, A., Pineau, R., Lachance, R., Pelchat, G., Jus, K., Pires, P., and Villeneuve, R. Epidemiology of tardive dyskinesia, Part I. *Dis. Nerv. Syste.* 37:210–214, 1976.
Klawans, H.L. The pharmacology of tardive dyskinesia. *Am. J. Psychiatry* 130: 82–86, 1973.
Kucharski, L.T., Smith, J.M., and Dunn, D.D. Tardive dyskinesia and hospital discharge. *J. Nerv. Ment. Dis.* 168:215–218, 1980.
Lai, H., Makous, W.L., Houta, A., and Lenog, H. Effects of ethanol on turnover and function of striatal dopamine. *Psychopharmacology* 61:1–9, 1979.
Moller, N.I., Fayalland, B., Pedersen, V. et al. Pharmacology of neuroleptics upon repeated administration. *Psychopharmacologia (Berl)* 34:95–104, 1974.
Mukherjee, S., Rosen, A.M., Cardenas, C., Varia, V., and Olarte, S. Tardive dyskinesia in psychiatric outpatients. *Arch. Gen. Psychiatry* 39:466–469, 1982.
Owen, F., Cross, A.J., Crow, T.J. et al. Increased dopamine receptor sensitivity in schizophrenia. *Lancet* 2:223–226, 1979.
Quitkin, F., Rifkin, A., Gochfeld, L., et al. Tardive dyskinesia: are first signs reversible? *Am. J. Psychiatry* 134:84–87, 1977.
Raymond, V., Beaulieu, M., Labrie, F., and Boissier, J. Potent antidopaminergic activity of estradiol at the pituitary level on prolactin release. *Science* 200: 1173–1175, 1978.
Schonecker, M. Ein eigentumliches syndrom im oralen bereich bei megaphen applikation. *Nervenarzt* 28:35, 1957.
Seeger, T., and Gardner, E. Enhancement of self-stimulation in rats and monkeys after chronic neuroleptic treatment: evidence for mesolimbic supersensitivity. *Brain Res.* 175:49–57, 1979.
Simpson, G.M., Varga, E., Lee, J.H., and Zoubok, B. Tardive dyskinesia and psychotropic drug history. *Psychopharmacology* 58:117–124, 1978.
Smith, J.M. Abuse of the antiparkinson drugs: a review of the literature. *J. Clin. Psychiatry* 41:351–354, 1980.
Smith, J.M., and Baldessarini, R.J. Changes in prevalence, severity, and recovery in tardive dyskinesia with age. *Arch. Gen. Psychiatry* 37:1368–1373, 1980.
Smith, J.M., and Dunn, D.D. Sex differences in the prevalence of severe tardive dyskinesia. *Am. J. Psychiatry* 136:1080–1082, 1979.
Smith, J.M., Kucharski, L.T., Eblen, C., Knutsen, E., and Linn, C. An assessment of tardive dyskinesia in schizophrenic outpatients. *Psychopharmacology* 64:99–104, 1979.
Smith, R.C., and Lucavathi, D.E. Behavioral and biochemical effects of chronic neuroleptic drugs: interaction with age. In: W.E. Fann, R.C. Smith, J.M. Davis, et al., Eds. *Tardive Dyskinesia: Research and Treatment.* Spectrum Publications, Jamaica, N.Y., 1980, pp. 65–88.

Smith, R.C., Strizich, M., and Klass, D. Drug history and tardive dyskinesia. *Am. J. Psychiatry* 135:1402-1403, 1978.

Staton, D., and Brumback, R. Neuroleptic-induced reinnervation sprouting in the central nervous system. *J. Clin. Psychiatry* 41:427-428, 1980.

Veith, K. Comparison of behavioral supersensitivity to apomorphine after fluphenazine dehydrochloride and fluphenazine decanoate treatment in rats. *Prog. Neuropsychopharmacol.* 1:289-295, 1977.

Villeneuve, A., Czaejust, T., and Cote, M. *Neuropsychobiology* 6:145-151, 1980.

Waddington, J., and Gamble, S. Neuroleptic treatment for a substantial proportion of adult life: behavioral suquelae of 9 months haloperidol administration. *Eur. J. Pharmacol.* 67:363-369, 1980.

Walters, J.R., and Roth, R.H. Dopaminergic neurons: an in vivo system for measuring drug interactions with presynaptic receptors. *Arch. Pharmacol.* 296: 5-14, 1976.

Yaryura-Tobias, J.A., Wolpert, A., Dana, L., and Merlis, S. The action of L-dopa on schizophrenic patients. *Curr. Ther. Res.* 12:528-531, 1970.

14

The Implications of Cerebral Ventricular Size for Neuroleptic Therapy of Schizophrenia

DANIEL R. WEINBERGER

The role of neuroleptic drugs in the treatment of schizophrenia is still evolving even after thirty years of experience with these agents. Early claims that neuroleptics were curative or specifically anti-schizophrenic have been tempered by adoption of more rigorous diagnostic and outcome measures and by increasing awareness of long-term toxicities. At the present time, the following conclusions about the therapeutic role of neuroleptic drugs seem justified: 1) they provide symptomatic benefit for most but not all psychotic patients and are rarely if ever curative; 2) they are more effective in ameliorating positive or accessory psychotic symptoms such as hallucinations, delusions, thought disorder and agitation then negative symptoms such as flat affect, withdrawal, diminished motivation, etc. (Crow, 1980); 3) their efficacy in treating positive psychotic symptoms is not restricted to schizophrenia but is diagnostically nonspecific. This is consistent with the widespread use of neuroleptics in patients with affective and organic psychoses.

For schizophrenic patients whose most disabling symptoms are "positive," these drugs offer marked benefit. Unfortunately, for many chronic schizophrenic patients, it is the negative symptoms that prove most disabling Such patients may live free of institutional care for longer periods while re   ng neuroleptic agents, but they often remain severely impaired.

The fact that some patients derive great benefit from neuroleptic therapy while others fail to do so is testimony to the biological and probably etiological heterogeneity of schizophrenia. It has prompted a search for factors or mech-anisms that might contribute to this broad spectrum of clinical responsiveness. A number of such factors have been proposed, including specific symptom profiles (Houlihan, 1977), pre-morbid social adjustment (Gittleman-Klein and Klein, 1969), various biochemical markers (Meltzer, 1979), EEG findings (Itil, 1980) and more recently cerebral ventricular size (Weinberger et al., 1980). In this presentation we review the implications of cerebral ventricular size for response to neuroleptic therapy in schizophrenia.

CEREBRAL VENTRICULAR SIZE IN CHRONIC SCHIZOPHRENIA

The claim that schizophrenic patients have larger cerebral ventricles than do normal individuals was first made over fifty years ago in a pneumoencephal-ography study (Jakobi and Winkler, 1927). Similar findings have been reported by other investigators using both pneumoencephalography (PEG) and recently computed tomography (CT). The evidence from PEG has been reviewed else-where (Weinberger and Wyatt, 1982a). It includes several controlled studies reporting large ventricles in schizophrenic patients, especially those with a chronic, unremitting form of illness. The evidence from CT is more extensive and more credible. Table 1 summarizes the results of recent controlled CT studies. These reports provide compelling evidence for what is probably one of the most consistently replicated biological findings in psychiatry. Only those studies meeting the following criteria were included in the table: blind compari-son of CT scans of schizophrenic and control subjects scanned on the same machine with identical procedures; and, use of quantitative measures for deter-mining ventricular size. These inclusion criteria obviate problems inherent in impressionistic CT "readings" and comparisons to controls from the literature or from different CT machines. A more detailed discussion of the reports cited is provided elsewhere (Weinberger et al., 1983).

The results of the studies listed support the following conclusions about ventricular size in schizophrenia:

1) Schizophrenic patients as a group have significantly larger cerebral ventricles than do healthy, normal individuals, including their own siblings and discordant twins.

2) In a minority of cases, the frequency of which varies probably accord-ing to the clinical characteristics of the sample, ventricular size outside the normal range for age is seen.

3) Ventricular enlargement is not the result of psychiatric treatment as it is found in first episode schizophreniform patients.

With the exception of only two controlled studies, the evidence is fairly consistent. What the two negative studies indicate most probably is that some samples of patients will by chance alone include only small ventricle patients. This is consistent with the fact that most schizophrenic patients do not have abnormal ventricular size. Even in those whose ventricles are enlarged, the degree of enlargement is mild (Weinberger et al., 1979a). Yet an unresolved issue is whether ventricular enlargement is a characteristic of a distinct subgroup of patients or whether ventricular size is normally distributed in schizophrenia with the entire distribution shifted upwards. There is support for both possibilities and neither can be excluded at the present time (Weinberger et al., 1983).

One approach that has been taken to the question of whether ventricular enlargement occurs in a distinct subtype is to treat this parameter as an independent variable and compare patients with and without it. The results have been surprisingly fruitful and suggest that patients with enlarged ventricles are more homogeneous and, in general, more severely impaired. Specifically, schizophrenic patients with enlarged ventricles have significantly more negative symptoms, more cognitive-neuropsychological deficits, more other neurological signs, and a different profile of biochemical markers (Weinberger and Wyatt, 1982b). These findings lend support for the notion that ventricular enlargement is a characteristic of a separate subgroup of patients. It is not conclusive evidence, however. It might also simply reflect a threshold phenomenon. In other words, patients might be more or less affected by a similar pathological process that produces large ventricles, but only in extreme cases do the clinical differences described become significant. This explanation also applies to differences in neuroleptic drug responsiveness to be reviewed next.

CEREBRAL VENTRICULAR SIZE AND RESPONSE TO TREATMENT

An association between ventricular enlargement and poor response to treatment was suggested by earlier PEG studies, especially a well-controlled study by Haug (1962). Another pneumoencephalographer, Huber, reported that ventricular enlargement found early in the course of illness predicted a poor outcome at follow-up twenty years later (Huber, 1979).

A recent CT study has provided further evidence for a link between ventricular size and response to neuroleptic drugs. Weinberger et al. (1980) studied twenty chronic schizophrenic inpatients on NIMH research wards. Each patient had completed a neuroleptic therapy response protocol involving a four week drug-free period and an eight week period of standard neuroleptic treatment. During these periods, clinical psychopathology ratings were compiled by blinded nursing staff. A comparison of ratings following the drug-free and treatment periods served as a quantitative measure of the degree of response. For the purposes of the study, patients were divided into two groups on the basis of the CT scans. One group (N = 10) consisted of patients whose ventricles were within

Table 1. Controlled CT Studies of Cerebral Atrophy

Study	Sample	Results
Johnstone et al. (1976)	17 chronic schizophrenics 8 normal controls	Larger cerebral ventricles in schizophrenics than in controls (p < .01)
Weinberger et al. (1979a,b)	60 chronic schizophrenics 62 normal controls	Ventricles and cortical sulci significantly larger in patients than in controls
Mundt et al. (1980)	68 chronic schizophrenics 69 symptomatic medical patients	No difference in linear measurements of third ventricle or frontal horn span
Weinberger et al. (1981)	10 chronic schizophrenics 12 non-schizophrenic controls (all siblings of the patients)	No abnormalities in siblings, ventricles of patients significantly larger
Pearlson and Veroff (1981)	22 schizophrenics 16 manic-depressives 35 psychiatric controls	11 schizophrenics with evidence of atrophy 4 manic-depressives with atrophy (varied with age) 0 controls with atrophy
Tanaka et al. (1981)	49 schizophrenics 38 medical controls	Significantly enlarged ventricles in patients over 40-years-old
Andreasen et al. (1982)	52 subchronic schizophrenics 47 psychiatric and neurologic controls	Ventricle size significantly increased in schizophrenic group with a bimodal distribution

Study	Sample	Findings
Okasha and Madkour (1982)	42 schizophrenics 39 normal controls	Significantly larger third and lateral ventricles in patients
Reveley et al. (1982)	22 normal MZ twinships 16 normal DZ twinships 7 MZ twinships discordant for schizophrenia	Schizophrenics significantly larger ventricles than normals and than their discordant co-twins
Takahashi et al. (1982)	169 schizophrenics 169 matched volunteers	Significantly larger ventricles and more cortical atrophy in patients
Nyback et al. (1982)	46 psychotic patients 41 schizophrenic 19 firstbreak patients 46 volunteer controls	Significantly larger third and lateral ventricles found in both acute and chronic psychotic patients
Nasrallah et al. (1982)	55 chronic schizophrenics 27 controls	Significantly larger ventricles in schizophrenic patients
Jernigan et al. (1982)	30 schizophrenics 30 volunteers	No significant difference in ventricular size or sulcal fluid volume
Weinberger et al. (1982)	35 schizophreniform patients 17 chronic schizophrenics 23 affective disorder patients 27 other psychiatric patients 26 neurological controls	Ventricular size increased significantly only in schizophreniform and chronic schizophrenic disorders

two standard deviations of the mean of a normal control sample and the other of patients whose ventricular size exceeded this limit. The groups turned out to be very well matched for a number of factors which might have affected drug-response, including age, age at onset of illness, years of illness and hospitalization, drug dosage, and plasma neuroleptic concentrations. After the four week drug-free period, the two groups did not differ significantly in mean psychopathology ratings. After drug therapy, however, the psychopathology ratings between the groups were significantly different. The small ventricular patients were less symptomatic and showed a more homogeneous response pattern. Among the large ventricles patients, response was variable with as many patients deteriorating as improving. The results of the study strongly suggested that ventricular size was a factor related to treatment response.

We are presently in the process of completing a second study of this phenomenon. To date, twenty-five new patients have been evaluated in a more rigorously controlled, double-blind design. All schizophrenic patients admitted to the NIMH research wards of the Adult Psychiatry Branch at Saint Elizabeths Hospital enter the study. After a two to four week acclimatization phase, each patient completes a six week placebo period and then six weeks of treatment with haloperidol at a dose of 0.4 mg/kg. Psychopathology ratings are completed daily by blinded nursing staff. Twenty-five new patients not included in the earlier study have completed this new study. Because we have liberalized our inclusion criteria for accepting patients in the research program, this study includes a broader clinical spectrum of patients who are generally less impaired than those previously studied in our laboratory. This change is reflected in the reduced frequency of patients whose ventricular size is outside the two standard deviation limit. Of the twenty-five patients who have completed the new study, six exceed this limit. If the data analysis is done as in the earlier study, the patient groups are lopsided. Nevertheless, the results, though preliminary, show a strong trend ($p < 0.1$) consistent with the findings from the first study. The difference is significant ($p < 0.05$) if covariance for initial values is performed. If the patients are divided for comparison into those above versus those below the mean for this sample, the results also are significant at the 0.05 level. It appears, therefore, that larger ventricles are associated with poorer response.

One other group of investigators have reported a study of ventricular size and treatment response and the results are similar. Schultz et al. (1982) studied 10 schizophrenic patients ill for less than two years with BPRS ratings before and after treatment. Six of ten patients had enlarged ventricles by criteria similar to those of Weinberger et al. (1980). The two worst responders had the largest ventricles, while the two best responders had the smallest. Furthermore, ventricular size and degree of response correlated at $r = 0.61$, $p = 0.06$, and mean response between the two groups was significant at the less than 0.1 level.

These studies obviously require further replication. In the meantime, they stand as evidence that ventricular size is a factor in the response of schizophrenic patients to neuroleptic therapy. This does not mean that patients with large ventricles will not respond to such treatment and should not receive neuroleptics. In fact, since the response difference between patients with larger and small ventricles is relative, not absolute, the findings have no direct clinical significance. The choice of drug treatment requires a clinical judgment, irrespective of enlarged ventricles. In this regard, the relationship of ventricular size and treatment response is more a research than clinically meaningful finding.

The research implications of the findings bear mainly on the dopamine hypothesis of schizophrenia. The findings suggest that the psychopathology of schizophrenic patients with large ventricle is less related to dopaminergic mechanisms. By contrast, small ventricles patients may be more homogeneous in terms of dopamine and psychopathology. A series of studies have supported this notion by showing that the dopamine hypothesis appears to be more relevant in patients with small ventricles. We have reviewed this area elsewhere (Weinberger and Wyatt, 1982b).

Finally, the drug response findings also support the hypothesis that schizophrenic patients with large ventricles are a separate subgroup. It is tempting to hypothesize, furthermore, that a specific pathological process related to the pathogenesis of schizophrenia underlies the CT abnormality and that dopaminergic mechanisms are a secondary phenomena. This idea is similar to the "two-factor theory" of schizophrenia proposed by Davis (1974). Against this idea, however, is the fact that nothing specific can be inferred from either ventricular enlargement or its relationship to treatment response. Ventricular enlargement itself is nonspecific and is found in association with numerous other conditions. It is not a lesion but a sign, a sign that something pathological has happened or is happening in the brain. The specific meaning of the sign can only be determined if its etiology is known.

Even its role in response to neuroleptics cannot be imputed to a specific process in schizophrenia. As discussed earlier, a threshold phenomenon cannot be ruled out. Ventricular enlargement may be only one of several risk factors for the pathogenesis of schizophrenia. As such, it might, particularly if extreme, affect treatment response even if not the critical pathogenic factor. This appears to be the case for Parkinson's disease where poor response to L-dopa has been associated with ventricular enlargement (Schneider et al., 1979). There is also one study of elderly patients with affective disorders that found on association between large ventricles and poor outcome (Jacoby et al., 1981).

These questions are fertile ground for further investigation. The available data permit the following conclusions, none of which have clear implications for clinical treatment: enlarged ventricles are associated with schizophrenia, enlarged ventricles are associated with several clinical parameters observed in schizophrenic patients, and ventricular size is a factor affecting the response of schizophrenic patients to neuroleptic drugs.

REFERENCES

Andreassen, N.C., Smith, M.R., Jacobs, C.G., et al. (1982). Ventricular enlargement in schizophrenia: Definition and Prevalence. *Am. J. Psychiatry* 139: 274-278.

Crow, T.J. (1980). Molecular pathology of schizophrenia: More than one disease process? *Br. Med. J.* 280:66-68.

Davis, J.M. (1974). A two factor theory of schizophrenia. *J. Psychiatr. Res.* 11: 25-29.

Gittleman-Klein, R., and Klein, D.F. (1969). Premorbid asocial adjustment and prognosis in schizophrenia. *J. Psychiatr. Res.* 7:35-53.

Houlihan, J.P. (1977). Heterogeneity among schizophrenic patients: Selective review of recent findings (1970-1975). *Schizophrenia Bull.* 3:246-258.

Huag, J.O. (1962). Pneumoencephalographic studies in mental disease. *Acta Psychiatr. Scand.* (Suppl. 165) 38:1-114.

Huber, G. (1979). Pure defect and its meaning for a somatosis hypothesis of schizophrenia. In *Biological Psychiatry Today*, J. Obiols, C. Ballus, E. Lonzales and J. Pujol, eds. Elsevier, North-Holland, pp. 345-350.

Itil, T.M. (1980). Computer-Analyzed electroencephalogram to predict the therapeutic outcome in schizophrenia, in *Perspectives in Schizophrenia Research*, C.F. Baxter, T. Melnechuk, eds., New York: Raven Press (1980), pp. 61-75.

Jacobi, W., Winkler, H. (1927). Encephalographische studien au chronisch schizophrenien. *Arch. Psychiat. Nervenkr.* 81:299-332.

Jacoby, R.J., Levy, T., Bird, J.M. (1981). Computed tomography and the outcome of affective disorders: A follow-up study of elderly patients. *Br. J. Psychiatry* 139:288-292.

Jernigan, T.L., Zatz, L.M., Moses, J.A., Berger, P.A. (1982). Computerized measures of cerebral atrophy in schizophrenics and normal volunteers. *Arch. Gen. Psychiatry* 39:765-770.

Johnstone, E.C., Crow, T.J., Frith, C.D. (1976). Cerebral ventricular size and cognitive impairment in chronic schizophrenia. *Lancet ii*:924-926.

Meltzer, H.E. (1979). Biology of schizophrenia subtypes: A review and proposal for method of study. *Schizophrenia Bull.* 5:460-479.

Mundt, C.H., Radie, W., Gluck, E. (1980). Computer tomographische untersuchungen der liqvorraume an chronisch schizophrenen patienten. *Nervenarzt* 51:743-748.

Nasrallah, H.A., Jacoby, C.G., McCalley-Whitters, M., Kuperman, S. (1982). Cerebral ventricular enlargement in sub-types of chronic schizophrenia. *Arch. Gen. Psychiatry* 39:774-777.

Nyback, H., Hindmarsch, T., Greitz, T., Sedvall, G. (1982). Computed tomography of the brain in patients with acute psychosis and in healthy volunteers. *Acta Psychiatr. Scand.* 65:403-414.

Okasha, O., and Modkour, O. (1982). Cortical and central atrophy in chronic schizophrenia: A controlled study. *Acta Psychiatr. Scand.* 65:29-34.

Pearlson, G.D., and Veroff, A.E. (1981). Computerized tomographic scan changes in manic-depressive illness. *Lancet ii*:470.

Reveley, S.M., Reveley, M.A., Clifford, C.A., Murray, R.M. (1982). Cerebral ventricular size in twins discordant for schizophrenia. *Lancet i*:540-541.

Schneider, E., Fischer, P.-A., Jacobi, P., Becher, H., Berger, M. (1979). Cerebral atrophy and long-term response to levodopa in Parkinson's disease. *J. Neurol.* 222:37-43.

Schultz, S.G., Sinicrope, P., Koller, M., Kishore, P., Friedel, R.O. (1982). Treatment response and ventricular brain ratio in young schizophrenic patients. Presented at the 37th Annual Meeting of the Soc. Biol. Psychiatr., Toronto, May 14, 1982.

Tanaka, T., Hazama, H., Kawahara, R., Kobayashi, K. (1981). Computerized tomography of the brain in schizophrenic patients. *Acta Psychiatr. Scand.* 63:191-197.

Takahashi, R., Inaba, K., Kato, N., Kumashiro, H., Nishimura, T., Okuma, T., Otsuki, S., Sakai, T., Sato, T., Shimazone, T. (1982). CT scanning and the investigation of schizophrenia. In *Biol. Psychiatry* (1981), B. Jansson, C. Perris, G. Struve, eds. Elsevier, North-Holland, Amsterdam, pp. 259-268.

Weinberger, D.R., Bigelow, L.B., Kleinman, J.E., Klein, S.T., Rosenblatt, J.E., and Wyatt, R.J. (1980). Cerebral ventricular enlargement in chronic schizophrenia: Association with poor response to treatment. *Arch. Gen. Psychiatry.*

Weinberger, D.R., DeLisi, L.E., Neophytides, A.N. and Wyatt, R.J. (1981). Familial aspects of CT abnormalities in chronic schizophrenic patients. *Psychiatry Res.* 4:65-71.

Weinberger, D.R., DeLisi, L.E., Perman, G., et al. (1982). CT scans in schizophreniform disorder and other acute psychiatric patients. *Arch. Gen. Psychiatry* 39:778-783.

Weinberger, D.R., Torrey, E.F., Neophytides, A.N. and Wyatt, R.J. (1979a). Lateral cerebral ventricular enlargement in chronic schizophrenia. *Arch. Gen. Psychiatry* 36:735-739.

Weinberger, D.R., Torrey, E.R., Neophytides, A.N. and Wyatt, R.J. (1979b). Structural abnormalities of the cerebral cortex in chronic schizophrenia. *Arch. Gen. Psychiatry* 36:935-939.

Weinberger, D.R., Wagner, R.J. and Wyatt, R.J. (1983). Neuropathological studies of schizophrenia: A selective review. *Schiz. Bull.* 9:193-212.

Weinberger, D.R. and Wyatt, R.J. (1982a). Cerebral morphology in schizophrenia: *In vivo* studies. In *Schizophrenia as a Brain Disease*, F. Henn, H. Nasrallah, eds. Oxford University Press, England, pp. 148-175.

Weinberger, D.R. and Wyatt, R.J. (1982b). Cerebral ventricular size: A biological marker for sub-typing chronic schizophrenia, in *Biological Markers in Psychiatry and Neurology*, P.I. Hanin, E. Usdin, eds. Pergamon Press, Ltd. New York, pp. 505-512.

15

Clinical Significance
of Neuroleptic Plasma Levels

Stephen H. Curry

In a related contribution in this volume, the desirable pharmacokinetic data base relevant to the use of neuroleptics in emergency psychiatry was reviewed and found to be deficient. In this paper, the relationship between neuroleptic plasma levels and response is reviewed, and proposals are made for further research. This area was last reviewed three or four years ago and this paper is concerned with bringing the older reviews up to date (Curry, 1980; Curry, 1982; Cohen et al., 1980; Kurland et al., 1980; Morselli and Zarifian, 1980; Tune and Coyle, 1981).

In considering the plasma level effect relationship, it is necessary to consider three areas: (1) occurrence of acute effects of little or no relevance to psychiatric illness; (2) the time course of plasma levels, the illness, and the drug response; and (3) the concept of a therapeutic range.

OCCURRENCE OF ACUTE EFFECTS

The acute effects of neuroleptic drugs include sedation, postural hypotension, anticholinergic effects and extrapyramidal symptoms. Together, these can give the patient a feeling of general malaise. A weak correlation of effects of this type and plasma levels of chlorpromazine was demonstrated in some of the earliest studies in the field. More recently, a strong relationship between fluphenazine plasma levels and patient reports of side effects was demonstrated in experiments comparing fluphenazine enenthate and fluphenazine decanoate. It is important to realize however that these studies concern effects which provide no

239

guide as to the future therapeutic outcome. They are believed to be mediated by mechanisms other than those involved in the antipsychotic effect of neuroleptic drugs, and attempts to assess changes in psychotic symptoms in relation to pharmacokinetic measurements after single doses have not been made.

TIME CONSIDERATIONS

The various studies which have examined the change in psychopathology with time after institution of neuroleptic drug therapy have shown a steady improvement in rating scores over a period of six weeks,. This effect is especially evident in newly diagnosed, relatively young schizophrenics. Although successful treatment sets in immediately after the dosing starts, most authorities agree that clinical improvement is rarely detected until two or three days of drug treatment have elapsed. It is important to realize that this has been noticed in patients given either a fixed dosage regimen for six weeks, or a regimen starting with low doses, followed by a gradual increase in dosage until clinical judgement indicates that the maximum possible therapeutic result is being obtained together with the minimal levels of unwanted effects. No studies have employed loading doses, largely because of the need to minimize unwanted effects, especially during the early stages of treatment. Higher doses are possible later because tolerance to these unwanted effects develops.

It also must be realized that, on all regimens (at least with chlorpromazine) enzyme induction causes the plasma level per unit of dose to decrease. If the dosage is unchanged, the mean plasma level declines from about the eighth day of treatment, settling to a relatively constant level by about six weeks after starting treatment. Thus clinical improvement can occur concomittantly with a reducing drug level. Attempts to explain this by means of active metabolite theories have been unsuccessful. Remarkably, this has led some psychiatrists to reject completely any theory of plasma level significance. They should have realized that as the disease improves there could be a diminished need for the drug. In other words, patient sensitivity varies as the illness progresses, and, not surprisingly, the longitudinal relationship within is complex.

THERAPEUTIC RANGES

In a general sense, there is a U-shaped relationship between therapeutic outcome and plasma levels of the drugs. However, the middle, useful range is very wide. At lower levels, patients are unsuccessfully treated. At higher levels, they either experience unwanted effects with bad to poor scores on psychiatric rating scales, or they actually experience induction of psychosis by the drugs, perhaps, due to massive central anticholinergic effects. Because of the time course considerations mentioned in the previous section, each patient is likely to be at a different point in the progression of illness and drug response, and this is the reason for the wide desirable range. Few studies in the field have controlled this factor. When it is controlled in the future, the desired range will probably become narrower, especially if future studies can be concerned with concentrations of the drugs in plasma water, rather than in whole plasma. These considerations may account for positive correlations between level and effect observed only in the first two weeks after instituting treatment.

SPECIFIC EXAMPLES

Chlorpromazine seems to have a desirable therapeutic range of 35 to 350 ng^{-1} ml in plasma. There is a spurious negative correlation between levels of chlorpromazine sulfoxide and clinical outcome, due to the fact that poor responders receive high doses, have high first-pass effects, and accumulate this metabolite. One group has reported a general lack of correlation and has emphasized the speed of response as the most important consideration (May et al., 1981; Sedvall, 1981; Van Putten et al., 1980; 1981).

Fluphenazine has a wide desirable range of 0.2-2.8 ng ml^{-1}, with a higher incidence of unwanted effects at higher levels, although one group of investigators expresses the general view of higher doses leading to higher levels and better results (Dysken et al., 1981; Sakalis and Traficante, 1981).

Haloperidol has a desirable range of 8-17.7 ng ml^{-1}, although it has been suggested that clinical effect requires trough or pre-dose levels of approximately 10 ng ml^{-1}, with peak, or post-dose levels of 20 ng ml^{-1}, causing a high incidence of extrapyramidal problems. There is also a strong correlation between haloperidol concentrations and prolactin levels. Furthermore, a correlation has been shown between acute dystonia and red cell levels, not suggesting that receptors for acute dystonia are found in red cells, but that red cells are a useful model (Evans, 1981; Itoh et al., 1980; Magliozzi et al., 1981; Meltzer et al., 1981; Rubin et al., 1980; Vaisanen et al., 1981).

None of the correlation studies have been conducted in relation to emergency psychiatry and rapid neuroleptization. However, there is a loading dose study reported in the literature. In this study, one group of patients received standard dosing and would have exhibited the standard plasma level rise towards steady state. A second group received a loading dose, so that drug exposure was much higher in the earlier days of treatment. Interestingly, both groups had approximately the same level after a while and approximately the same BPRS score. Unfortunately, no ratings were conducted at a time relevant to emergency psychiatry.

Among the other drugs, with butaperazine, chronic non-responders had lower peak levels compared with newly admitted schizophrenics, who showed better responses. A U-shaped clinical pharmacokinetic relationship with red cells and not plasma has been noted (Casper et al., 1980). With thioridazine, there is no correlation with level or effects and prolactin (Crammer, 1980; Papadopoulos et al., 1980). Also, with this drug, correlations between levels and effects are weak, but there is evidence for a "sulforidazine barrier." Sulforidazine is an important metabolite of thioridazine. Above 0.135 ng ml^{-1}, five out of six patients were successfully treated. Below this level, nine out of ten were poor responders. Finally, thiothixene levels after a test dose were positively correlated with future outcome as assessed by the BPRS (Bolvig-Hannsen et al., 1981; Yesavage, 1982).

CONCLUSION

Existing information has little relevance to emergency psychiatry. Basic research is needed into the kinetics of neuroleptic drugs in the emergency room, and of pharmacological responses including manifestations of antipsychotic effects as a function of pharmacokinetic variables. The techniques for this now exist, and the objective of clarification of these problems should be pursued immediately.

REFERENCES

Bolvig-Hannsen, L., Larsen, F.F., and Vestergard, P. Plasma levels of perphenazine (Trilafon) related to development of side effects. *Psychopharmacol.* 74:306-309 (1981).
Casper, R., Garver, D.L. Dekirmenjian, H., Chang, S., and Davis, J.M. Phenothiazine levels in plasma and red blood cells. *Arch. Gen. Psychiatry* 37:301-395 (1980).
Cohen, B.M., Lipinski, J.F., Pope, H.G., Harris, P.Q., and Altesman, R.I. Neuroleptic blood levels and therapeutic effect. *Psychopharmacol.* 70:191-193 (1980).
Crammer, J.L. Antipsychotic agents: Thioridazine; pharmacokinetics, plasma levels, and clinical response. In: *Psychotropic Drugs: Plasma Concentration and Clinical Response.* G.D. Burrows and T.R. Norman, eds. New York, Marcel Dekker 1981, pp. 303-318.
Curry, S.H. Methodological pitfalls; the influence of experimental design on results. In: *Drug Concentrations in Neuropsychiatry* (Ciba Foundation). Amsterdam, Excerpta Medica (1980), pp. 35-49.
Curry, S.H. Assessment of Psychotropic Drugs Following Acute Doses: I. *Pharmacodynam. Pharmacokinet.* These proceedings, in press, (1982).
Curry, S.H. Applied clinical pharmacology of schizophrenia. In: *Schizophrenia; Diagnosis and Treatment.* S.R. Hirsch and P.B. Bradley, eds. Oxford, OUP in press (1982).
Dysken, M.W., Javaid, J.I., Chang, S.S., Schaffer, C., Shaid, A., and Davis, J.M. Fluphenazine pharmacokinetics and therapeutic response. *Psychopharmacol.* 73:205-210 (1981).

Evans, L. Butyrophenones: plasma levels and therapeutic effect. In: *Psychotropic Drugs: Plasma Concentration and Clinical Response*. G.D. Burrows and T.R. Norman, eds. New York, Marcel Dekker, 1981, pp. 243–286.

Itoh, H., Yage, G., Ohtsuka, N., Iwamura, K., and Ichikawa, K. Serum level of haloperidol and its clinical significance. *Prog. Neuropsychopharmacol.* 4:717–183 (1980).

Kurland, A.A., Nagaraju, A., and Hanlon, T.E. The dopamine radioreceptor assay—a clinical application. *J. Clin. Pharmacol.* 20:191–193 (1980).

Magliozzi, J.R., Hollister, L.E., Arnold, K.V., and Earle, G.M. Relationship of serum haloperidol levels to clinical response in schizophrenic patients. *Am. J. Psychiatry* 138:365–367 (1981).

May, R.R.A., Van Putten, T., Jenden, D.J., Yale, D., and Dixon, W.J. Chlorpromazine levels and the outcome of treatment in schizophrenic patients. *Arch. Gen. Psychiatry*, 38:202–207 (1981).

Meltzer, H.Y., Busch, D.A., and Fang, V.S. Effect of neuroleptics on serum prolactin levels in relation to clinical response and neuroleptic blood levels. In: *Clinical Pharmacology in Psychiatry*. E. Usdin, ed. New York, Elsevier, 1981, pp. 251–168.

Morselli, P.L., and Zarifian, E. Clinical significance of monitoring plasma levels of psychotropic drugs. In: *Drug Concentrations in Neuropsychiatry* (Ciba Foundation). Amsterdam, Excerpta Medica (1980), pp. 115–139.

Papadopoulos, A.S., Chand, T.G., Crammer, J.L., and Lader, S. A pilot study of plasma thioridazine and metabolites in chronically treated patients. *Br. J. Psychiatry* 126:591–596, 1980).

Rubin, T.T., Forsman, A., Neykants, J., Owman, R., Tower, B., and Michiels, M. Serum haloperidol determinations in psychiatric patients. *Arch. Gen. Psychiatry* 37:1069–1074 (1980).

Sedvall, G. Correlations between clinical biochemical and pharmacokinetic data in chlorpromazine-treated patients. In: *Clinical Pharmacology in Psychiatry*. E. Usdin, eds. New York, Elsevier, 1981, pp. 243–249.

Sakalis, G., and Traficante, L. Antipsychotic agents: Fluphenazine. In: *Psychotropic Drugs: Plasma Concentration and Clinical Response*. G.D. Burrows and T.R. Norman, ed. New York, Marcel Dekker, 1981, pp. 287–301.

Tune, L. and Coyle, J.T. Acute extrapyramidal side effects: serum level of neuroleptics and anticholinergics. *Psychopharmacology* 75:9–15 (1981).

Tune, L.E., Creese, I., Depaulo, J.R., Slavney, P.R., and Snyder, S.H. Neuroleptic serum levels measured by radioreceptor assay and clinical response in schizophrenic patients. *J. Nerv. Ment. Dis.* 169:60–63 (1981).

Vaisanen, K., Vuikari, M., Rimon, R., and Raisanen, P. Haloperidol, thioridazine and placebo in mentally subnormal patients—serum levels and clinical effects. *Acta Psychiat. Scand.* 63:262–265 (1981).

Van Putten, T., May, P.R.A. and Jenden, D.J. Does a plasma level of chlorpromazine help?: *Psychol. Med.* 11:729–734 (1981).

Van Putten, T., May, P.R.A., Jenden, D.J., Cho, A.K., and Yale, C., Plasma and saliva levels of chlorpromazine and subjective response. *Am. J. Psychiatry* 137:1241–1242 (1980).

Yesavage, J.A., Becker, J. Werner, R.D., et al. Serum level monitoring of thiothixene in schizophrenia: acute single dose levels at fixed doses. *Am. J. Psychiatry* 139:174–178 (1982).

Only recent publications are listed. For older literature, see Curry, 1980 and citations in publications listed.

16

The Clinical Utility
of Plasma Neuroleptic Levels

BRUCE M. COHEN

INTRODUCTION

Determinations of neuroleptic levels in blood are now available through a variety of commercial laboratories. As there is great interest and increasing clinical use of these levels, it is important to ask how they can be interpreted. Do they correlate with clinical effects? Theoretically, there is little reason to expect a strong correlation. There are too many confounding factors separating a level in blood from neuroleptic action in brain. Has any utility been demonstrated for neuroleptic levels? In fact, when correlations between blood levels of neuroleptic and effect have been sought in clinical studies, the results of even the most careful studies available have been equivocal. For these reasons, detailed later, the skeptical use of blood levels of neuroleptic must be advised until larger and better studies are completed.

THEORETICAL CONSIDERATIONS

The advantages of knowing neuroleptic levels in blood, if such levels correlate with or predict clinical effects, are clear. The blood level of medication, rather than dose, which is a poor predictor of response (Baldessarini, 1977), could be used to adjust the medication regimen into the therapeutic range. This could be done early in treatment, thereby eliminating the waiting otherwise necessary in evaluating the efficacy of a given neuroleptic dose. Furthermore,

245

blood levels could be used to identify instances in which neuroleptic doses were excessive and toxic. Without direct evidence of an excess of drug in tissue, such toxicity (especially that due to akathisia, akinesia, and confusion) can be mistaken for symptoms of the underlying illness (Baldessarini, 1977). Finally, long-term toxicity (e.g. tardive dyskinesia) which may be due to excess exposure, might be reduced.

However, it is important to recall that the range of levels which clinical laboratories report for the purpose of comparison are usually the average neuroleptic levels seen in a sampling of patients. They do not represent the results of carefully designed studies of the relationship between blood levels and clinical effect. Can they be taken as an estimate of the therapeutic range? To do so, one must assume that there is a meaningful relationship between neuroleptic level in blood and clinical effect.

While it seems obvious that very low levels of drug should be associated with little therapeutic effect, moderate levels should be associated with a good therapeutic effect and tolerable side effects, and high levels should be associated with toxicity, there is a surprisingly small likelihood of such a correlation being generally true. For such a correlation to be true, the following conditions must all be met:

   1) Drug measured in blood must be a good reflection of drug at its active site in brain. If it is not, then there is no reason why levels in blood should predict clinical effects.

Unfortunately, neuroleptic distribution is complex, and drug in blood bears no simple physical relationship to drug in brain. Drug in blood is usually measured as total plasma or erythrocyte bound neuroleptic. Each is related to neuroleptic in brain only through the fraction of drug which is free in plasma (Mayer and Guttman, 1968; Freedberg et al., 1979). Free neuroleptic in plasma is a small part of total plasma neuroleptic and cannot be reliably measured. The relationship of free drug to the often measured bound drug is dependent on multiple plasma proteins which are known to vary from person to person and to change through time (Piafsky et al., 1978). In turn, free drug in plasma has a poorly established relationship with drug in brain. The relationship of drug in brain to drug at its active site is unknown. How much drug is available at the active site may depend most highly on what is in local tissue stores (e.g. lipids) (Bickel, 1974). This pool of drug need not be in equilibrium with drug in blood or even in the rest of the brain. Thus, no stable relationship between drug measured in blood and its activity in brain is to be expected.

   2) Metabolites must either not be important in drug effect or must not be variable in amount or distribution between patients or across time.

Alternatively, it must be possible to estimate metabolites in blood and weigh their importance. If metabolites are important, but their concentration, distribution, and activity cannot be adequately estimated, then what is measured in blood will bear little relationship to what is active in brain.

Unfortunately, most neuroleptics appear to have important active metabolites, and even techniques which can detect the presence of these metabolites cannot account for their distribution (Bickel, 1974; Lader, 1976). Thus, what is measured in blood may be a poor reflection of what is active in brain.

3) Drug sensitivity must be similar between patients and remain similar through time. If sensitivity is not a constant, the same blood or brain level of medication may have very different effects in different individuals or even the same individual at different times.

Unfortunately, evidence from animal studies (Campbell et al., 1980) and observations on patients (Baldessarini, 1977) suggest that sensitivity to the effects of neuroleptics is quite variable both from individual to individual and from one time to another. Thus, no meaningful comparison of neuroleptic levels can be expected, and it may not be possible to establish a therapeutic range.

4) Neuroleptic drugs must have a relatively direct effect related to drug concentration at their site of action. If the effects of neuroleptics are indirect (e.g. due to compensatory mechanisms in the brain as has been suggested for some psychoactive agents) then transient levels in the blood or even at the active site may be irrelevant to the degree of drug effect.

Unfortunately, there is little reason to think that neuroleptic effects are direct, especially as these effects are not immediate on drug institution and as symptoms may not reappear soon after withdrawal (Baldessarini, 1977). Thus, a blood or even tissue level of neuroleptic may bear little relation to ultimate drug effect.

5) Blood levels of a drug and its active metabolites, as sampled at a particular time, must bear a good relationship to total exposure to drug. That is, there must be something reliable and representative about a blood level.

Unfortunately, the actual events which occur following drug ingestion are that blood levels rise and fall strikingly. In addition, drug absorption, distribution, and metabolism are quite likely in considerable flux (Cooper et al., 1976). Thus, no sampling time may be a representative sampling time.

Clearly, there is little a priori reason to assume that blood levels predict clinical effects. On the positive side, when the above considerations have been tested, some evidence appears that a blood level drawn many hours after a dose reflects the total of drug absorbed (Davis et al., 1978; Cooper et al., 1976) and that there is a relationship between drug in blood and drug in brain (Jorgensen et al., 1969; Janssen and Allewijn, 1969; Curry et al., 1970; Cohen et al., 1980). However, regarding the bulk of these conditions, there is little to suggest that they are fulfilled. One would be tempted to predict that any relationship of blood level to ultimate clinical effect would be modest at best and hard to demonstrate against the variability of metabolism, distribution, and sensitivity expected between individuals and across time.

It is important to realize that there need be no correlation of neuroleptic blood levels to clinical effects. This keeps one more objective in interpreting studies of such correlations. Still, empirical findings must be examined on their own merit, and there are many studies of neuroleptic levels in blood to be considered.

STUDIES OF THE RELATIONSHIP OF
NEUROLEPTIC BLOOD LEVELS TO CLINICAL EFFECT

Since assays for neuroleptics in blood first became available, there has been a continuing stream of studies attempting to relate blood levels during treatment to therapeutic outcome. These now number well over one hundred. The studies and their findings have been well reviewed by others (Davis et al., 1978; Cooper et al., 1976; May and Van Putten, 1978; Gelder and Kolokowska, 1979). In general, the bulk of the evidence from over a decade of work is contradictory. No consistent correlations are found between blood levels of neuroleptics or their metabolites and therapeutic or side effects.

Is it correct, then, to conclude that there is no demonstrable correlation between blood levels and therapeutic effect. At this time, the answer is no, because the design of most of these studies could have obscured any such correlation (Davis et al., 1978; May and Van Putten, 1978). Most studies were too small and used inhomogeneous groups of patients. The patients were often already in treatment when they entered the studies and many were chronically ill and were apparent poor responders or nonresponders to medication. Almost all of the studies used flexible dose regimens and relatively high doses of medication. Therefore, the bulk of these studies can offer no clear evidence for or against the correlation of blood levels during treatment and clinical effects.

In fact, there are studies which have taken other approaches which imply that such correlations may exist. Studies in animals and patients receiving acute (single) doses of medication provide some of this evidence. In the animal studies, which are few and done with haloperidol, because it may have no active metabolites, blood levels, brain levels, and drug effects on behavior all follow one another quite closely (Campbell et al., 1980; Ohman et al., 1977), a promising finding. Similarly, a small number of studies with patients consistently show that blood levels achieved after a single dose of medication correlate highly with immediate response (Gottschalk et al., 1975; Gottschalk et al., 1976) and eventual response (Gottschalk et al., 1976; May et al., 1979; Sakurai et al., 1980; May et al., 1981; Yesavage et al., 1981) to medication. Furthermore, a few studies on individual patients indicate that patients with very low or high blood levels can be identified and that both groups of patients show improvement when their levels are brought closer to the average (Davis et al., 1978; Curry et al., 1970; Cohen et al., 1980). Taken together, these findings imply that there may be a measurable relationship between blood level and clinical effect which could be demonstrated in properly designed studies.

Before asking if there are such studies, it is worthwhile to review just what design is needed for a study to give meaningful information on the correlation sought. Some of these important aspects of design can be outlined as follows (Davis et al., 1978; May and Van Putten, 1978).

Patients

A) Patients should be drug responders and should not be spontaneous remitters. It has been estimated that roughly 25% of psychotic patients do not respond to medication and that another 25% will remit spontaneously during study (Gottschalk, 1979). In these groups the drug is having no effect or is not responsible for any change seen. Studying blood levels in these patients is as irrelevant as studying penicillin levels in patients with viral pneumonia. Drug free or placebo observation periods are necessary to reduce the number of spontaneous remitters in the study. The use of acutely rather than chronically ill patients is necessary to limit the number of non-responders. Ideally, only patients who once showed a response to medication or who eventually show such a response (this can be determined on follow-up) might be used in the study.

B) Patients should be drug free before study to eliminate the confounding effects of prior treatment. This is especially difficult to accomplish in most settings as patients rarely reach the hospital ward until after some treatment is given in the community or the emergency ward.

C) Patients should be adequately homogeneous by diagnosis or, at least, by syndrome so that the same drug effect is being studied in all subjects. Similarly, homogeneity by age or sex may be necessary to limit variability in drug distribution and metabolism.

D) An adequate number of patients should be studied so that one can find a correlation if it exists or, of equal importance, rule out a meaningful correlation with some certainty if it does not. Small numbers make any such determination unreliable.

Treatment

A) The dose of medication to be used in each patient must be chosen before the patient is evaluated and the study begins. It must be fixed during the study. *This may be the single most important, controllable way in which most studies fail.* If dose is tailored to the individual patient's needs, most patients who are drug responders will receive adequate doses, their blood levels will all be in the therapeutic range, and they will show clinical improvement. Since all of these people will be on the "flat" plateau of the blood level vs. clinical effects curve (see Figure 1), any apparent correlation between level and effect will be lost. Even worse, any patient who is not responsive to medication will receive high doses and have high blood levels but will not improve, while spontaneous remitters will receive low doses, have low blood levels and appear to have a marked drug response. In this way, a negative correlation between blood level and effect may falsely be generated (see Figure 1).

B) The length of the study must be adequate to insure that any drug effect is clearly seen. For neuroleptics, this means that dose should be fixed for

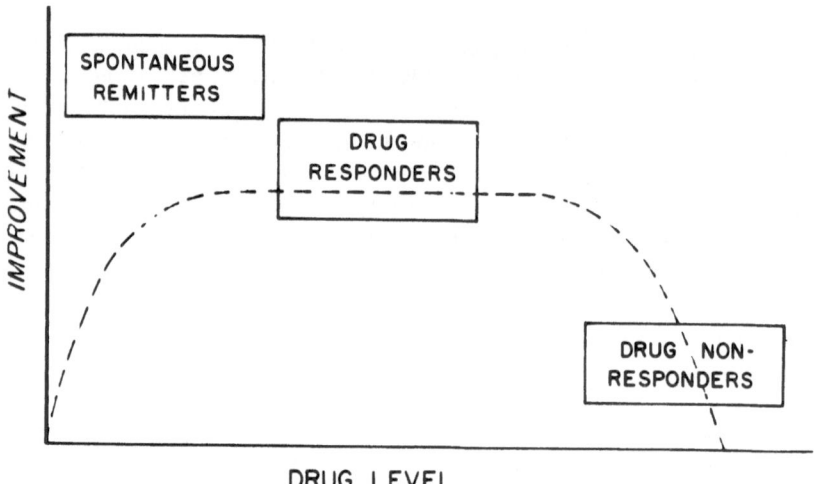

Figure 1. Blood level of drug vs. clinical improvement: an expected curve and the effect of using a flexible drug regimen. The dotted line in the figure represents what one might hope to see in the graphing of improvement vs. the blood level of drug measured in a large group of patients. If a correlation of blood level and improvement exists, less improvement should be seen when blood levels which are very low or very high than at moderate blood levels. The boxes show where in a flexible dose study patients who are spontaneous remitters, true drug responders, or true drug non-responders, respectively, will cluster. See text for details.

at least two weeks. Parenthetically, it should be noted that in studies involving short treatment, one is studying the rate of response as much as the degree of response. A full response may take weeks or even months.

C) Not only the dose of neuroleptic, but also the dose of any concomitant medications should be fixed during the study to avoid the confounding effects of drug interactions.

D) Dose must not be set so high that the lower end of the blood level to clinical response curve is lost. That is, a dose should be selected which will produce improvement in some, but not all patients. This caution is especially important for neuroleptics, which appear to have a very broad therapeutic range. Doses which are standard in North America probably put most patients well into the therapeutic range. The use of these "moderate" doses will limit the number of patients with low blood levels and little consequent improvement; most patients will be on the "plateau" of Figure 1 and it will be impossible to see the correlation between drug level and improvement. Oddly, in practice many studies fix a minimum dose (which is never very low) but few fix a maximum dose.

Measures

A) Blindness is required between those who rate clinical improvement and those who measure blood levels of drug.

B) Ratings of clinical state must be done by reliable and valid means. Well standardized scales should be used and if there are multiple raters, inter-rater reliability should be tested and reported.

C) Assaying of drug level must be done by reliable and valid means. Many clinicians, not being familiar with laboratories, assume that assay techniques themselves are consistent and accurate. Actually, tests of their reliability and validity in the past have been disappointing (Turner et al., 1976; McCormick et al., 1978).

D) Sample handling must be careful and appropriate. For example, many neuroleptics are light sensitive and blood drawn for a neuroleptic determination must be kept in the dark. As another example, the Becton-Dickinson Vacutainer tubes used for many years in blood-drawing caused a profound change in the protein binding of many drugs (Cotham and Shand, 1975; Brunswick and Mendels, 1977), including neuroleptics (Baldessarini et al., 1979). Blood drawn into such tubes could not be used for determining plasma or erythrocyte levels of drug because a variable amount of drug redistributed from the former to the latter after exposure to the stopper.

E) Drug metabolites may have to be measured as, for some drugs, they may contribute the bulk of active neuroleptic in blood and tissue (Davis, et al., 1978; Cohen et al., 1979; Javaid et al., 1980). Unfortunately, which metabolites are active and which are not is not clearly known for any drug. There are techniques (radioreceptor assays, see Synder, 1981; Cohen and Lipinski, 1981) that can simultaneously monitor all active drugs in a specimen, but these techniques cannot separately determine one drug species from another and, therefore, individual differences in distribution between parent compound and metabolites cannot be accounted for. This is an area requiring more research using a variety of assay techniques concurrently.

F) The sampling time, or time when blood is drawn must be appropriate. It should be recalled that there is no steady state drug level but that levels are probably most variable in the first few hours after drug ingestion during the absorption peak. It is probably best to sample for neuroleptics, which have long half lives, at greater than eight hours after ingestion and twelve hours is often chosen as a convenient time (Davis, 1978).

It is clear that performing a study satisfying all of the above criteria would require quite an effort and take an extended period of time. Probably no such studies have ever been done. However, there are a few studies which satisfy some of these criteria and which at least used a fixed dose of medication and a relatively appropriate population of patients. Ten such studies found in a survey of relevant papers published in English are noted in Table 1 and are briefly described below.

The study of Sakalis et al. (1972), updated by Lader (1976), contained 32 patients with heterogeneous diagnoses. All had "functional" psychosis, some were chronically ill and may not have been adequately responsive to medication. Patients were drug free for one month before study. Chlorpromazine was given for four to six weeks at 400 mg/d. Plasma levels were measured by gas chromatography in samples drawn during the absorption peak, two hours after a dose. Improvement was rated by the IMPS. The investigators found a trend for improvement to correlate with plasma level, $r = 0.32, 0.1 > p > 0.5$.

Garver et al. (1977) and, in a replication study, Casper et al. (1980) studied a total of 34 patients (10 in the first study, 24 in the second) with RDC schizophrenia, any type. Thus the patient group was probably heterogeneous. All patients were either acutely ill or suffering a relapse of chronic psychosis. Patients were drug free for two to three weeks after admission. Fixed, randomly chosen doses of butaperazine between 10 and 80 mg/d were administered for 12 (first study) or 14 (second study) days. Antiparkinson medication was employed as necessary and not at fixed doses. Drug levels were determined in plasma and erythrocytes by fluorometry with blood drawn twelve hours after ingestion several times between days 5 and 14. Improvement was monitored by the NHSI. The investigators found a significant curvilinear correlation between drug levels in erythrocytes and improvement, with erythrocyte butaperazine levels between 30 and 60 mg/ml being best. There was a trend for a similar curvilinear relationship between plasma levels and improvement.

Table 1. Fixed Dose Studies Relating Blood Levels of Neuroleptic to Improvement

Group	#	Patients diagnosis	Drug	Assay	Correlation: blood levels to improvement
Sakalis et al., 1972 Lader, 1976	32	Functional psychosis	CPZ	GC	Trend
Garver et al., 1977 Casper et al., 1980	34	RDC schizophrenia	BPZ	Fluor.	Plasma: trend (curvilinear) RBC: yes (curvilinear)
Vanderheeren et al., 1977	10	Acute schizophrenia	THZ	TLC	Impression: high mesoridazine in improvers
Wode-Helgodt et al., 1978	48	Acute Psychosis	CPZ	GCMS	Yes (modest) at 2 weeks Trend at 4 weeks
Clark et al., 1978	13	Chronic schizophrenia	CPZ	Fluor.	No
Cohen et al., 1980	16	Acute psychosis	THZ	RRA	Plasma: yes RBC: yes
Hansen, et al., 1981	13	Acute psychosis	PPZ	GC	Yes
Dysken et al., 1981	29	Acute psychosis	FPZ	GLC	Trend (curvilinear)
May et al., 1981	48	Functional psychosis	CPZ	GCMS	No
Van Putten et al., 1982	34	Functional psychosis	THX	RRA	Yes (modest)

The table summarizes the characteristics and findings of ten fixed dose studies of the relationship of neuroleptic levels in blood to clinical improvement. Under "correlation," a "yes" indicates a statistically significant ($p<0.05$) correlation of blood level to improvement was found, "trend" indicates the authors of the above studies felt that a correlation had been found but it failed to reach statistical significance, "no" indicates no correlation was found. See the text for details on these studies. Abbreviations are as follows: CPZ = chlorpromazine, BPZ = butaperazine, THZ = thioridazine, PPZ = perphenazine, FPZ = fluphenazine, THX = thiothixene, GC = gas chromatography, Fluor = fluorometry, TLC = thin layer chromatography, GCMS = gas chromatography will mass spectroscopy, RRA = radioreceptor assay, GLC = gas-liquid chromatography.

Vanderheeren et al. (1977) studied 10 "acute schizophrenics," diagnosed without formal criteria. Fifteen patients were initially in the study, but three dropped out and data was lost on two. Thioridazine, 400 mg per day, was given for one to four months. Plasma levels of drug were determined by thin-layer chromatography on samples drawn during the absorption peak at three hours after ingestion. Ratings of improvement were impressionistic and no statistical analysis of the results was done due to the small numbers. The authors had the impression that patients who improved had higher mesoridazine levels in plasma.

Wode-Helgodt et al. (1978) studied 44 patients with mixed diagnoses, all of whom were acutely psychotic. Patients received one to seven days of placebo before active medication. Four of the original 48 patients had to be dropped from the study due to an inadequate early response or side effects requiring a dose change. Patients received fixed, randomly assigned doses of chlorpromazine, 200 to 600 mg per day, for two (44 patients) to four (38 patients) weeks. Plasma and CSF levels were determined by gas chromatography with mass spectrometry on samples drawn 12 hours after drug ingestion after one to four weeks of drug had been given. Clinical improvement was rated by CPRS. Patients with plasma levels over 40 ng/ml or CSF levels over 1 ng/ml did best. At two weeks, the correlation between plasma level and improvement was modest but significant with $r = 0.39$, $p < 0.05$. At four weeks, there was only a trend towards a correlation.

Clark et al. (1978, 1976) studied 13 long-term institutionalized chronic schizophrenic patients. Of an original 18 patients, 5 were lost for reasons not clearly specified. Patients had been on pineal extract as part of a previous study, and had not received neuroleptics for 12 weeks. Chlorpromazine dose was fixed at 200 mg/M^2 (roughly 300 mg/d) or 600 mg/M^2 (roughly 900 mg/d). Blood levels (whether plasma, whole blood, etc. is not stated) were done by fluorimetry on samples drawn somewhat early, at six hours after drug ingestion. Clinical rating was by a combination of the NOSIE, the BPRS, and a global impression. It is unclear how many of these chronic patients worsened off neuroleptics or improved on neuroleptics. Therefore, it is unclear if they were an appropriate population to study. There was no correlation between chlorpromazine, chlorpromazine sulfoxide, or their ratio and "behavioral change."

Cohen et al. (1980, 1981) studied 16 patients with mixed diagnoses but either an acute psychosis or an acute exacerbation of chronic psychosis. Patients were drug free for at least one month prior to study and were drug free after admission for several days to a week to allow for spontaneous remission. Thioridazine was given in fixed doses, 200 or 400 mg/d, with dose determined before patients were seen. Treatment was for two weeks. Plasma and erythrocyte levels were estimated by radioreceptor assay in blood drawn twelve hours after drug ingestion four times between days four and fourteen. Clinical rating was by

BPRS and GAS and all patients were shown, on long term follow-up, to be eventual drug responders (though not necessarily responders to their original dose of thioridazine). Neuroleptic activity in plasma and erythrocytes correlated highly with one another and equally well with clinical improvement; for plasma, r_s = 0.88, N = 16, p < 0.005.

Hansen et al. (1981) studied 13 patients, all acutely psychotic but with various diagnoses. Twenty-one patients began the study, but only thirteen survived the first week on the fixed dose. Perphenazine was given at 24 to 48 mg/d, depending on the patients presenting clinical condition, but was fixed after the first dose for four weeks. Antiparkinson medication was used as necessary. Plasma levels were determined by gas chromatography in blood sampled seven hours after drug ingestion. Ratings were done by BPRS and CPRS. Nine patients with blood levels over 2 nmol/l showed 50-85% improvement and four patients with levels below 1.5 nmol/l showed only 0-20% improvement. The authors do not provide a calculation for the correlation of levels vs. improvement, but r_s appears to be about 0.7 with p < 0.05 for all patients taken together.

Dysken et al. (1981) studied 29 patients with mixed diagnoses who were acutely psychotic or suffering an acute exacerbation of a chronic psychosis. Five patients received a diagnosis of schizoaffective disorder, depressed. Patients were medication free one week or more prior to study. Dose selection was from 5, 10, or 20 mg of fluphenazine/day, but one patient apparently received 40 mg/day. Antiparkinson medication was used as necessary. The patients were studied for two weeks. Plasma levels were determined by gas-liquid chromatography on blood drawn 12 hours after ingestion on days 8, 11, and 15. Clinical improvement was monitored by the NHSI. There was an apparent curvilinear relationship between blood level and improvement with three patients showing no improvement having levels greater than 2.8 ng/ml and two patients with no improvement and one with poor improvement having levels less than 0.2 ng/ml. A quadratic regression could be fit to the data with p < 0.02.

May et al. (1981) studied 48 patients with mixed diagnoses, all having a "functional psychosis of the schizophrenic type." Most of these patients were chronically ill and may not have been appropriate for study. Patients had received "no recent medication" and had a two to seven day drug free period in the hospital. They received chlorpromazine, 3 mg/lb/d (roughly 450 mg/d) for four weeks, but some patients were treated with lower doses due to side effects. Plasma levels were determined by gas chromatography with mass spectrometry in samples drawn 12 hrs after ingestion at four weeks of treatment. Clinical improvement, the degree of which is unclear, was rated by BPRS and MACC. No consistent correlation of level to improvement was found.

Van Putten et al. (1982, 1983) studied 34 generally chronic, mostly schizophrenic patients. Again, the number of patients who were drug responders is unclear. A formal diagnosis of schizophrenia was not required. Patients were drug free for two weeks or more prior to study. Patients received thiothixene at 0.2 mg/lb/d (roughly 30 mg/d) fixed for four weeks, but eleven patients received substantially lower doses due to drug sensitivity. Antiparkinson medications were used as necessary. Plasma level was estimated by radioreceptor assay on blood drawn twelve hrs after ingestion. Clinical improvement was rated by the CGI, NOSIE, and BPRS. There was a modest but significant correlation between level and improvement with patients having over 40 "neuroleptic units" in blood doing best.

In reviewing these ten studies several things are obvious. First, there are very few of them and even fewer are of any one drug. The most widely used drug was chlorpromazine and it was employed in only four studies of which only two used the same assay technique. In addition, all of the studies are small, some exceedingly so. Patients tend to be rather heterogeneous diagnostically and to include the chronically ill who may be poor responders to neuroleptics. Doses of medication tend to be moderately high and only sometimes truly fixed. Clearly, it is too early to draw any conclusion although the presence of some modest correlations of blood level of drug to effect is at least heartening.

CONCLUSIONS

What is to be done now? Large (possibly collaborative) studies are needed using the design elements discussed above. Such studies might concentrate on determining the lower end of the drug level to drug effect curve first. Unfortunately, given the experience so far in this area, it seems unlikely that such studies can be done. In particular, it is very difficult to find the large numbers of appropriate patients needed for these studies. In addition, it is hard to keep patients on fixed doses for even two weeks in the face of poor improvement. However, if such patients are dropped from the study or their dose is changed there will be little chance of defining the relationship of drug level to response.

While waiting for the results of more and better studies, what should clinicians do? At the present, a clinician cannot assume that a blood level of neuroleptic has any clear meaning, since no such meaning has been shown. Again, it is important to recall that the range of levels a laboratory will provide for comparison is usually a compilation of average levels, *not* a therapeutic range. Such averages may vary by lab, assay technique, patient population, and even with time. The relationship of these levels to drug effect is unknown and not likely direct. In addition, as poor as studies are of short term response, there are no adequate studies of the worth of a blood level sampled during long term treatment, when most blood may be drawn for neuroleptic determination in clinical practice.

For now, there is no place for the routine clinical use of blood levels, and clinical judgement regarding dose and the monitoring of side effects and therapeutic effects remains the best guide to treatment. The sparing use of blood levels to help confirm clinical judgement may be appropriate. However, the clinician must recall that it is the unusual patient in whom he is most likely to want a blood level, and it is just this patient for whom the level may be least interpretable. A comparison to average levels may not be appropriate. Finally, it should be noted that blood levels can be interpreted many ways. For example, a low level can mean non-compliance, low absorption, rapid metabolism, spontaneous remission of the illness, that the patient is highly responsive or sensitive to medication, or that the dose is inadequate. Ultimately, the distinction between these and similar possibilities will be made on clinical grounds. The clinician will probably have a good idea of which is true before a level is drawn.

BIBLIOGRAPHY

Baldessarini, R.J. (1977). Antipsychotic Agents. In: *Chemotherapy in Psychiatry*, Harvard University Press, Cambridge, MA.

Baldessarini, R.J., Cohen, B.M., Herschel, M., Campbell, A. and Lipinski, J.F. (1979). Radioreceptor assay for neuroleptics. *American Psychiatric Association New Research*, Abs. NR36.

Bickel, M.H. (1974). Binding of phenothiazines and related compounds to tissue and cell constituents. In: Forrest, I.S., Carr, C.J. and Usdin, E. (eds.), *The Phenothiazines and Structurally Related Drugs*. New York, Raven Press, pp. 435–443.

Brunswick, D.J. and Mendels, J. (1977). Reduced levels of tricyclic antidepressants in plasma with vacutainers. *Commun. Psychopharmacol.* 1:131–134.

Campbell, A., Herschel, M., Cohen, B.M. and Baldessarini, R.J. (1980). Tissue levels of haloperidol by radioreceptor assay and behavioral effects of haloperidol in the rat. *Life Sci.* 27:633–640.

Casper, R., Garver, D.L., Dekirmenjian, H., Chang, S. and Davis, J.M. (1980). Phenothiazine levels in plasma and red blood cells. *Arch. Gen. Psychiatry* 37:301–305.

Clark, M.L., Kaul, P.N. and Whitfield, C.R. (1978). Chlorpromazine kinetics and clinical response. *Psychopharm. Bull.* 14:43–45.

Clark, M.L. and Kaul, P.N. (1976). A preliminary report on clinical response and blood levels of chlorpromazine and its sulfoxide during chlorpromazine therapy in chronic schizophrenic patients. In: Gotschalk, L.A. and Merlis, S. (eds.), *Pharmacokinetics of Psychoactive Drugs*, New York, Spectrum Publications, pp. 191–197.

Cohen, B.M., Lipinski, J.F., Pope, H.G. and Harris, P.Q. (1980). Neuroleptic blood levels of patients on thioridazine and clinical improvement. *Psychopharmacology* 70:191-194.

Cohen, B.M. and Baldessarini, R.J. (1981). Assay of haloperidol (letter). *Am. J. Psychiatry* 138:1513-1514.

Cohen, B.M., Herschel, M. and Aoba, A. (1979). Neuroleptic, antimuscarinic, and antiadrenergic activity of chlorpromazine, thioridazine, and their metabolites. *Psychiatry Research* 1:199-208.

Cohen, B.M., Herschel, M., Miller, E.M. and Baldessarini, R.J. (1980). Radioreceptor assay of haloperidol tissue levels in the rat. *Neuropharmacology* 19:663-668.

Cohen, B.M. and Lipinski, J.F. (1981). Radioreceptor assays and blood levels of neuroleptics. In: Usdin, E. (ed.), *Neuroreceptors – Basic and Clinical Aspects.* Wiley and Sons, New York, pp. 199-214.

Cohen, B.M., Lipinski, J.F., Harris, P.Q., Pope, H.G. and Friedman, M. (1980). Clinical use of the radioreceptor assay for neuroleptics. *Psychiatry Research* 2:173-178.

Cooper, T.B., Simpson, G.M. and Lee, H.H. (1976). Thymoleptic and neuroleptic drug plasma levels in psychiatry: current status. *Int. Rev. Neurobiol.* 19:269-309.

Cotham, R.N. and Shand, D. (1975). Spuriously low plasma propranalol concentrations resulting from blood collection methods. *Clin. Pharmacol. Ther.* 18:535-538.

Curry, S.H., Derr, J.E. and Maling, H.M. (1970). The physiological disposition of chlorpromazine in the rat and dog. *Proc. Soc. Exp. Biol. Med.* 134:314-318.

Curry, S.H., Marshall, J.H.L., Davis, J.M. and Janowsky, D.A. (1970). Chlorpromazine plasma levels and effects. *Arch. Gen. Psychiatry* 22:289-296.

Davis, M.M., Erickson, S. and Dekirmenjian, H. (1978). Plasma levels of antipsychotic drugs and clinical response. In: Lipton, M.A., DiMascio, A. and Killiam, K.F. (eds.), *Psychopharmacology: A Generation of Progress.* Raven Press, New York, pp. 905-916.

Dysken, M.W., Javaid, J.I., Chang, S.S., Schaffer, C., Shahid, A. and Davis, J.M. (1981). Fluphenazine pharmacokinetics and therapeutic response. *Psychopharmacology* 73:205-210.

Freedberg, K.A., Innis, R.B., Creese, I. and Snyder, S.H. (1979). Antischizophrenic drugs, differential plasma protein binding and therapeutic activity. *Life Sci.* 24:2467-2474.

Garver, D.L., Dekirmenjian, H., Davis, J.M., Casper, R. and Ericksen, S. (1977). Neuroleptic drug levels and therapeutic response: preliminary observations with red blood cell bound butaperazine. *Am. J. Psychiatry* 134:304-307.

Gelder, M. and Kolakowska, T. (1979). Variability of response to neuroleptics in schizophrenia. *Comp. Psychiatry* 20:397-408.

Gottschalk, L.A. (1979). A preliminary approach to the problems of relating the pharmacokinetics of phenothiazines to clinical response with schizophrenic patients. In: Gottschalk, L.A. (ed.), *Pharmacokinetics of Psychoactive Drugs, Further Studies,* Spectrum Publications, New York, pp. 63-81.

Gottschalk, L.A., Biener, R., Noble, E.P., Birch, H., Wilbert, D.E., and Heiser, J.F. (1975). Thioridazine plasma levels and clinical response. *Compr. Psychiatry* 16:323-337.

Gottschalk, L.A., Dinovo, E., Biener, R., Birch, H., Syben, M. and Noble, E.P. (1976). Plasma levels of mesoridazine and its metabolites and clinical response in acute schizophrenia after a single intramuscular drug dose. In: Gottschalk, L.A. and Merlis, S. (eds.), *Pharmacokinetics of Psychoactive Drugs.* New York, Spectrum, pp. 171–190.

Hansen, L.B., Larsen, N.E. and Vestergard, P. (1981). Plasma levels of perphenazine related to development of extrapyramidal side effects. *Psychopharmacology* 74:306–309.

Janssen, P.A.J. and Allewijn, F.T.N. (1969). The distribution of the butyrophenones, haloperidol, trifluperidol, moperone, and clofluperol in rats, and its relationship with their neuroleptic activity. *Arzneimforsch.* (Drug Res.) 19:199–208.

Javaid, J.F., Pandey, G.N., Duslek, B., Hu, H.-Y. and Davis, J.M. (1980). Measurement of neuroleptic concentrations by GLC and radioreceptor assays. *Comm. Psychopharmacology* 4:467–475.

Jorgensen, A., Hansen, V., Larsen, U.D. and Khan, A.R. (1969). Metabolism distribution and excretion of flupenthixol. *Acta Pharmacol. Toxicol.* 27:301–313.

Lader, M. (1976). Monitoring plasma concentrations in neuroleptics. *Pharmakopsych.* 9:170–177.

May, P.R.A., Tokar, J.T., Davis, J.M., Yale, C. and Dekirmenjian, H. (1979). Plasma thioridazine and therapeutic response in schizophrenia. In: Gottschalk, L.A. (ed.), *Pharmacokinetics of Psychoactive Drugs, Further Studies,* Spectrum Publications, New York, pp. 97–114.

May, P.R.A. and Van Putten, T. (1978). Plasma levels of chlorpromazine in schizophrenia. *Arch. Gen. Psychiatry* 35:1081–1087.

May, P.R.A., Van Putten, T., Jenden, D.J., Yale, C. and Dixon, W.J. (1981). Chlorpromazine levels and the outcome of treatment in schizophrenic patients. *Arch. Gen. Psychiatry* 38:202–207.

Mayer, M. and Guttman, D. (1968). The binding of drugs by plasma proteins. *J. Pharm. Sci.* 895–918.

McCormick, W., Ingelfinger, J.A., Isakson, G. and Goldman, P. (1978). Errors in measuring drug concentrations. *N. Engl. J. Med.* 299:1117–1121.

Ohman, R., Larsson, M., Nilsson, I.M., Engle, J. and Carlsson, A. (1977). Neurometabolic and behavioural effects of haloperidol in relation to drug levels in serum and brain. *Naunyn-Schmiedebergs Arch. Exp. Pathol. Pharmak.* 299:105–114.

Piafsky, K.M., Borga, O., Odar-Cederlof, I., Johansson, C. and Sjoqvist, F. (1978). Increased plasma binding of propranalol and chlorpromazine mediated by disease induced elevations of plasma α acid glycoprotein. *N. Engl. J. Med.* 279:1435–1439.

Sakalis, G., Curry, S.H., Mould, G.P. and Lader, M.H. (1972). Physiologic and clinical effects of chlorpromazine and their relationship to plasma level. *Clin. Pharmacol. Ther.* 13:931–946.

Sakurai, Y., Takahashi, R., Nakahara, T. and Ikenaga, H. (1980). Prediction of response to and actual outcome of chlorpromazine treatment in schizophrenic patients. *Arch. Gen. Psychiatry* 37:1057–1062.

Smith, R.C., Crayton, J., Dekirmenjian, H., Klass, D. and Davis, J.M.: Blooa levels of neuroleptic drugs in nonresponding chronic schizophrenic patients. *Arch. Gen. Psychiatry* 36:579–584.

Snyder, S.H. (1981). Dopamine receptors, neuroleptics and schizophrenia. *Am. J. Psychiatry* 138:460–464.

Turner, W.J., Turano, P. and Badzinski, S. (1976). An attempt to establish quality control in determination of plasma chlorpromazine by a multi-laboratory collaboration. In: Gottschalk, L.A. and Merlis, S. (eds.), *Pharmacokinetics of Psychoactive Drugs*, New York, Spectrum Publications, New York, pp. 33–42.

Vanderheeren, F.A.J. and Muusze, R.G. (1977). Plasma levels and half lives of thioridazine and some of its metabolites. *Eur. J. Clin. Pharmacol.* 11:135–140.

Van Putten, T., May, P.R.A., Marder, S.R. and Wilkins, J.N. (1982). Plasma level of thiothixene by radioreceptor assay and clinical outcome. *Psychopharm. Bull.* 18:99–101.

Van Putten, T., May, P.R.A., Marder, S.R., Wilkins, J.N. and Rosenberg, B.J. (1983). Plasma levels of thiothixene by radioreceptor assay: clinical usefulness. *Psychopharmacology* 79:40–44.

Wode-Helgodt, B., Borg, S., Fryo, B. and Sedvall, G. (1978). Clinical effects and drug concentrations in plasma and cerebrospinal fluid in psychotic patients treated with fixed doses of chlorpromazine. *Acta Psychiat. Scand.* 58:149–173.

Yesavage, J.A., Holman, C.A., Cohn, R. (1981). Correlation of thiothixene serum levels and age. *Psychopharmacol.* 74:170–172.

17

Neuroregulators and Schizophrenia: A Look at the Dopamine and Endorphin Hypotheses

JACK D. BARCHAS, ROY KING, AND PHILIP A. BERGER

INTRODUCTION

The development of the concept of neuroregulators, substances which might act as neurotransmitters or as neuromodulators in the functioning of neural networks, has proved to be particularly important for psychiatry by providing a framework for new conceptions of mental illness. The neurotransmitters and neuromodulators function in different ways (Barchas et al. 1978) yet it is clear that these materials may be directly involved in severe disorders and may alter functioning through individual and joint actions. Strong evidence supports the notion that various medications which are used in treatment alter neuroregulator mechanisms. In this brief review we will consider two of the several dozen systems which have been postulated and discuss aspects of them as they apply to schizophrenia. One, the dopamine hypothesis of a relative excess of dopamine in schizophrenia is perhaps the most powerful and generally accepted notion of that disorder—yet the hypothesis remains unproven and can be reformulated to take into account recent concepts regarding the physiology of the dopaminergic neural unit as it can be described mathematically. The other system is the opioid peptide system, really a set of systems, for which hypotheses are still loosely described. For the opioid peptides we attempt to describe some of the current evidence for involvement in schizophrenia, the ways in which the substances are being studied, and some directions for future research which may be related to schizophrenia or other serious mental disorders.

THE DOPAMINE HYPOTHESIS OF SCHIZOPHRENIA

Brief Description of the Hypothesis and its Current Status

The dopamine hypothesis centers about the notion that a relative excess of dopamine is involved in the symptoms of schizophrenia. The hypothesis can be viewed as having two components: 1) neuroleptics act through dopamine and 2) schizophrenia is caused by a relative excess of dopamine. In point of fact the two components are separate. The evidence for the first is strong, that for the second weak and now demanding new approaches to the problems.

There are a number of categories of evidence that antipsychotic medications might act by blocking dopamine receptors. Evidence for this view has been developed by many investigators (for review see Berger and Barchas, 1981). The evidence includes the following: neuroleptics can cause extrapyramidal symptoms, a result which would be expected of an antidopaminergic action. Neuroleptics increase dopamine turnover, an important finding (Carlsson and Lindquist, 1963) that can be explained as a feedback mechanism and is to be expected if dopamine receptor mechanisms are blocked. The electrical effects of dopamine on dopamine neurons is blocked by neuroleptics. Neuroleptics block stereotyped behavior due to amphetamines in animals, a form of behavior which is believed to occur through dopamine mechanisms. Neuroleptics block dopamine sensitive adenylate cyclase. Neuroleptics block dopamine receptors when studied in brain homogenates and the capacity to have this effect on receptors seems to correlate with antipsychotic effects. Neuroleptics increase prolactin concentrations, normally prolactin secretion is known to be inhibited by dopamine, again an action of neuroleptics on a dopamine receptor.

Taking the evidence together there is strong evidence that most neuroleptics act by altering dopamine mechanisms. Yet despite that strong evidence that neuroleptics act by blocking dopamine transmission, the evidence for the other side of the coin, that schizophrenia is a disease of a relative excess of dopamine, is still unproved although the evidence is suggestive. Thus, drugs which decrease dopamine, such as AMPT, or drugs which enhance dopamine, like amphetamines, each have the predicted effect on schizophrenia. AMPT may have some effect in decreasing schizophrenic symptoms while amphetamines can mimic a psychotic state.

Perhaps most striking has been the failure to demonstrate a specific change in dopamine mechanisms in brain material or CSF from schizophrenics. Thus, there is no consistent change in dopamine metabolites in CSF (Berger, Faull, et al., 1981), no change in the activity of the enzymes involved in the formation of dopamine (Wyatt et al., 1978), and no changes in the amount of dopamine in brains from schizophrenics.

The issues regarding the dopamine hypothesis have been extremely stimulating of research. They have resulted in the development of a series of effective treatments. Nevertheless it is necessary to approach the hypothesis in new ways. One of those is better understanding of the basic science mechanisms of the dopamine system including processes of regulation of the system. Such information applies to all aspects of the system including its receptors and post-synaptic mechanisms which are now appropriately receiving considerable attention. Through such studies one would hope that more specific medications with fewer side effects might be developed.

At the same time there is also a need for study of dopamine regulation in other ways. While discovered by Udenfriend and his colleagues almost 20 years ago, it is only recently that the rate limiting enzyme in the formation of dopamine, tyrosine hydroxylase, has been purified and characterized from brain (Raese et al., 1977; Edelman et al., 1981). It is becoming clear that the enzyme has complex regulation with the capacity to respond to activation with marked activation (a process of some interest in light of the known susceptibility of schizophrenics to stress). Indeed, it is likely that the enzyme is rapidly activated and deactivated (Lazar, Lockfeld et al., in press) and may be activated by neuroleptic administration (Lazar, Mefford et al., in press). The complex regulatory processes involving tyrosine hydroxylase and the known genetic controls on the enzyme (Kessler et al., 1972; Ciaranello et al., 1972; Barchas et al., 1974) raise the question as to whether any of the activation-deactivation processes are also controlled genetically or influenced in terms of their set-point by environmental factors in development. For example, one could well imagine individuals who might overrespond to stress, underrespond, or continue to respond in the absence of stress. Processes such as these may require investigation in relation to schizophrenia.

Investigation of better means of testing the dopamine hypothesis should develop from improved knowledge at a basic science level. Thus, studies of "dopamine" receptors in the brains of schizophrenics can now be made more specific to various subtypes of receptors. Tyrosine hydroxylase activity which appears to be normal in schizophrenics might be studied in terms of activation-deactivation. Improved methods of analysis of dopamine and its metabolites and studies of turnover are enhanced by developments in analytical neurochemistry including mass spectrometry (Faull et al., 1983) and high performance liquid chromatography (Mefford et al., in press). Ultimately improved biochemical and analytical chemical studies, combined with an ability to study dopaminergic systems in a more totally integrated manner using neurophysiological tools should provide new ways of viewing the dopamine hypothesis and investigating dopamine in relation to schizophrenia and other diseases.

Mathematical Models of the Dopamine Neuronal System –
Towards a New Dopamine Hypothesis of Schizophrenia

A recent model of schizophrenia incorporates the dynamic physiology of dopaminergic neurons into a mathematical analysis of dopamine neurophysiology and neurochemistry (King et al., 1981). Rather than postulating the cause of schizophrenic symptoms to be simple functional excess of dopamine, it proposes that the dopamine neuron undergoes an instability in its action that is reflected in a disorganization of its firing over time and space. The early descriptive psychiatrists such as Bleuler (Bleuler, 1950) and Leonhard (Leonhard, 1979), noted that schizophrenics often show a profound discoordination of thought, movement, and affect. A patient could, for instance, simultaneously manifest euphoria and fear, or feel both a surge and a poverty of thoughts at the same time or vacillating abruptly over periods of minutes. Other schizophrenics may sense the left half of their bodies as inert and the right half invigorated. This desynchronization of behavior was also noted by Ellinwood in cats treated chronically with amphetamine (Ellinwood et al., 1974).

Until the last decade most physiological models of neurochemistry were linear. Such linear systems usually manifest a single stable equilibrium that under external perturbation returns homeostatically to that equilibrium. This observation formed the basis of Claude Bernard's principle of "le milieu interieur". However, the many biological systems that involve long feedback delays and nonlinear response curves will be better described by nonlinear dynamics. In general, nonlinear systems under increasing nonlinearities or feedback will bifurcate or branch into several equilibrium states, rhythmic oscillations, or even turbulent chaotic activity. The dopaminergic system fulfills the criteria of a system which can be better described by nonlinear dynamics because (King et al., 1981) there is a complicated system of strong local dendrito-dendritic inhibitory feedback and long-loop striatal nigral feedback for dopamine neurons of the substantia nigra; (King et al., in press) dopamine synthesis paradoxically increased over baseline at both low and high firing rates (Nowycky and Roth, 1978). This U-shaped curve of dopamine synthesis vs firing requires a nonlinear response curve; the activation of dopamine synthesis requires a 20–30 minute delay to occur. The revised dopamine hypothesis incorporates these properties, in addition to the neuronal feedback loops and long-term regulation of dopamine receptor number.

The model predicts several interesting observations. Because of the activation of dopamine synthesis at low firing rates, the dopamine feedback loop can become unstable and a simple homeostatic equilibrium in dopamine activity can bifurcate into two separate domains of stability. One of these retains its stability firing at a relatively low rate while the other can bifurcate further into oscillatory and erratic activity over a period of 20–30 minutes. Mathematically, these phenomena require an activation of dopamine synthesis of a factor of at least 3–4, while experimentally the activation has been measured to be between 4 and 5.

Drug effects fit with this model. Modifications of a dopaminergic system such as the addition of amphetamine, or high dose apomorphine which lead to an increased effectiveness of dopamine at the synapse will, when incorporated into the model, lead to the production of this aberrant chaotic activity. Likewise, drugs which decrease the amount or efficacy of dopamine at the synapse such as the neuroleptics or a α-methyl-para-tyrosine will renormalize erratic and unstable activity.

Anatomical and physiological evidence suggests that there are several loosely coupled dopaminergic nuclei including those dopamine neurons of the left and right substantia nigras and the ventral tegmental areas. The model predicts that one might simultaneously find one dopaminergic nuclei in a relatively high firing chaotic state while the other dopaminergic nucleus would be in a stable low firing state. With the long-term changes in dopamine receptor number that attempt to maintain a constant dopaminergic output, other behaviors will occur. For instance, these can be oscillations between a relatively stable low firing dopaminergic state and chaotic high firing dopaminergic state with a period of days to weeks concurrent with the time course of dopamine receptor changes. In addition, two dopamine nuclei could alternately discharge rapidly and discharge slowly over the same time period. Finally, on a much faster time scale of seconds, the feedback delays in neuronal firing caused by the activation time of the dopaminergic receptor will also generate interesting phenomena. With increasing effectiveness of dopamine at the synapse, a stable dopamine firing pattern will bifurcate into bursts of oscillations, with a frequency of .3–4 hertz.

Most of the psychophysiological findings in schizophrenia show a large intrasubject variability in measures of evoked potentials, attention, and raw EEG (Cromwell, 1978); perhaps these rapid instabilities create this increased variability. Thus, much of the fluctuating, discoordinated and unpredictable behavior of schizophrenics over seconds, minutes, and days might be explained by this new hypothesis of dopaminergic instability. Genetic changes in the activation of tyrosine hydroxylase, the rate-limiting enzyme in dopamine synthesis, dopamine receptor sensitivity or other neuronal systems which impinge upon and modulate the dopaminergic networks could all lead to this erratic dopamine behavior.

OPIOID PEPTIDES IN SCHIZOPHRENIA

The discovery of endogenous opiate-like peptides, the endorphins, has opened a new approach to the study of schizophrenia. A major research effort focuses on the possible role of the endorphins in schizophrenia. This area of research is at its earliest phases and there is controversial evidence for both an excess and a deficiency of endorphin activity in schizophrenia (Watson et al., 1979; Verebey et al., 1978; Berger, Akil et al., 1982).

The first of the opiate peptides discovered were methionine (met-) and leucine (leu-) enkephalin, both pentapeptides (Hughes, 1975; Hughes et al., 1975). The sequence of the amino acids in met-enkephalin is contained within the pituitary peptide, *beta*-lipotropin (beta-LPH). Met-enkephalin is beta-LPH 61-65; leu-enkephalin has the same sequence, except that its terminal amino acid is leucine instead of methionine. Other endorphins also are contained in the sequence of beta-LPH, including beta-endorphin (beta-LPH 61-91) (Li et al., 1976; Bradbury et al., 1976) and *gamma*-endorphin (beta-LPH 61-77) (Ling et al., 1976). A heptapeptide related to met-enkephalin is also present in the brain, met-enkephalin-arg[6]-phe[7] (Boarder et al., in press). Although there are structural relationships between these peptides, they are not derived from one another, indeed enkephalin biosynthetic pathways may be quite different than those for *beta*-endorphin. Most recently still another group of opioid peptides have been described, dynorphin and alpha-neo-endorphin, and it has just been demonstrated that these two latter peptides are present in the same neuronal system in the brain (Weber et al., 1982).

Evidence for a Relative Deficiency of Endogenous Opioids in Schizophrenia

There is some evidence for a relative deficiency of endorphins in schizophrenia but it is a matter of some controversy. For example, while the stiffness resulting from beta-endorphin administration in rats has been interpreted by some as similar to the symptoms of catalepsy produced by neuroleptics (Jacquet et al., 1976), not all investigators agree (Segal et al., 1978).

It is true that there have been statements in the psychiatric literature for over 100 years suggesting positive effects of exogenous opiates on schizophrenic symptoms (Berger, 1978), but there have been no double-blind studies. Such a double blind study would have a number of intrinsic difficulties. Nevertheless there have been investigations of agonist-like substances and the results are of interest. A met-enkephalin analog, FK 33-824, has been studied in a single blind study and reported to decrease psychotic symptoms in eight schizophrenic patients (Jorgensson et al., 1979). Such studies, stimulated by essential single blind studies, using other analogs as well as double blind conditions will be of importance.

Considerable interest has been attracted to the endorphin-like peptide des-tyrosine-gamma-endorphin, a peptide structurally related to beta-endorphin but devoid of opiate activity. This substance has been reported to decrease schizophrenic symptoms in six patients studied in a single-blind design and in eight patients studied in a double-blind design (Verhoeven et al., 1979). It is reported by members of the group that performed these studies that the substance may be present endogenously. Studies dealing with this topic are now ongoing in several centers.

Another opioid agonist that appropriately needs investigation is beta-endorphin itself. A beneficial effect was reported with beta-endorphin in three of four schizophrenic patients given 15 intravenous doses from 1.5 to 9 mg in a single-blind design (Kline et al., 1977, 1979). The report stimulated considerable interest and because of the potential significance of the findings a series of studies were undertaken to test the finding. A study was undertaken on the Stanford Mental Health Clinical Research Center designed to test the effects of intravenously administered beta-endorphin on psychotic behavior and to obtain some information on pharmacokinetics and physiological effects of the substance (Berger, Watson et al., 1980).

For the study ten male subjects were studied. Each subject was diagnosed by Research Diagnostic Criteria (RDC), based on a semistructured admission interview by a psychiatrist (Spitzer et al., 1978), as either chronic schizophrenia (undifferentiated, three patients; paranoid, four patients; disorganized one patient) or chronic schizoaffective disorder, depressed type (two patients). Particular attention was devoted to diagnostic categories and interrater agreement. All subjects were medication free for at least two weeks prior to the study. After a two-week stabilization period, subjects received a single weekly injection on the same day for three weeks. The first saline injection would be for an acclimatization period. The next two injections, given in random order, were either saline control or 20 mg beta-endorphin. Both the patients and those involved in drug administration and patient rating were blind to the content of the injections.

One aspect of the study involved examination of the pharmacokinetics of beta-endorphin. Concentrations of the substance are 100 times higher if the substance is administered from an albumin coated syringe. In our patients a kinetic curve with two components with half-lives of 15 minutes and 39 minutes was obtained. This information should be of interest to others who administer beta-endorphin for various purposes.

Physiological parameters also revealed changes. Thus, prolactin was markedly elevated after beta-endorphin administration, a change that would be expected since morphine is known to induce marked elevations in prolactin. When EEG responses were monitored there were changes in the alpha frequency range (8–12 Hz) following injection of either morphine or beta-endorphin. After morphine, the amount of alpha increased rapidly and remained high for at least 50 minutes. Beta-endorphin produced a rise in alpha activity which was similar to but faster than that produced by morphine, but the increase lasted less than 30 minutes. Saline injections did not produce any changes in alpha activity (Pfefferbaum et al., 1979).

Despite the evidence of physiological effects of beta-endorphin, clinical responses were not dramatic. It should be noted that neither the research or nursing staff nor the patients could distinguish the response to beta-endorphin from the response to saline. The BPRS did suggest a statistically significant improvement but the improvement is not apparent clinically. The Stanford Study did not reveal the improvement noted in the single blind study noted earlier. Nevertheless there is reason to study beta-endorphin further for the Stanford Study used only a single dose. In addition several other potential opioid peptide agonists related to other peptides would also seem worthy of study.

Evidence for a Relative Excess of Endogenous Opioids in Schizophrenia

Several lines of argument and evidence support the view that some aspects of schizophrenia might reflect a relative excess in activity of one or more or the various endorphins. A catatonic-like behavior has been described in rats given beta-endorphin (Bloom et al., 1976). Of particular interest are reports of endorphins in the cerebrospinal fluid. There is still considerable controversy regarding exactly what endorphin-like compounds are present in the CSF. This area of basic research must be furthered for clinical investigation to proceed appropriately. Nevertheless, work has been initiated in relation to clinical states. There are reports of elevations in the concentrations of endorphin fractions other than beta-endorphin and enkephalin in cerebrospinal fluid of some unmedicated schizophrenic patients. In those patients, there is evidence of that the increased concentrations return toward normal when these patients are medicated (Wahlstrom et al., 1976; Terenius et al., 1976; Lindstrom et al., 1978). It is unclear what the materials are and whether they are causal or secondary but the finding is of interest and requires further explication. In addition, elevated CSF concentrations of beta-enorphin also have been described in some schizophrenic patients (Domschke et al., 1979).

Another line of work that suggests a relative increase in endorphin like materials in schizophrenia stems from investigations using endorphin antagonists, in this case naloxone. Naloxone is a powerful opiate antagonist and is safe for clinical use although relatively short acting. A series of controlled double-blind studies have reported evidence of improvement in some schizophrenic symptoms following intravenous naloxone administration (Watson et al., 1978; Emrich et al., 1977; Davis et al., 1979; Lehmann et al., 1979). In terms of specific symptoms, it should be noted that two of the studies report decreased hallucinations. One study reports decreased unusual thought content. Another study reports general improvement in psychotic behavior after naloxone administration. Perhaps because of lower doses of naloxone not all investigators have been able to confirm this finding (Janowsky et al., 1977; Volavka et al., 1977; Kurland et al., 1977). Such a difference in results by dose are interesting since naloxone reverses the effects of morphine and heroin at low doses and with a short duration of action. Strikingly some of the changes in schizophrenic patients which we have observed lasted for some hours. If there are multiple receptors for opioid peptides it is unclear at what receptors naloxone is acting, if indeed it is acting at such receptors in this instance, for the drug can alter other neurochemical systems, possibly through an opioid mechanism. Nevertheless, there is considerable reason to believe that the mechanism may involve opioid peptides and does require further investigation (Barchas et al., 1980). In this case both the receptor and the nature of the possible endogenous ligand on which naloxone would be acting must be investigated.

Another direction of research that has been used to support the idea that some aspects of schizophrenia might represent a relative excess of one or another endorphin came from the reported improvement in schizophrenic symptoms following hemodialysis. The investigators proposed that the result was secondary to the removal of leucine-5-beta-endorphin (Palmour et al., 1979; Wagemaker et al., 1977). There are serious problems with these studies. The nature of the patients and their diagnoses was not clear and videotapes of some of the patients were not convincing in terms of the diagnosis of the patients. The hemodialysis trial was not double-blind and therefore hemodialysis was not proven to be the effective modality if the patients improved. It should be noted that the theoretical base of the studies in terms of the proposed nature of the endogenous substance that was being dialyzed is also in question. The existence of elevated concentrations of leucine-5-beta-endorphin in either the dialysate (Lewis et al., 1979; Ross et al., 1979) or the plasma of schizophrenic patients has not been confirmed. Indeed there is at this time no evidence that such a substance exists from any basic science investigation. At the time the study was undertaken it was believed that the enkephalins originated from beta-endorphins and the investigators presented a view that they had found the precursor for leu-enkephalin. It is now recognized that the precursors for the materials may be completely different. Thus, the evidence from dialysis cannot be taken as evidence supporting an endorphin hypothesis of schizophrenia.

Directions for Future Studies Involving Opioid Peptides

Possibilities for future research dealing with opioid peptides in relation to schizophrenia are exciting. First, in research dealing with schizophrenia increasing attention will need to be paid to possible subtypes of the disorder. While this notion is frequently noted most clinical studies are of such restricted populations that it would be difficult to be able to observe subtypes of the disorder. The development of psychiatric clinical research centers is an important step in that direction for they permit multiple diagnostic measures and observation of patients free of medications. While there are very few such centers it may be that by achieving a degree of cooperation sufficient patient numbers could be achieved for meaningful evaluation of potential subtypes on various biochemical measures.

Studies of opioid peptides will require several different types of approaches. On the one hand there is a need to determine exactly what compounds are actually present physiologically. For some of the materials there is now strong evidence of multiple forms (Evans, Weber et al., 1981; Weber, Evans et al., 1981) and we do not yet know the role of those various forms. As described at the beginning of the discussion dealing with opioid peptides there also are now recognized to be a number of different substances. Some of them have received little study although they are powerful in certain test systems and potentially of significance. Several of the systems seem to be colocalized. The possibility that neuroregulators derived from the same nerve cell are working in cooperative, antagonistic, or mixed manners must be considered.

The issue of what classes of opioid peptides might be present is still quite unresolved. While attention has focused on the enkephalins and beta-endorphin other substances such as the heptapeptide related to the enkephalins may be significant and are present in substantial amounts in brain. Still other groups of materials give promise of potential behavioral roles such as dynorphin which is present in a generally recognized form as dynorphin$_{1-17}$ but of which another form is actually present in substantially greater amounts, dynorphin$_{1-8}$ (Weber, Evans et al., in press). Both of these will require investigation as will alpha-neo-endorphin with which they are colocalized in the brain. These materials are quite exciting because they are opioid-like, indeed more powerful than beta-endorphin in some test systems, yet have an anatomical localization quite distinct from beta-endorphin.

Thus, for the study of schizophrenia one must make a plea for more basic information regarding the nature and characteristics of endogenous opioid peptide agonists and antagonists—identification of putative neuroregulators. At the same time there is a need for further investigation of the nature of the receptors and the pattern of their interaction with various ligands. An understanding of the genetic aspects involving these processes should prove extremely valuable (see review Barchas and Sullivan, 1982). That type of knowledge is already developing in terms of the molecular genetics related to some of the opioid peptides and can be expected to continue to provide a new view of the substances which are present and the ways in which they are derived.

A theme of the conference is the development of new treatment approaches. In the case of the opioid peptides and mental disorders it will be essential to obtain basic information. That information should translate relatively quickly into applied clinical studies, many of which can go on contemporaneously with the efforts in basic science. Indeed this area of research has highlighted the constant interplay between areas of scientific effort at a basic and clinical level.

The development of means of identifying the various opioid peptides will make it possible to determine if there are changes in their concentrations or relative balance in brain tissue or cerebrospinal fluid from patients. It will also be possible, knowing their structures, to develop more effective agonists and antagonists to the various putative ligands. It is now clear that there are a great many substances for which such synthetic derivatives must be considered. This search for ligands will be enhanced by a better understanding of the possible multiple receptors (Akil et al., 1980; Hewlett et al., 1981) which should facilitate the development of receptor subtype specific agents. That effort has been extremely beneficial in other areas of medicine and should prove equally valuable in relation to whatever forms of mental or neurological disorders involve various opioid peptides.

Still further into the future would be the development of agents which would alter aspects of the biosynthesis or metabolic processing and inactivation (Sullivan et al., 1980) of opioid peptides. Information regarding the biosynthesis and metabolic inactivation of opioid peptides is essential for developing means by which they might be altered pharmacologically. Such agents might be structurally quite different than opioid peptides and not act on their receptors but rather on other mechanisms ranging from the genone to inactivating enzymes.

In the earlier section of this review we discussed the dopamine hypothesis. Ultimately there is a need to be able to consider whether any of the subtypes of schizophrenia involves an alteration in the balance between different neuroregulators. Such hypotheses have been made in terms of dopamine with a number of other transmitters such as GABA, acetylcholine, and norepinephrine. At the same time, it is of interest that a number of opioid peptides are found in areas of the brain that are associated with dopaminergic function (Weber, Roth et al., 1982). There are numerous possibilities for interactions between these systems. One might postulate that a dopaminergic alteration occurs secondary to a change in opioid peptides and that current treatment is directed to the correction of the dopaminergic change rather than to the lesion in the opioid system. Conversely, a change in dopaminergic systems as described for the new mathematical model presented in this paper might be involved in a change in endorphin systems which would alter various basic drive and behavioral states which are associated with the schizophrenia syndrome.

Through various types of biological approaches one can expect to see developed a new generation of types of biological tests and assessment devices. While one cannot be certain that these will have relevance to schizophrenia there is sufficient evidence to continue intensive efforts. In the opiate peptides we are dealing with a group of substances that may have relevance to very basic behaviors and drives. Since those are processes which are disturbed in the group of illnesses we refer to as schizophrenia, as well as in the group of illnesses we refer to as depression and affective disorders (Barchas et al., in press), it is apparent that further work dealing with opioid peptides is an exciting intellectual quest as well as being of potential clinical significance.

ACKNOWLEDGEMENTS

Our work dealing with schizophrenia has been supported by the National Institute of Mental Health through clinical program project award MH 23861, and through mental health clinical research center award MH 30854, as well as a grant from the Scottish Rite Schizophrenia Research Program, and an award from the Veterans Administration.

REFERENCES

Aage, J., Fog, R., and Veilis, B. (1979). Synthetic enkephalin analogue in treatment of schizophrenia. *Lancet* 1:935.

Akil, H., Watson, S.J., Barchas, J.D., et al. (1979). Beta-endorphin immunoreactivity in rat and human blood: radioimmunoassay comparative levels and physiological alterations. *Life Sci* 24:1659-1666.

Akil, H., Hewlett, W.A., Barchas, J.D. and Li, C.H. (1980). Binding of tritiated β-endorphin to rat brain membranes: characterization and opiate properties. *Eur. J. Pharmacol.* 64:1-8.

Barchas, J.D., Akil, H., Elliott, G.R., Holman, R.B., and Watson, S.J. (1978). Behavioral neurochemistry: neuroregulators in relation to behavioral states and mental disorders. *Science* 200:964-973.

Barchas, J.D., Ciaranello, R.D., Dominic, J.A., Deguchi, T., Orenberg, E.K., Stolk, J.M., Renson, J., and Kessler, S. (1974). Genetic differences in mechanisms involving neuroregulators. *J. Psychiatr. Res.* 11:347-360.

Barchas, J., Madden, J., Weber, E., Evans, C.J., and Berger, P.A. (in press). Endorphins and depression: potential for new approaches. In W. Burrows, ed., *Frontiers in Depression*.

Barchas, J.D. and Sullivan, S. (1982). Opioid peptides as neuroregulators: Potential areas for the study of genetic-behavioral mechanisms. *Behav. Genetics* 12:69-91.

Berger, P.A. (1978). Investigating the role of endogenous opioid peptides in psychiatric disorders. Peptides and behavior: A Critical Analysis of Research Strategies. *Neurosci Res Program Bull* 16:585-599.

Berger, P.A. and Barchas, J.D. (in press). Drugs and schizophrenia. In K. Melmon, ed., *Current Topics in Drug Therapeutics*, Amsterdam: Elsevier.

Berger, P.A., Akil, H., Watson, S.J. and Barchas, J.D. Behavioral pharmacology of the endorphins. *Ann. Rev. Medicine,* in press.

Berger, P.A., Faull, K.F., Kilkowski, J., Anderson, P.J., Kraemer, H., Davis, K.L. and Barchas, J.D. CSF monoamine metabolites in depression and schizophrenia. *Am. J. Psychiatry* 137:174-180, 1980.

Berger, P.A., Watson, S.J., Akil, H., Elliott, G.R., Rubin, R.T., Pfefferbaum, A., Davis, K.L., Barchas, J.D. and Li, C.H. β-endorphin and schizophrenia. *Arch. Gen. Psychiatry* 37:635–640, 1980.

Bleuler, E. (1950). *Dementia Praecox or the Group of Schizophrenias*. New York: International Universities Press.

Bloom, F., Segal, D., Ling, N. et al. (1976). Endorphins: profound behavioral effects in rats suggest new etiological factors in mental illness. *Science* 194:630–632.

Boarder, M.R., Lockfeld, A.J. and Barchas, J.D. Measurement of methionine-enkephalin[ARG^6,PHE^7] in rat brain by specific radioimmunoassay directed at methionine-sulphoxide enkephalin [ARG^6,PHE^7]. *J. Neurochem.*, in press.

Bradbury, A.F., Felber, W.F., Smith, D.G. et al. (1976). Lipotropin C-fragment: an endogenous peptide with potent analgesic activity, in Kosterlitz, H.W. (ed.): *Opiates and Endogenous Opioid Peptides*. Amsterdam, Elsevier/North-Holland, pp. 9–17.

Carlsson, A. and Lindquist, M. (1963). Effect of chlorpromazine or haloperidol on formation of 3-methoxytyramine and normetanephrine in mouse brain. *Acta Pharmacol. Toxicol.* 20:140–144.

Ciaranello, R.D., Barchas, R., Kessler, S. and Barchas, J.D. Catecholamines: strain differences in biosynthetic enzyme activity in mice. *Life Sci.* 11: 565–572, 1972.

Cromwell, R. (1978). Attention and information processing. A foundation for understanding schizophrenia. In Wynne, L., Cromwell, R., Matthysse, S. eds., *The Nature of Schizophrenia*. New York: Wiley Pub., pp. 219–225.

Davis, G.C., Bunney, W.E., Jr., Buchsbaum, M.S. et al. (1979). Use of narcotic antagonists to study the role of endorphins in normal and psychiatric patients, in Usdin E., Bunney, W.E., Jr., Kline N.S. (eds.): *Endorphins in Mental Health Research*. London, Macmillan Press, pp. 393–406.

Domschke, W., Dickschas, A., Mitznegg, P. (1979). CSF beta-endorphin in schizophrenia. *Lancet* 1:1024.

Edelman, A.M., Raese, J.D., Lazar, M.A., and Barchas, J.D. (1981). Tyrosine hydroxylase from brain: Phosphorylation of the enzyme by cyclic AMP-dependent protein kinase. *J. Pharmacol. Exp. Ther.* 216:647–653, 1981.

Ellinwood, E., Sudilovsky, A., and Nelson, L. (1974). Behavior and EEG analysis of chronic amphetamine effect. *Biol. Psychiatry* 8:169–176.

Emrich, H.W., Cording, C., Piree, S.: Indication of an antipsychotic action of the opiate antagonist naloxone. *Pharmakopsychiatr Neuropsychopharmakol* 10:265–270, 1977.

Evans, C.J., Weber, E. and Barchas, J.D. (1981). Isolation and characterization of α-N-acetyl β-endorphin(1–26) from the rat posterior/intermediate pituitary lobe. *Biochem. Biophys. Res. Commun.* 102:897–904.

Faull, K.F. and Barchas, J.D. Mass spectrometric analysis of neurotransmitters and their metabolites. In: *Methods of Biochemical Analysis*, Vol. 29, D. Glick, ed. John Wiley & Sons, New York, pp. 325–383.

Faull, K.F., Kraemer, H.C., Barchas, J.D. and Berger, P.A. (1981). A review: clinical application of the probenecid test for measurement of monoamine turnover in the CNS. *Biol. Psychiatry* 16:879–899.

Hewlett, W.A., Akil, H. and Barchas, J.D. (1981). Differential interactions of dynorphin(1-13), β-endorphin, and enkephalin-related peptides at μ and δ sites in different brain regions. In *Advances in Endogenous and Exogenous Opioids*. Proceedings of International Narcotic Research Conference, July 1981, Kyoto, Japan, Kodansha Lt., Tokyo.

Hughes, J., Smith, T.W., Kosterlitz, H.W. et al. (1975). Identification of two related pentapeptides from the brain with potent opiate agonist activity. *Nature* 258:577-579.

Hughes, J. (1975) Isolation of an endogenous compound from the brain with pharmacological properties similar to morphine. *Brain Res* 88:295-308.

Jacquet, Y.F., Marks, N. (1976). The C-fragment of beta-lipotropin: An endogenous neuroleptic or antipsychotrogen. *Science* 194:632-636.

Janowsky, D.S., Segal, D.S., Bloom, F. (1977). Lack of effect of naloxone on schizophrenic symptoms. *Am. J. Psychiatry* 134:926-927.

Kessler, S., Ciaranello, R.D., Shire, J.G.M. and Barchas, J.D. (1972). Genetic variation in catecholamine-synthesizing enzyme activity. *Proc. Nat. Acad. Sci.* 69:2448-2450.

King, R., Raese, J.D. and Barchas, J.D. (1981). Catastrophe theory of dopaminergic transmission: A revised dopamine hypothesis of schizophrenia. *J. Theoret. Biol.* 92:373-400.

King, R., Raese, J., Huberman, B.A. and Barchas, J.D. (in press). Dopamine neuronal instability: a model for the schizophreniform psychoses. *Psychopharm. Bull.*

Kline, N.S., Lehmann, H.E. (1979). Therapy with beta-endorphin in psychiatric patients, in Usdin E., Bunney, W.E., Jr., Line, N.S. (eds.): *Endorphins in Mental Health Research*. London, Macmillan Press, pp. 500-517.

Kline, N.S., Li, C.H., Lehmann, H.E. et al. (1977). Beta-endorphin-induced changes in schizophrenic and depressed patients. *Arch. Gen. Psychiatry* 34:1111-1113.

Kurland, A.A., McCabe, O., Hanlon, T.E. et al. (1977). The treatment of perceptual disturbance in schizophrenia with naloxone hydrochloride. *Am. J. Psychiatry* 134:1408-1410.

Lazar, M.A., Lockfeld, A.J., Truscott, R.J.W. and Barchas, J.D. Tyrosine hydroxylase from bovine striatum: catalytic properties of the phosphorylated and nonphosphorylated forms of the purified enzyme. *J. Neurochem.*, in press.

Lazar, M.A., Mefford, I.N. and Barchas, J.D. Tyrosine hydroxylase activation: Comparison of *in vitro* phosphorylation and *in vivo* administration of haloperidol. *Biochem. Pharmacol.*, in press.

Lehmann, H., Vasavan Nair, N.P., Kline, N.S. (1979). Beta-endorphin and naloxone in psychiatric patients: clinical and biological effects. *Am. J. Psychiatry* 136:762-766.

Leonhard, K. (1979). *The Classification of Endogenous Psychoses*. New York: Irvington Publishers.

Lewis, R.V., Gerber, L.D., Stein, S. et al. (1979). On beta$_H$-Leu^5-endorphin and schizophrenia. *Arch. Gen. Psychiatry* 36:237.

Li, C.H. and Chung, D. (1976). Isolation and structure of an untriakontapeptide with opiate activity from camel pituitary glands. *Proc. Natl. Acad. Sci. USA* 73:1145-1148.

Lindstrom, L.H., Widerlov, E., Gunne, L.M. et al. (1978). Endorphins in human cerebrospinal fluid: clinical correlations to some psychotic states. *Acta Psychiatr. Scand.* 57:153-164.

Ling, N., Burger, R., Guillemin, R. (1976). Isolation, primary structure, and synthesis of alpha-enkephalin and gamma-endorphin, two peptides of hypothalamic-hypophysio origin with morphinomimetic activity. *Proc. Natl. Acad. Sci. USA* 73:3942-3946.

Mefford, I.N., Jurik, S., Noyce, N. and Barchas, J.D. Analysis of catecholamines, metabolites and sulfate conjugates in brain tissue and plasma by high performance liquid chromatography with electrochemical detection. In T. Nagatsu, ed., *Methods in Biogenic Amine Research*, Amsterdam: Elsevier/North-Holland, in press.

Nowycky, M. and Roth, R. (1978). Dopaminergic neurons: role of the presynaptic receptor in the regulation of transmitter biosynthesis. *Prog. Neuro-Psychopharmacol.* 2:139-158.

Palmour, R., Ervin, F., Wagemaker, H. et al. (1979). Characterization of a peptide from the serum of psychotic patients, in Usdin, E., Bunney, W.E., Jr., Kline, N.S. (eds.): *Endorphins in Mental Health Research*. London, Macmillan Press, pp. 581-593.

Pfefferbaum, A., Berger, P.A., Elliott, G.R. et al. (1979). Human EEG response to beta-endorphin. *Psychiatry Res* 1:83-88.

Raese, J.D., Edelman, A.M., Lazar, M.A. and Barchas, J.D. (1977). Bovine striatal tyrosine hydroxylase: multiple forms and evidence for phosphorylation by cyclic AMP-dependent protein kinase. In: *Structure and Function of Monoamine Enzymes.* E. Usdin, N. Weiner and M.B.H. Youdim (Eds.), New York: Marcel Dekker, pp. 383-400.

Ross, M., Berger, P.A., Goldstein, A. (1979). Plasma beta-endorphin immunoreactivity in schizophrenia. *Science* 200:974-981.

Segal, D.S., Browne, R.G., Arnsten, A. et al. (1978). Behavioral effects of beta-endorphin. In van Ree, J.N., Terenius, L. (eds.): *Characteristics and Function of Opioids: Developments in Neuroscience.* Amsterdam, Elsevier/North-Holland, pp. 413-414.

Spitzer, R.L., Endicott, J. and Robins, E. (1978). Research diagnostic criteria: rationale and reliability. *Arch. Gen. Psychiatry* 35:773-782.

Sullivan, S., Akil, H., Blacker, D. and Barchas, J.D. (1980). Enkephalinase: Selective inhibitors and partial characterization. *Peptides* 1:31-35.

Terenius, L., Wahlstrom, A. and Lindstrom, L. et al. (1976). Increased levels of endorphins in chronic psychosis. *Neurosci. Lett.* 3:157-162.

Verebey, K., Volavka, J. and Clouet, D. (1978). Endorphins in psychiatry. *Arch. Gen. Psychiatry* 35:877-888.

Verhoeven, W.M., van Praag, H.M. and van Ree, J.M. et al. (1979). Improvement of schizophrenic patients treated with (Des-Tyr[1])-gamma-endorphin (DTgammaE). *Arch. Gen. Psychiatry* 36:294-298.

Volavka, J., Mallya, A. and Baig, S. et al. (1977). Naloxone in chronic schizophrenia. *Science* 196:1227-1228.

Wagemaker, H. and Cade, R. (1977). The use of hemodialysis in chronic schizophrenia. *Am. J. Psychiatry* 134:684-685.

Wahlstrom, A., Johansson, L. and Terenius, L. (1976). Characterization of endorphins (endogenous morphine-like factors) in human CSF and brain extracts. In Kosterlitz, H.W. (ed.): *Opiates and Endogenous Opioid Peptides.* Amsterdam, Elsevier/North-Holland, pp. 49-56.

Watson, S.J., Berger, P.A. and Akil, H. et al. (1978). Effect of naloxone on schizophrenia: reduction in hallucinations in a subpopulation of subjects. *Science* 201:73–75.

Watson, S.J., Akil, H. and Berger, P.A. et al. (1979). Some observations on the opiate peptides and schizophrenia. *Arch. Gen. Psychiatry* 36:220–223.

Weber, E., Evans, C.J. and Barchas, J.D. (1981). Acetylated and nonacetylated forms of β-endorphin in rat brain and pituitary. *Biochem. Biophys. Res. Commun.* 103:982–989.

Weber, E., Evans, C.J. and Barchas, J.D. Opioid peptide dynorphin: predominance of the aminoterminal octapeptide fragment in rat brain regions. *Nature,* in press.

Weber, E., Roth, K.A. and Barchas, J.D. Immunohistochemical distribution of α-Neo-endorphin/dynorphin neuronal systems in rat brain: evidence for colocalization. *Proc. Natl. Acad. Sci.,* in press.

Wyatt, R.J., Erdelyi, E., Schwartz, M., Herman, M. and Barchas, J.D. (1978). Difficulties in comparing catecholamine-related enzymes from the brains of schizophrenics and controls. *Biol. Psychiatry* 13:317–334.

18

Future Research Directions in the Treatment of Schizophrenia

RICHARD JED WYATT AND LYNN E. DeLISI

INTRODUCTION

Most clinicians agree that the current treatments for schizophrenia, while advanced from what were available 30 years ago, are far from ideal. At present, our treatments fall into three categories: the psychological, the social, and the biological. While there is some evidence that appropriate psychosocial treatments can diminish the burden of schizophrenia, relatively few clinicians now argue that they can alter the basic course of the disorder. Similarly, the biological treatments (particularly the neuroleptic drugs) can markedly reduce schizophrenia's morbidity. No one argues, however, that they cure.

In this paper we discuss research for treatments that will probably be tried in the next few years. Because of the nature of this symposium (Guidelines for the Use of Psychotropic Drugs) we shall not discuss social or psychological treatments of schizophrenia. It is important to note, however, that several fairly simple concepts are coming from psychosocial studies that may make the schizophrenic's environment less toxic (Goldstein et al., 1978; Brown et al., 1972; Leff and Vaughn, 1981).

Nonetheless, it seems to us that ultimately the treatment, or better, the prevention, of schizophrenia will result from biological research. It is important to note that, to date, many of the successful biological treatments introduced into psychiatry have not been derived from any fundamental knowledge of the disorder. They have sprung from intuitive minds that have not always applied linear reasoning. Our sense is that this is unlikely to continue. We see improvements in treatment coming from hypothesis testing—relying on careful experimentation. We think that meticulous design is particularly required for schizophrenia research, given our feeling that this syndrome is more than a single disease. If schizophrenia is more than a single entity, the beneficial effects of specific treatments or preventions, aimed at one of the diseases that make up the syndromes, may be diluted or overlooked.

Toward this end, we and others are trying to determine the biological subtypes of schizophrenia. We are approaching this task in much the same way—and we hope with similar success—as investigators have with mood disorders over the last 15 years. For example, Weinberger, in his paper presented at this meeting, discusses data reporting biological differences between schizophrenic patients with normal and enlarged cerebral ventricles. It is still unclear, however, if ventricular size will delineate an etiologically different subgroup or several subgroups or a continuum of schizophrenic patients. These data may have important implications, particularly for pharmacological treatments. More clearly describing which patients one might want to maintain on neuroleptics, given neuroleptics' known propensity to produce tardive dyskinesia, would be a marked treatment improvement.

Meaningful biological subtyping of schizophrenia is, however, still in its infancy. Here we describe some evidence that viruses may be associated with some forms of schizophrenia and potential treatments if viruses are involved. We then discuss diseases that masquerade as schizophrenia. Investigations of clozapine and clozapine-like drugs are described, and, finally, some problems in evaluating new ideas for the treatment of schizophrenic patients are raised.

VIRUS AND SCHIZOPHRENIA

History is replete with examples suggestive of associations between outbreaks of infectious disorders and psychoses. Reports from ancient and pre-renaissance times indicate coincidence of epidemic illnesses (e.g., plague) with dementia-like disorders (Torrey, 1980; Berrios, 1981). Benjamin Rush, in an historical treatise on madness, noted that, "This disease sometimes appears in a typhus form . . ." and ". . . now and then pervades a whole country in the form of an epidemic . . ." such as in England in the years 1355 and 1373, in France, and Italy in 1374 and again in England in 1719. Rush also described "a striking instance of the union of madness with common fever" in patients during one such epidemic (Rush, 1810). Karl A. Menninger, also, identified a psychosis associated with the influenza outbreak of 1918-1919 (Menninger, 1928). Menninger subsequently noted that the acute confusional psychoses occurring after the influenza outbreak of 1889-1892 could also be diagnosed as acute schizophrenia, with similar syndromes occurring during outbreaks of other major infections (i.e., tuberculosis, typhus, typhoid fever and cholera) (Menninger, 1928).

In addition, there are several examples of known viral diseases that are, at least initially, diagnostically similar to schizophrenia. The rare Russian tick-born encephalitis, endemic to the Yakut Republic of the USSR, is said to be, in its chronic form, indistinguishable from classical schizophrenia (Petrov, 1970). Other, more common viral encephalides are also either initially confused with schizophrenia or develop post-encephalitic dementia-like sequelae. The Russian investigator, Malis (1961), was the first to propose that a virus that is present in the body for a long time in a latent state could produce symptoms of schizophrenia. Subsequent Russian literature, particularly in the late 1950s to 1960s, focused heavily on a viral etiology of schizophrenia (Morozov, 1954; Mar, 1957; Korsakova, 1973).

Recent establishment of the existence of "slow viral infections" (viruses having an incubation period of years to decades prior to producing symptoms) have led a few Western researchers to propose an etiologic similarity between neurodegenerative disorders and schizophrenia (Torrey and Peterson, 1973; Gajdusek, 1978; Crow, 1978). The first human slow virus disease discovered was Kuru, a neurological disorder endemic to New Guinea and transmitted by cannibalism. Kuru, however, is unlike schizophrenia because it results in massive brain degeneration and ultimately death. Other diseases, also thought to be of slow-virus origin, such as Creutzfeld-Jacob disease and perhaps even multiple sclerosis, have clearly associated neurodegenerative changes. In addition, some conventional viruses, such as measles, can also produce neurodegenerative disorders, such as subacute sclerosing panencephalitis, many years after the initial contact.

Indirect support for the viral hypothesis has come from epidemiological studies of schizophrenia. The seasonality of schizophrenic births, a peak in late winter and early spring that coincides with the peak incidence of some viral infections, such as measles and rubella, has been described (Hare et al., 1973; Torrey et al., 1977; Pulver et al., 1981). The uneven prevalence of schizophrenia throughout the world, also, is a pattern similar to the occurrence of some known viral diseases (Torrey, 1973).

Further support for this hypothesis has grown out of the application of specific immunological techniques. Serum and CSF immunoglobulins, often elevated in viral diseases, have been found in some studies to be increased in schizophrenic patients (Strahilevitz et al., 1976; Torrey et al., 1978; Gowdy, 1980). This finding is not, however, consistent (DeLisi et al., 1981) and the type of immunoglobulin elevated varies. Further studies of viral specific antibodies support the possibility that these elevations are a consequence of viral infection. Increased serum antibody titers to herpes simplex type I virus were reported in one study (Halonen et al., 1974), although not subsequently confirmed (Rimon et al., 1979). In addition, an elevation of the ratio of CSF to serum IgG antibody titers has been reported for both measles (Torrey et al., 1978) and cytomegalovirus (CMV) (Albrecht et al., 1980). An antibody ratio two standard deviations or more above the control mean is considered suggestive of local central nervous system antibody production. Sixty-eight percent of schizophrenic patients sampled had increased CMV ratios. The titer ratios reported, however, can be deceiving. An absolute increase in CSF antibodies was not actually found in the latter study, but rather a decrease in serum antibodies contributed to the altered titres. In a more recent communication, however, Torrey et al. (1982) report absolute increases in CSF CMV IgM antibodies in a small subgroup of both chronic schizophrenic and bipolar patients, and none in controls. Since increased IgM is specifically suggestive of active viral infection, this last finding warrants further exploration and confirmation in other groups of schizophrenic patients.

Tyrrell et al. (1979) demonstrated degenerative cytopathic changes in tissue cultures inoculated with CSF from about one-third of sampled schizophrenic subjects as well as over two-thirds of subjects with serious nervous system diseases. This effect, however, was not serially transferred from culture to culture and no viral particles were detected by electron microscopy. Although the agent appears similar in size and in chemical characteristics to RNA type viruses, CSF inoculated into several animals failed to produce disease or cytopathic brain changes after more than one year of incubation. Further exploration of this finding is warranted, though, for if these cytopathic alterations are indeed virally induced, the failure to prove its existence may be a result of not yet obtaining the proper physical conditions for its growth and maintenance.

Additional significant findings have emerged from several post-mortem neurohistologic studies. Fisman (1975) described "encephalitic-like" lesions in seven of 10 schizophrenic brains. These lesions were concentrated in the area of the trigeminal nucleus for which the herpes virus has a predilection. Sequiera et al. (1979), using herpes-simplex type I nucleic acid sequences, in a hybridization technique, demonstrated the viral genome in a small number of human post-mortem brain specimens from chronic psychotics. They did not, however, have necropsy material from healthy subjects for comparison and note that this may be a normally expected autopsy finding similarly seen in other primates.

Stevens (1982) recently examined histologic sections from a number of brain regions from 25 schizophrenic and 28 non-schizophrenic patients, all between ages 21 and 54. Three-quarters of the brains from the schizophrenic patients had patchy fibrillary gliosis most marked in the periventricular, and periaqueductal structures, as well as basal forebrain. Gliosis and other microscopic changes were equally evident in the control brains, although occurring in different regions. The finding of gliosis in limbic related structures in the schizophrenic patients is consistent with earlier neuropathological work as well as with the enlarged ventricles found in some schizophrenic patients (Weinberger and Wyatt, 1982) and is further evidence consistent with viral produced changes.

In subsequent preliminary work, Stevens et al. (unpublished data) attempted to identify specific viruses likely to be associated with the gliosis. Brains from patients with a chronic schizophrenic illness were immunoreactive to specific CMV antigens, while they were non-reactive to herpes simplex antigens. Although the reaction was also present in three of thirteen controls, in the controls the reaction was shown to be nonspecific, having cross-reactivity with other antigens. Contrary to Stevens' findings, Aulakah et al. (1981), using a cytomegalovirus (^{3}H)-DNA probe, which should hybridize to any CMV virus present, were unable to detect cytomegalovirus related genetic information in the autopsied brains from six schizophrenic patients. This line of research requires continued work before any consistent finding will emerge.

A major criticism of studies supportive of the viral hypothesis of schizophrenia is that long term neuroleptic treatment of chronic schizophrenic patients, as well as long term hospitalization, alters immunity. These patients may simply be less resistant to viral infections. The viral manifestations could be an effect, rather than a cause, of the illness and its treatment.

Treatment Considerations

Despite a number of inconsistencies, the evidence for a viral presence in, at least, a subgroup of schizophrenic-like illnesses is gaining sufficient strength to consider the experimental use of antiviral agents in appropriate patients. While the clinical course of schizophrenia is variable, the chronic form often develops slowly with acute exacerbations, then remissions, before following a chronic downhill course. If schizophrenic symptoms are virally induced and the virus is in some way actively producing changes causing the disorder, antiviral agents might be appropriately prescribed. If schizophrenia is a relatively stable disorder, however, and the hypothetical viral agent has done its damage by the time the patient is first diagnosed, there may be little to treat.

Criteria for patient selection, such as evidence of increased antibody titers and production, need to be established prior to the initiation of antiviral agents, since these agents may not be without side effects. Although the newest of these drugs appear to have minimal toxicity when used in acute situations, the effects of chronic use are unknown. In life threatening situations such as herpes-simplex encephalitis, the risk is negligible compared with potential benefits. In schizophrenia, however, benefit/risk ratios must be determined in order not to produce more damage than the disorder itself causes. Also, prophylactic use of a drug entailing some risk, without specifically knowing the viral agent being treated, will be difficult and costly and could cause considerable side effects (as occurred from the swine flu vaccination program). Presumably, a specific drug will have been studied in patients with diseases in which the viral etiology is well established. From these studies the toxic effects of the antiviral agent should be known. If a schizophrenic viral-like agent is potentially responsive to a specific antiviral drug not extensively studied in man, then at least good toxicology profiles should be available from animal studies.

Since it is expected that only a subgroup of the acute schizophrenias may be virally induced, one would suspect that the illness in others would be due to other etiologies. Complete spontaneous recovery might be expected in some of these cases. While there is little data pertaining to prediction of the long-term course of acute schizophrenic disorders, there is good data to suggest that neuroleptics and a supportive environment (Astrachan et al., 1974; Tuma et al., 1978) can greatly decrease the morbidity during the first few years. There must be, therefore, clear criteria to separate the potential viral etiology patients from the rest. This will require quick and specific tests to determine those most at risk.

Giving an antiviral agent must be viewed as treatment related research. Mechanisms will have to be developed to deal appropriately with issues of consent. For the chronic or remitting schizophrenic, urgency may be somewhat less important. If a hypothetical virus is responsible for acute exacerbations of schizophrenia, similar perhaps to the occurrence of herpes simplex perioral lesions, then it might be appropriately identified during one episode and treated during the next. While treatment is in the research stage, this will give the scientist-clinician both the time and the opportunity to obtain consent from the patient. Obviously, this is the ideal situation provided that the time lost does not result in an ultimate worsening of the patient's state. At present there are four main antiviral strategies that researchers might employ.

1. Use of available antiviral agents should be investigated. For example, acycloguanosine (Acyclovir)—recently found effective in herpes simplex encephalitis (Saral et al., 1981) or adenine arabinoside (Vidarabine)—have been shown to be effective in herpes simplex and CMV infections (Phillips et al., 1977). These act primarily by inhibiting the production of viral DNA, and unlike previously used antiviral agents, these drugs exhibit little toxicity against healthy cells.

2. Use of interferon, which is a substance naturally produced in response to a viral infection, might be considered. Synthetic interferon is now being used for clinical research trials in cancer patients. Not only is it a point inhibitor of viral replication, but also cellular proliferation and enzymatic activity specific to the immune response (Borden, 1979; Marx, 1979). Recent success has been reported in reducing exacerbations of multiple sclerosis with interferon use over a six-month period (Jacobs et al., 1981). The use of interferon for treatment for CNS disorders, however, may be hampered by its inability to cross the blood-brain barrier, thus requiring intrathecal injections. Nevertheless, Cantell et al. (1980) reported some initial improvement in four schizophrenic patients with

subcutaneous interferon injections. While Cantell et al. (1980) advocate further investigation of the usefulness of interferon for treating psychosis, they also note its high potential for causing granulocytopenia and bone marrow toxicity.

3. Use of transfer factor, a substance conveying specific immunoreactivity to individuals previously unresponsive to a particular antigen, is another possibility. Although it has not appeared effective for the treatment of CNS disorders such as multiple sclerosis (Graybill, 1974), there is at least some evidence of its effectiveness in some cytomegalic viral infections (Jones et al., 1981).

4. Ultimately, a vaccine, even if the viral agent is not clearly isolated, may be developed from specific factors isolated from the blood of patients who develop schizophrenia. Alternatively, in the future, those identified as particularly at risk, may have available to them pooled gamma-globulin from completely recovered acute schizophrenics that may be beneficial in a similar manner to gamma-globulin prophylaxis for people exposed to viral hepatitis.

New approaches to the treatment of viral-like infections have been steadily appearing in recent years. Coinciding with these advances may be the appearance of a new subgroup of schizophrenia defined by evidence of a specific viral etiology. As we investigate further viral associations to the schizophrenic syndrome and delineate patients to which a viral etiology might apply, our treatment strategies for this potential subgroup of patients will become clearer.

DISEASES THAT MAY MASQUERADE AS SCHIZOPHRENIA

There have been a number of diseases that have, at times, been clinically indistinguishable from schizophrenia. Through increased medical knowledge over the last century, we have gradually identified specific pathologic determinants for a number of these diseases so that they are now rarely, if ever, confused with schizophrenia. Syphilis, mental retardation, and pellagra are examples of some that were misdiagnosed at various times. There are still today, however, a number of disorders that, at least in their early phases, appear to be schizophrenia, and are subsequently re-diagnosed, such as Huntington's disease. As our knowledge expands, we undoubtedly will continue to separate other distinct disorders from the diagnostic category of schizophrenia. It is particularly important to differentiate these syndromes from classical, neuroleptic responsive schizophrenia so that other, more specific treatments may be applied.

Phenylketonuria (PKU)

One disease that has, for a long time, been recognized as behaviorally similar to schizophrenia is phenylketonuria. PKU is one of the heritable syndromes, or "inborn errors of metabolism" and when unrecognized and untreated, leads to mental retardation. PKU is an autosomal recessive disorder, classically characterized by a deficiency in hepatic phenylalanine hydroxylase, although a deficiency of an enzyme cofactor, dihydropteridine, may be present in a variant form. PKU homozygosity appears in approximately one out of 20,000 births, and the frequency of PKU heterozygosity is close to 2% (Thalhammer et al., 1975). While it is usually detectable by massive urinary screening efforts in infants, occasionally milder forms may go unnoticed until adulthood and present as a schizophreniform illness (Perry et al., 1973).

Although controversial, some family studies suggest, also, an association of PKU heterozygosity with an increased risk for development of schizophrenia (Folling, 1934; Penrose and Comb, 1935; Thompson, 1957). Poisner (1960) reported elevated plasma phenylalanine concentrations in some schizophrenic patients, and Lippman (1958) found decreased tolerance to phenylalanine loading in 13 of 50 schizophrenics. We have been unable, however, to confirm these findings either by oral or intravenous phenylalanine loading tests in a group of chronic schizophrenic patients (Potkin et al., 1983).

If other studies find that PKU and PKU heterozygosity significantly contributes to the genetic aspects of schizophrenia, screening for this syndrome among psychiatric hospital admissions might be of considerable importance. Logic suggests that reduction in dietary phenylalanine may be an effective treatment alternative to the use of neuroleptics for these patients. Furthermore, detection of PKU in women of childbearing age may warrant both genetic counseling and dietary treatment during pregnancy. If warranted, such screening could contribute to prevention of possible fetal nervous system damage and perhaps later psychiatric problems in individuals who do not themselves have PKU.

Treatment of PKU with low phenylalanine diets in early childhood is well established, but the point at which dietary restriction is no longer necessary remains controversial (Scriver and Clow, 1980). While adults with PKU, previously removed from phenylalanine restrictive diets, may appear to have no deleterious effects, they may be at increased risk for development of psychiatric symptoms. More research is needed to determine the usefulness of low phenylalanine diets, as well as supplementary dihydropteridine (or an analog), for the treatment and prevention of neuropsychiatric problems in this group.

Phenylethylamine (PEA), the product of the decarboxylation of phenylalanine, is present in increased amounts in the urine of PKU subjects, heterzygotes for PKU, as well as some schizohprenic patients (Jeste et al., 1981; Potkin et al., 1979; Reynolds et al., 1978; Fischer et al., 1972; Hackney, 1967). PEA is of particular interest because of its chemical and behavioral similarity to amphetamine, which under some circumstances can produce a psychosis similar to paranoid schizophrenia.

Recently, a subgroup of hospitalized delusionally depressed patients with an atypical bipolar disorder have been reported to have unusually high 24-hour urinary PEA excretion (Karoum et al., 1982). While these patients had little response to conventional antidepressant medication, one of them improved dramatically on an open trial of carbidopa (Linnoila et al., in press). Carbidopa, a peripheral decarboxylase inhibitor, acts by decreasing phenylalanine conversion to PEA. Whether carbidopa is beneficial for the treatment of schizophrenia or other psychiatric patients has not yet been determined. This initial case report may serve to initiate other experimental treatments of psychiatric patients with increased PEA.

CLOZAPINE AND CLOZAPINE-LIKE ANTIPSYCHOTICS

Clozapine, a di-benzodiazepine derivative with a piperazinyl side-chain, is a novel neuroleptic with properties unlike classical neuroleptics. It has no cataleptic action, and fails to block apomorphine and amphetamine induced stereotypies in animals (Stille et al., 1971a, and 1971b; Al-Shabibi and Doggett, 1980). Despite clear antipsychotic efficacy, there is a remarkable lack of extrapyramidal side effects in patients receiving clozapine (DeMaio, 1969; Shopsin et al., 1979), a finding that many clinicians feel will increase compliance among their patients. Perhaps most important, though, is that no cases of tardive dyskinesia have yet been reported with clozapine use.

At one time, many clinicians felt it was necessary for antipsychotic agents to be given in doses high enough to produce extrapyramidal effects in order to be efficacious. These drugs became known as the neuroleptics (from the Greek: neuro=nerve, lepsis=a taking hold), which literally means drugs that produce neurological symptoms. Because of the association between extrapyramidal side effects and antipsychotic potency, potential antipsychotics were screened for production of catalepsy and blocking of apomorphine induced stereotypies. This process excluded those drugs unlikely to produce extrapyramidal symptoms. That clozapine has clear antipsychotic activity, and does not appear to produce these symptoms, makes use of this agent enticing.

The research into various neuropharmacologic actions of clozapine has proved interesting. Although controversial, there may be an association of clozapine's lack of extrapyramidal effects with a reduction in cholinergic neuronal firing in the brain (Haubrich et al., 1975; Burki et al., 1975; Miller and Hiley, 1974). Also, clozapine only weakly produces dopamine receptor blockade and accelerates dopamine metabolism at very high doses (Burki et al., 1975). This may explain its failure to elevate serum prolactin concentrations in a manner similar to actions of other neuroleptics (Kane et al., 1981; Meltzer et al., 1979).

In carefully controlled studies, clozapine was found to have antipsychotic potency approximating that of chlorpromazine (Shopsin et al., 1979; Nikkanen et al., 1974; Ackenheil et al., 1974). Also, there is some evidence of antidepressant and anxiolytic effects as well (Shopsin et al., 1979; Nahunek et al., 1975). Whether or not clozapine actually relieves the so called negative symptoms of schizophrenia—i.e., anhedonia, avolition, affective flattening, alogia and attentional deficits—remains unclear. Conventional neuroleptics appear to be of little benefit in treating these symptoms.

Clozapine had been in use for a few years in many European and Asian countries until a serious side effect became evident (Amsler et al., 1977). A sudden outbreak of granulocytopenia and agranulocytosis in Finnish patients in 1975 appeared to be related to clozapine treatment. Of 13 cases with agranulocytosis, eight died due to secondary infection. The granulocytopenia (white cell count below $3,200/\mu l$, granulocytes below 1,600) and agranulocytosis (none or very few granulocytes in the peripheral blood) appeared to be due to toxic (metabolic) rather than allergic phenomena.

In toxic agranulocytosis, drugs such as the phenothiazines are thought to inhibit stem cell DNA synthesis during first exposure in specific, predisposed individuals. This results in a reduction in bone marrow production of granulocytes. An investigation of the incident failed to discover any factors present in individuals that were suggestive of a particular predisposition towards development of this reaction. Since there was no obvious way to determine individuals at risk, the drug was taken off the market (Amsler et al., 1977) and, therefore, never became commercially available in Canada or the United States.

Clozapine is still available, however, in The People's Republic of China. The Chinese manufacture it themselves and claim highly successful results. They do not believe it produces tardive dyskinesia and have seen no serious blood dyscrasias resulting from its use. Since a predisposition towards development of serious blood dyscrasias appears not to be present among the Chinese, it would be useful to carry out careful studies in China. In a country with a population of a billion people multiple studies could be performed to determine in which patients this drug is most efficacious and if, indeed, it does not produce tardive dyskinesia. Such studies would provide valuable information concerning the risk/benefit ratio for this agent. To date, positive clinical experience suggests that development of a similar drug, not producing blood toxicity, would be of considerable benefit.

Loxapine, perlapine, RMI-81,582, sulpirimide, metoclopramide and trebenzomine are examples of antipsychotics chemically or pharmacologically related to clozapine. Both loxapine and perlapine, while structurally similar to clozapine, appear to have properties similar to classical neuroleptics. Sulpirimide and metoclopramide, two substituted benzamides with antipsychotic action also produce all the side effects characteristic of conventional neuroleptics.

RMI-81,582, a morphanthridine compound, similar to clozapine in that it produces few extrapyramidal symptoms and no increase in prolactin release, was removed from further clinical testing because of toxicity in dogs (Meltzer et al., 1980). Trebenzomine, however, in one initial report of use in schizophrenic and schizoaffective patients, appears hopeful as a new antipsychotic agent, and warrants further clinical trials (Meltzer et al., 1980). Psychiatric improvement in an initial study was not accompanied by any extrapyramidal symptoms or increment in serum prolactin concentrations.

Melperone, a butyrophenone, is also a clozapine-like drug with antipsychotic properties. Unlike the structurally related haloperidol, it has only a minimal incidence of extrapyramidal symptoms (although greater than clozapine), and results in only very small transient rises in prolactin secretion. While its use thus far has been primarily limited to elderly patients in Europe, there have been no reports of associations of this drug with tardive dyskinesia.

A number of pharmaceutical companies are said to be developing other such drugs. The absence of clozapine produced extrapyramidal symptoms could have considerable implications for future pharmacologic screening of useful antipsychotics. It now has been suggested that clozapine-like drugs, i.e., ones that do not increase prolactin or produce extrapyramidal symptoms, should be screened for in several existing classes of drugs and that pharmaceutical companies should reevaluate their methods of drug selection for antipsychotic action (Shopsin et al., 1979; Meltzer et al., 1980).

In summary, the findings that clozapine and clozapine-like drugs appear to have considerable therapeutic potential, do not appear to exert conventional neuroleptic side effects, or produce tardive dyskinesia, have significant therapeutic implications. Further investigations, however, of possible clozapine-produced side effects must be completed before this drug or related compounds can be generally prescribed. If clozapine or analogs are found not to produce tardive dyskinesia or other serious effects, these drugs could add considerably to the pharmacopeia of schizophrenia.

DEALING WITH NEW IDEAS

An enormous problem for clinicians treating schizophrenic patients is knowing how to evaluate the numerous claims for treatments and cures. Not only is it difficult to know which ones to take seriously initially, but if one attempts to verify a claim and fails, there is no standard criteria for when to stop investing money, time, and patient welfare on any one particular inquiry. Unfortunately, somewhere buried in these sundry claims a useful treatment for subgroups of schizophrenics may be found, as was the case with lithium treatment for manic-depressive disorder.

Cade, in 1949, wrote about lithium's effect on mania in a relatively obscure medical journal (Cade, 1949). For a variety of reasons, it was not until 1969 that lithium was introduced for the treatment of manic-depressive patients in the United States. Since that time, manic-depressive disorder has been managed successfully in an increasing number of patients. It is fair to assume that during the delay between Cade's publication and the widespread use of the drug, for many, there was undue suffering and considerable financial hardship (Reifman and Wyatt, 1980).

Shortly after Cade published his reports on lithium and mania, there was a series of what were considered, for their time, well designed and executed studies performed with niacin and nicotinamide for the treatment of schizophrenia (Hoffer et al., 1957). Hoffer et al. (1957) claimed that oral doses of 1 g of niacin every 24-hours made 11 of 18 chronic schizophrenics "well" while the remainder improved significantly. Subsequent to these claims, an expensive series of well controlled studies was carried out in several countries, attempting to replicate the Hoffer and Osmond report. In general, no therapeutic response was found (APA, 1973; Bann et al., 1977). The proponents of these treatments, claimed that the nonreplicating studies were improperly performed. They continue to advocate these and other vitamins and minerals in large doses for the treatment of schizophrenia. Because of the difficulty in performing well controlled studies administering mega amounts of multiple vitamins to large groups of patients, this issue remains unresolved (Pauling, et al., 1973; Wyatt, 1974).

Today some of the most interesting reading, with regard to new treatments in psychiatry, appears in the *Journal of Orthomolecular Psychiatry*. Specifically published are hypotheses, anecdotes and case histories claiming success with one or another dietary substance, elimination of a substance or a desensitization technique. If there is a "new lithium" described in that journal or a similar publication, it may be difficult to recognize its importance. We hope that by raising this issue we may stimulate others to try and cope with the problem rationally. Certainly, many patients and their families, in addition to clinicians, need constructive advice on this topic.

DISCUSSION

We have now discussed a few new directions that will probably be taken by the academic and pharmaceutical communities in the next few years. We have also suggested developing an increased sensitivity to diseases that might be misdiagnosed as schizophrenia. Finally, we have touched briefly on what we feel is a vitally important research goal; to subdivide the schizophrenias into what we hypothesize are a number of disease entities. If schizophrenia can be divided into meaningful subgroups, then more rational treatments and preventions will certainly follow. This has been seen repeatedly in most other medical fields. Separating one kind of pneumonia from another led to rational and successful treatment and the current distinctions that are being made in the diagnosis of cancer are beginning to lead to its prevention and successful treatment. By more clearly subtyping the schizophrenias, those treatment innovations that are developed can be applied more appropriately.

REFERENCES

Ackenheil, M., Beckman, H., Greil, W. (1974). Antipsychotic efficacy of clozapine in correlation to changes in catecholamine metabolism in man. In: *Phenothiazines and Structurally Related Drugs*. Ed. by Forrest, I.S., Cair, C.J. and Usdin, E., Raven Press, New York.

Albrecht, P., Torrey, E.F., Boone, E., Hicks, J.T., Daniel, N. (1980). Raised cytomegalovirus antibody level in cerebrospinal fluid of schizophrenic patients. *Lancet* ii:769–772.

Al-Shabibi, V.M.H. and Doggett, N.S. (1980). Clozapine's anti-acetylcholine property modulates its anti-stereotypic action in the mesolimbic system communications. *J. Pharm. Pharmacol.* 32:359–361.

Amsler, H.A., Teerenhovi, L., Barth, E. Hayula, K. and Vuopio, P. (1977). Agranulocytosis in patients treated with clozapine. A study of the Finnish. Epidemic *Acta. Psychiatr. Scan.* 56:241–248.

APA Task Force on Vitamin Therapy in Psychiatry Megavitamin and Orthomolecular Therapy in Psychiatry, Washington, D.C., 1973.

Astrachan, B.M., Brauer, L., Harrow, M., Schwartz, C. (1974). Symptomatic outcome in schizophrenia. *Arch. Gen. Psychiatry* 31:155–160.

Aulakh, G.S., Kleinman, J.E., Aulakh, H.S., Albrecht, P., Torrey, E.F. and Wyatt, R.J. (1981). Search for cytomegalovirus in schizophrenic brain tissue. *Proc. Soc. Exp. Biol. Med.* 167:172–174.

Bann, T.A., Lehman, H.E., Deutsch, M. (1977). Negative findings with megavitamins in schizophrenic patients: Preliminary report. *Commun. Psychopharmacology* 1:119–122.

Berrios, G.E. (1981). Delirium and confusion in the 19th century: A conceptual history. *Br. J. Psychiatry* 139:439–449.

Borden, E.C. (1979). Interferons: Rationale for clinical trials in neoplastic disease. *Ann. Intern. Med.* 91:472–479.

Brown, G.W., Birely, J.L.T. and Wing, J.K. (1972). Influence of family life on the course of schizophrenic disorders: A replication. *Br. J. Psychiatry* 121: 241–258.

Burki, H.R., Eichenberger, E., Sayers, A.C., White, T.G. (1975). Clozapine and the dopamine hypothesis of schizophrenia, a critical appraisal. *Pharmakopsychiat.* 8:115–121.

Cade, J.F.J. (1949). Lithium salts in the treatment of psychotic excitement. *Med. J. Aust.* 36:349–352.

Cantell, K., Pulkkinen, E., Elosuo, R. and Suominen, J. (1980). Effect of interferon on severe psychiatric diseases. *Ann. Clin. Res.* 12:131-132.

Crow, T.J. (1978). Viral causes of psychiatric disease. *Postgrad. Med. J.* 54:763-
767.

DeLisi, K.E., Weinberger, D.R., Neckers, L.M., Potkin, S.G., Shiling, D. and
Wyatt, R.J. (1981). Quantitative determination of immunoglobulin concentrations in CSF and plasma of schizophrenic patients. *Br. J. Psychiatry*
139:513-519.

DeMaio, D. (1969). Preliminary clinical evaluation of a new neuroleptic agent
HF-1854. In: *The Present Status of Psychotropic Drugs: Pharmacological
and Clinical Aspects.* Amsterdam, Exerpta Medica Foundation, pp. 485-
488.

Fischer, E., Spatz, H., Saavedra, J.M., Reggiani, H., Mira, A. and Heiler, B.
(1972). Urinary elimination of phenylethylamine. *Biol. Psychiatry* 5:139-
147.

Fisman, M. (1975). The brain stem in psychosis. *Br. J. Psychiatry* 126:414-422.

Folling, A. (1934). Uber ausscheidong von phenylbrenztrauben saure in den harn
als stobbwech-seianomalie in verbindurg mit imbezillitat. *Physiol. Chem.*
127:169-176.

Gajdusek, D.C. (1978). The possible role of slow virus infection in chronic
schizophrenic dementia. *Birth Defects,* VIV:81-87.

Goldstein, M.J., Rodnick, E.H., Evans, J.R., May, P.R.A., Steinberg, M.R.
(1978). Drug and family therapy in the aftercare of acute schizophrenics.
Arch. Gen. Psychiatry 35:1169-1177.

Gowdy, J.M. (1980). Immunoglobulin levels in psychotic patients. *Psychosomatics* 21:751-756.

Graybill, J.R. (1974). Transfer factor in diseases of the central nervous system.
Adv. Neurol. 6:107-126.

Hackney, I.M. (1967). Autistic behavioral patterns in phenylketonuria children.
Can. Psychiatr. Assoc. J. 12:333-334.

Halonen, P., Rimon, R., Arochonka, K., Jantti, V. (1974). Antibody levels to
Herpes simplex Type I, measles and rubella viruses in psychiatric patients.
Br. J. Psychiatry 125:461-465.

Hare, E.H., Price, J.S., Slater, E. (1973). Mental disorder and season of birth.
Nature 241:480.

Haubrich, D.R., Wang, P.F.L., Herman, R.L. and Clody, D.E. (1975). Acetylcholine synthesis in rat brain: Dissimilar effects of clozapine and chlorpromazine. *Life Sci.* 17:739-748.

Hoffer, A., Osmond, H. and Callbeck, M.J. (1957). Treatment of schizophrenia
with nicotinic acid and nicotinamide. *J. Clin. Exp. Psychopathol.* 18:131-
158.

Jacobs, L., O'Malley, J., Freeman, A., Ekes, R. (1981). Intrathecal interferon
reduces exacerbations of multiple sclerosis. *Science* 214:1026-1028.

Jeste, D.V., Doongaji, D.R., Panjwani, D., Datta, M., Potkin, S.G., Karoum, F.,
Thatle, S., Sheth, A.S., Apte, J.S. and Wyatt, R.J. (1981). Cross-cultural
study of biochemical abnormality in paranoid schizophrenia. *Psychiatry
Res.* 5:341-352.

Jones, J.F., Jeter, W.S., Fulgeneti, V.A., Minnich, L.L., Pritchett, R.F., Wedg-
wood, R.J. (1981). Treatment of childhood combined epstein-barr virus/
cytomegalovirus infection with oral bovine transfer factor. *Lancet* ii:
122-124.

Kane, J.M., Cooper, T.B., Sachar, E.J., Halpern, F.S., Bailine, S. (1961). Clozapine: Plasma levels and prolactin response. *Psychopharmacology* 73:184–187.

Karoum, F., Linnoila, M., Potter, W.Z., Chuang, L.W., Goodwin, F.K. and Wyatt, R.J. (1982). Fluctuating high urinary phenylethylamine excretion rates in some bipolar affective disorder patients. *Psychiatry Res.* 6:215–222.

Korsakova, S.S. (1973). (translated). *Psychopharmacology Bull.* 9:59.

Leff, J. and Vaughn, C. (1981). The role of maintenance therapy and relatives' expressed emotion in relapse of schizophrenia: A two-year follow-up. *Br. J. Psychiatry* 139:102–104.

Linnoila, M., Karoum, F., Potkin, S.G., Wyatt, R.J. and Potter, W.Z. (in press). Amelioration of psychosis with carbidopa: A case report. *Br. J. Psychiatry*.

Lippman, R.W. (1958). The significance of heterozygosity for hereditary metabolic errors related to mental deficiency (oligomentia). *Am. J. Ment. Defic.* 63:320–324.

Malis, G.I. (1961). *Research on the Etiology of Schizophrenia.* Translated by Basil Haith, New York, Consultant Bureau.

Mar, G.I., Svyadoshch, A.M. and Korsakov, J. (1957). *J. Neuropathol. Psych.* 57:1098.

Marx, J.L. (1979). Interferon (I): On the threshold of clinical application. *Science* 244:1183–1186.

Meltzer, H.Y., Goode, D.J., Schyve, P.M., Young, M., Fang, V.S. (1979). Effect of clozapine on human serum prolactin levels. *Am. J. Psychiatry* 136:1550–1555.

Meltzer, H.Y., Fang, V.S., Young, M.A. (1980). Clozapine-like drugs. *Psychopharmacology Bull.* 16:32–35.

Menninger, K.A. (1925). Schizophrenia syndrome as product of acute infectious disease. Association for Research in Nervous and Mental Disease Proceedings, 1928, 5:182–203.

Miller, R.J., Hiley, C.R. (1974). Anti-muscarinic properties of neuroleptics and drug-induced Parkinsonism. *Nature* (London) 248:596–597.

Morozov, V.M. (1954). Virus etiology of schizophrenia: Experimental study. *Zh. Neuropat. Psikhiat.* 54:732–734.

Nahunek, K., Svetka, J., Misurec, J. (1975). Klinicke zkusenosti s clozapinem. *Cesk. Psychiatr.* 71:11–20.

Nikkanen, P., Achte, K., Haskari, M. (1974). Results of a double blind study comparing clozapine and chlorpromazine in the treatment of schizophrenia. *Psychiatria Feumica*:307–313.

Pauling, L., Robinson, A.B., Oxley, S.S. (1973). Subjects and controls. In: *Orthomolecular Psychiatry Treatment of Schizophrenia*, Hawkins, D. and Pauling, L. (eds.), San Francisco, W.H. Freeman, Co., pp. 18–34.

Penrose, L.S., Camib, M.D. (1935). Inheritance of phenylpyruvic amentia (phenylketonuria). *Lancet*:192–194.

Perry, T.L., Hansen, S., Tischler, B., Richards, F.M., Sokol, M. (1973). Unrecognized adult phenylketonuria. *N. Engl. J. Med.* 289:395–398.

Petrov, P.A. (1970). V. vilyuisk encephalitis in the Yakut Republic (U.S.S.R.). *Am. J. Trop. Med. Hyg.* 19:146–150.

Phillips, C.A., Fanning, W.L., Gump, D.W., Phillips, C.F. (1977). Cytomegalovirus encephalitis in immunologically normal adults. Successful treatment with vidarabine. *JAMA* 238:2299–2300.

Poisner, A.M. (1960). Serum phenylalanine in schizophrenia: Biochemical genetic aspects. *J. Nerv. Ment. Dis.* 131:74–76.

Potkin, S.G., Karoum, F., Chuang, L., Cannon-Spoor, H.E., Phillips, I. and Wyatt, R.J. (1979). Phenylethylamine in paranoid chronic schizophrenia. *Science* 206:470–471.

Potkin, S.G., Cannon-Spoor, H.E., DeLisi, L.E., Neckers, L. and Wyatt, R.J. (1983). Plasma phenylalanine, tyrosine, and tryptophan in schizophrenia. *Arch. Gen. Psychiatry* 40:749–752.

Pulver, A.E., Sawyer, J.W., Childs, B. (1981). The association between season of birth and the risk for schizophrenia. *Am. J. Epidemiol.* 144:735–749.

Reifman, A. and Wyatt, R.J. (1980). Lithium: A brake in the rising cost of mental illness. *Arch. Gen. Psychiatry* 37:385–388.

Reynolds, G.P., Seakins, J.W.T., Grey, D.O. (1978). The urinary excretion of 2-phenylethylamine in phenylketonuria. *Clin. Chem. Acta.* 83:33–39.

Rimon, R., Halonen, P., Puhakka, P., Laitinen, L., Marttila, R. and Salmela, L. (1979). Immunoglobulin antibodies to Herpes simplex Type I detected by radioimmunoassay in serum and cerebrospinal fluid of patients with schizophrenia. *J. Clin. Psych.* 40:241–243.

Rush, B. (1810). Medical inquiries and observations upon the diseases of the mind. In: *Documentary History of Psychiatry*, Goshen, C.E. (ed.). New York, Philosophical Library, Inc., 1967, pp. 266–276.

Saral, R., Burns, W.H., Laskin, O.L., Sautos, G.W., Lietman, P.S. (1981). Acyclovir prophylaxis of herpes simplex-virus infections. *N. Engl. J. Med.* 305:63–67.

Scriver, C.R. and Clow, C.L. (1980). Phenylketonuria: Epitome of human biochemical genetics. *N. Engl. J. Med.* 303:1394–1400.

Sequiera, L.W., Carrasco, L.H., Curry, A., Jennings, L.C., Lord, M.A., Sutton, R.N.P. (1979). Detection of herpes simplex viral genome in brain tissue. *Lancet* ii:609–612.

Shopsin, B., Klein, H., Aaronson, M., Collora, M. (1979). Clozapine, chlorpromazine, and placebo in newly hospitalized acutely schizophrenic patients: A controlled double-blind comparison. *Arch. Gen. Psychiatry* 36:657–664.

Stevens, J.R. (1982). Neuropathology of schizophrenia. *Arch. Gen. Psychiatry* 39:1131–1139.

Stille, G., Ackerman, H., Eichenberger, E., Lauener, H. (1971a). The pharmacological properties of a potent neuroleptic compound from the dibenzodiazepine group. *Int. J. Neuropharmacol.* 4:375–383.

Stille, G., Lauener, H., Eichenberger, E. (1971b). The pharmacology of 8-chlor-11-(4'-methyl)-piperazineo)-5H-dibenzo(b,e)(1,4) diazepine (clozapine). *Farmaco (Prat)* 26:603–625.

Strahilevitz, M., Fleishman, J., Fischer, G., Harris, R. and Narasimhachari, N. (1976). Immunoglobulin levels in psychiatric patients. *Am. J. Psychiatry* 133:772–777.

Thalhammer, O., (1975). Frequency of inborn errors of metabolism, especially PKU, in some representative newborn screening centers around the world: A collaborative study. *Humangenetik* 30:273–286.

Thompson, J.H. (1957). Relations of phenylketonuric patients. *J. Ment. Defic. Res.* 1:67–78.

Torrey, E.F., Yolken, R.H., Winfrey, C.J. (1982). Cytomegalovirus antibody in the CSF of schizophrenic patients detected by enzyme immunoassay. *Science* 216:892–894.

Torrey, E.F. and Peterson, M.R. (1973). Slow and latent viruses in schizophrenia. *Lancet* ii:22–24.

Torrey, E.F., Torrey, B.B., Peterson, M.R. (1977). Seasonality of schizophrenia births in the United States. *Arch. Gen. Psychiatry* 34:1065–1070.

Torrey, E.F., Peterson, M.R., Brannon, W.L., Carpenter, W.T., Post, R.M. and van Kammen, D.P. (1978). Immunoglobulins and viral antibodies in psychiatric patients. *Br. J. Psychiatry* 132:342–348.

Torrey, E.F. (1980). Schizophrenia and civilization. New York, Aronson.

Tyrrell, D.A.J., Parry, R.P., Crow, T.J., Johnstone, E., Ferrier, I.N. (1979). Possible virus in schizophrenia and some neurological disorders. *Lancet* i:839–841.

Tuma, A.H., May, P.R.A., Yale, C., Forsythe, A.B. (1978). Therapist characteristics and the outcome of treatment in schizophrenia. *Arch. Gen. Psychiatry* 35:81–85.

Weinberger, D.R. and Wyatt, R.J. (1982). Cerebral ventricular size: A biological marker for subtyping chronic schizophrenia. *Biological Markers in Psychiatry and Neurology*, Hanin, P.I. and Usdin, E. (eds.), New York, Pergamon Press, pp. 505–512.

Wyatt, R.J. (1974). Comment. *Am. J. Psychiatry* 131:1258–1262.

SECTION III

Anxiety

Hints for Clinicians

The issues on clinical aspects are described by Dr. E. Sellers (Chapter 19, following).

19

Summary of the Guidelines for the Use of Psychotropic Drugs in the Treatment of Anxiety

Edward M. Sellers

With a reasoned approach to treatment, acute and chronic anxiety can be diminished by medications, particularly the benzodiazepines, which despite publicity to the contrary, are neither panacea nor poison (Lader, 1981).

At present much discussion in the popular and scientific press about the treatment of anxiety seems based on the diametrically opposed belief systems of "pharmacologic calvinism" and "psychotropic hedonism" (Klerman, 1972). Such moral stances towards prescribing medication for relief of anxiety need to be recognized as irrelevant to the development of rational guidelines for treatment. Optimal patient care of any kind depends on proper assessment; thoughtful selection of treatment; frequent monitoring of clinical response; periodic revision of treatment and continuity of care. The treatment of anxiety disorders should be no different. However, the ubiquitous occurrence of "anxiety" in both normal life and mental disorders, its ephemeral nature, its inherent distressing quality and the frequent admixture of depression create special problems for pharmacotherapy. The consequence is a complexity that often produces a gap between desirable and actual clinical practice.

The purpose of this section is to narrow the gap between benchtop and bedside. The following chapters review the areas of new research findings (Paul), methodology (Raskin), applied pharmacokinetics (Linnoila) and practical implications (Lader). Perhaps the single most important conclusion from this whole section for the clinician is that the pharmacotherpay of anxiety will undergo major changes in the next five years. Reasons for predicting such developments include: the identification of benzodiazepine receptors and of endogenous ligands with high affinity for such receptors; the discovery of β-carbolines that mimic anxiety in animals; the synthesis of specific benzodiazepine receptor antagonists; the identification of non-benzodiazepine chemical structures with affinity for "benzodiazepine" receptors; the demonstration that some triazolo benzodiazepines have "anti-depressant" activity (Paul); finally a change in the conceptual clinical framework as a consequence of the widespread use of the DSM-III classification system for mental illness (Williams, 1980).

Notwithstanding such future developments current treatment of anxiety disorders would be improved by widespread application of well-established principles of pharmacotherapy (Sellers, 1978; Jacob, 1979; Rosenbaum, 1982; Sellers, 1981). The following guidelines and recommendations arise out of the following chapters.

GUIDELINES AND RECOMMENDATIONS

Clinical Practice

1. Anxiolytics should be reserved for the symptomatic relief of severe symptoms, not for minor transient complaints. They are not of proven efficacy in obsessive-compulsive disorders, phobic disorders, or depressive illness for which other drugs are more effective.

2. Diagnose and treat any underlying disorders before settling for symptomatic relief.

3. Benzodiazepines are the drugs of choice in generalized anxiety disorder since they are effective and safe and produce less physical dependence than other central depressant drugs.

4. Avoid benzodiazepines when the patient has a history of drug or alcohol abuse.

5. Keep doses modest to prevent psychological impairment. Be familiar with the need for gradual withdrawal with much support and encouragement when abuse does occur or when discontinuing after long-term use. Monitor the possibility of dependence when patients are on long courses of treatment. The risk of dependence is significant after four to six months of habitual use.

6. Limit amount of drugs prescribed to that required in the interval between visits. Usual therapy should be 2–6 weeks followed by a re-evaluation of the need for a drug.

7. Warn patients that sedation may occur, especially early in treatment and immediately after each drug dose; and that interactions with alcohol and other depressants are frequent, major and hazardous.

8. Warn patients to keep the drugs for themselves and not to offer them to other people, nor to allow children access to them.

9. Emphasize that the drugs are only part of an overall strategy for management and treatment.

10. Short and intermediate half-life barbiturates and drugs such as glutethimide, ethchlorvynol, meprobamate, methyprylon, paraldehyde, etc., have no role in the treatment of anxiety (or insomnia). The prescribing of these drugs should cease and all should be removed from hospital formularies.

11. Antipsychotic drugs (neuroleptics) e.g., chlorpromazine, thioridazine, and trifluorperazine should not be used in the treatment of anxiety except by specialists with a full appreciation of the limited role of these drugs and their serious and sometimes irreversible side effects.

12. Nominally antidepressant drugs (e.g., tricyclics) may produce sedation but are not appropriate for patients with primary anxiety disorders.

13. Monoamine oxidase inhibitors may be the drugs of choice in some patients with phobic disorders. New MAO inhibitors with specificity for central nervous system MAO-B may circumvent the risks of tyramine reactions.

14. Beta-adrenoceptor antagonists may provide symptomatic relief for the somatic elements of anxiety. These drugs have little long term therapeutic role however, since the need for this effect without other therapy directed at the underlying problem is extremely rare.

15. The clinician need be familiar with only one drug from each of 3 groups of benzodiazepines:
  - Long acting, e.g., chlordiazepoxide, chlorazepate, diazepam, flurazepam, flunitrazepam, prazepam.
  - Intermediate, e.g., alprazolam, lorazepam, oxazepam, temazepam.
  - Short-acting, e.g., triazolam.
  - Long acting benzodiazepines are indicated for generalized anxiety disorders; intermediate acting benzodiazepines may be best used in anticipation or treatment of episodic anxiety disorders; short acting benzodiazepines are best used in the treatment of acute anxiety and insomnia.

16. Serum concentration measurements of MAO inhibitors, benzodiazepines, β-blockers, and tricyclics in generalized anxiety disorder, phobic, and panic disorders, obsessive-compulsive and post-traumatic stress disorders are only useful for kinetic studies and for monitoring patient-compliance in treatment failures. In the clinical setting, serum drug concentration measurements cannot substitute for consistent, systematic monitoring of clinical effects of drugs. The drug dose should be titrated to achieve the desired response with an acceptable

level of side effects. Since such measurements have no predictive therapeutic usefulness analytical services for these drugs should not be made available to clinicians who are not engaged in treatment research.

Research

1. Notwithstanding the usefulness of DSM-III and of various research-based diagnostic criteria, the search should be continued for standardized valid and reliable techniques to assess and follow patient response during therapy.

2. Priorities for investigators could include: development of operational diagnostic entry criteria to trials; use of trial designs with increased power so small sample sizes can be effectively used; development of quasi-experimental design and development of better methods of separating depression and anxiety in patient selection. Quasi-experimental designs are particularly relevant to field settings where quality of care is a concern. They blend a search for useful information with standardized approaches to clinical care.

3. Normative data on existing rating scales is needed on patients falling into the different DSM-III anxiety disorder diagnostic categories.

4. Patient risk factors associated with abuse of anxiolytics need to be identified as do explicit tactics for withdrawal of patients dependent on such drugs.

5. The comparative efficacy of behavioural and other non-pharmacologic treatments versus drug therapy of anxiety disorders should be determined.

Education and Training

1. Specific steps should be taken to clarify for clinicians and trainees the confusion resulting from the many benzodiazepines currently marketed.

2. For the clinician criteria-based audit procedures of the treatment of anxiety seem feasible.

3. University teaching programs in family and community medicine and psychiatry should have teachers with sufficient expertise to ensure proper training in the clinical pharmacology and therapeutic use of drugs in the treatment of anxiety.

4. The role of benzodiazepines in treatment of anxiety disorders vis a vis antidepressants, MAO inhibitors and serotonin uptake blockers and new agents is presently under detailed re-examination. Clinicians will need to engage in considerable revision of their knowledge and clinical practice in the next few years. Continuing medical education workshops should be conducted to ensure clinicians remain abreast of this rapidly changing field.

REFERENCES

Lader, M. Review: Benzodiazepines—panacea or poison. *Aust. N.Z. J. Psychiatry* 15:1–9, 1981.

Klerman, G.L. Psychotropic hedonism vs Pharmacological calvinism. Hasting Centers Center Report. *Inst. Soc. Ethics Life Sci.* 2:1–3, 1972.

Paul, S. Relevance of pathophysiology to pharmacotherapy. Presented at the International Symposium on Guidelines for the Use of Psychotropic Drugs. Toronto, May 1982.

Raskin, A. Clinical trial methodology: Issues for the Psychopharmacologic treatment of anxiety disorders. Chapter 21, this volume.

Linnoila, M. Pharmacokinetics and Drug Concentration Measurement: Relevance to Treatment of Anxiety Disorders. Chapter 22, this volume.

Lader, M. The efficacy and safety of drugs to treat anxiety. Chapter 20, this volume.

American Psychiatric Association: *Diagnostic and Statistical Manual of Mental Disorders. DSM-III.* Williams J.B.W. (ed.) (Third Edition), Washington, D.C., APA, 1980.

Sellers, E.M. Review Article: Clinical pharmacology and therapeutics of benzodiazepines. *Can. Med. Assoc. J.* 118:1533–1538, 1978.

Jacob, M.S., Sellers, E.M. Use of drugs with dependence liability. *Can. Med. Assoc. J.* 121(6):717–724, 1979.

Rosenbaum, J.F. The drug treatment of anxiety. *N. Engl. J. Med.* 306:401–404, 1982.

Sellers, E.M. Therapeutic monograph on anxiolytic sedative drugs. *Can. Med. Assoc. J.* 124(11):1439–1446, 1981.

The Efficacy and Safety of Drugs to Treat Anxiety

MALCOLM LADER

INTRODUCTION

The use of drugs and other substances to produce tranquillity is as old as mankind itself—alcohol, cannabis, and opiates being the main historical agents. In the present century the pharmaceutical industry has discovered and developed other anxiolytic/sedative agents, the foremost being the barbiturates and the benzodiazepines. Unfortunately, problems of dependence and abuse have always accompanied the use of such psychotropics. Hence, the introduction of new and supposedly safer drugs in this class has been eagerly welcomed followed by the desuetude of previous remedies.

The benzodiazepines represent the latest and most effective class of tranquilizers. This class of drugs is now undergoing a critical reevaluation and in particular their dependence potential is now being thoroughly investigated. For example, the WHO has recommended placing the benzodiazepines on Schedule 4 of the Psychotropic Drug Convention. However, until real substitutes materialize the benzodiazepines are likely to continue to be extensively prescribed.

ANTI-ANXIETY DRUGS

Anxiolytics/Sedatives

Sedatives like chloral hydrate and paraldehyde were developed in the last century. Chloral hydrate, in more acceptable solid formulations, still has some therapeutic usefulness but paraldehyde is unpleasant to take, liable to be abused, and may induce psychotic states.

The last of the important 19th century sedatives were the barbiturates. Side effects of drowsiness, tolerance to therapeutic effects, dangers when taken in overdose, and of physical and psychological dependence with consequent dangerous withdrawal syndromes, led to a growing dissatisfaction with these drugs.

Meprobamate was introduced as the first of the modern "Tranquilizers" (Berger, 1963). Unfortunately, its advantages over the barbiturates proved illusory. It was still dangerous in overdosage and likely to be associated with dependence. It is still used, finding its widest application in combination with an analgesic in the management of painful muscle and joint injuries. Other non-barbiturate hypnotics and sedatives were developed including glutethimide, methyprylon, and ethchlorvynol. The eager acceptance of these drugs reflected growing dissatisfaction with the barbiturates, but, in turn, these barbiturate substitutes proved equally disappointing.

Antipsychotic Drugs

Antipsychotic drugs (neuroleptics) such as chlorpromazine, thioridazine, and trifluoperazine have been advocated to treat anxiety. The suggested dose is quite low, typically half or less of the usual antipsychotic dose. Even at this low dosage, the antipsychotic drug may be poorly tolerated by the anxious patient because autonomic side effects such as dry mouth and dizziness too closely resemble his own symptoms. Even more upsetting are extrapyramidal symptoms such as restlessness (akathisia) and mild parkinsonism with paucity of voluntary movements and a coarse tremor. Such unwanted effects are usually uncommon at the low doses used but do occur and may be overlooked. Of more concern is the possibility of tardive dyskinesia.

The chief advantages of antipsychotic drugs in the management of anxiety are that dependence on these drugs is virtually unknown and overdoses are relatively safe. Accordingly, the chief indication for their use is as a short-term adjunct to nonpharmacological therapies in patients with a history of dependence on other CNS depressant drugs such as alcohol or the barbiturates.

Tricyclic Antidepressants

Several of these drugs such as amitriptyline, doxepin, and mianserin have useful secondary sedative properties and are the treatment of first choice in depressed patients with anxiety or agitation. Many clinical trials have established that the sedative properties of many tricyclic antidepressants are useful therapeutically in anxious patients. Nevertheless, these drugs are inappropriate for patients with primary anxiety states because of their range of side-effects, dangers in overdose and interactions with other drugs. The sedative antidepressants can be used to treat insomnia in depressed patients by giving the bulk of the daily requirements as a night-time dose. Caution is needed in the elderly and in the middle-aged with a history of cardiac disease because of the cardiotoxicity of some of these antidepressants such as amitriptyline.

Monoamine Oxidase Inhibitors

These drugs are used to treat atypical depressives but are controversial, some psychiatrists using them routinely and others avoid their use as attended by too many side effects. Some patients with phobic anxiety respond very well to full doses of phenelzine or tranylcypromine but "free-floating" anxiety is not usually helped.

Beta-Adrenoceptor Antagonists

Many bodily symptoms in patients with anxiety states are mediated by the sympathetic nervous system (Lader, 1974). In particular, palpitations, tremor, and gastrointestinal upset are mediated through over-activity of beta-adrenergic sympathetic neurones. Consequently, blockade of this activity by means of beta adrenoceptor antagonists might be expected to help patients with anxiety, especially those with the above symptoms. The results of clinical trials have consistently indicated that only those symptoms mediated by the beta division of the sympathetic nervous system are helped by administration of drugs such as propranolol and sotalol (Tyrer, 1980). Somatic symptoms such as headache not mediated that way or general psychological symptoms are not usefully improved. Whether a patient finds relief on a beta-blocker depends on his symptom profile. Patients with predominant complaints of palpitations, trembling, and gastrointestinal hurry are often much improved. Even so the improvement may be limited to those symptoms alone and general anxiety symptoms may be unchanged.

THE BENZODIAZEPINES

Pharmacological Aspects

Pharmacokinetic differences certainly exist among the various benzodiazepine derivatives, but nevertheless, their mode of action is assumed to be the same and qualitatively their pharmacological effects are similar.

Pharmacokinetics

Two aspects of the pharmacokinetics of the benzodiazepines are important, namely, the speed of the onset of action and the duration of action (Shader and Greenblatt, 1977). The speed of onset of action depends on the mode of administration, the speed of availability of the drug, the rapidity of absorption and the penetration time to the brain. Thus, diazepam is rapidly absorbed when taken orally and enters the brain quickly: it can give prompt relief of acute panic states. Lorazepam is also rapid in its entry to the brain and can be used intravenously as premedication. By contrast, oxazepam is slowly absorbed and takes some time to penetrate to the brain.

The metabolic half-lives of the benzodiazepines also vary greatly. A key compound is N-desmethyldiazepam (nordiazepam), the major active metabolite of diazepam. Its half-life is very long, typically over 100 hours. Consequently, it cumulates over the first month of treatment reaching higher plasma and body concentrations than the parent compound, diazepam (Mendelli et al., 1978). N-desmethyldiazepam is also the major metabolite of clorazepate, medazepam, prazepam, ketazolam, and to some extent chlordiazepoxide. The clinical actions of these drugs are very similar because they share this common, major metabolite.

Lorazepam, oxazepam and temazepam have half-lives of around 6–18 hours, so they tend not to cumulate appreciably. These compounds are appropriate to allay acute, shortlived anxieties and for use as hypnotics. Triazolam is even shorter-acting, its half-life being less than 4 hours. Flurazepam, the most popular hypnotic in the United States, has a similar short half-life but it has an active metabolite with a prolonged action. It is thus rather inappropriate as an hypnotic unless sedation during daytime is also required (Greenblatt et al., 1975). Nitrazepam, an hypnotic widely used in Europe, has a moderately long half-life of about 30 hours so it accumulates on repeated use as a nightly hypnotic.

Clinical Pharmacology

The benzodiazepines in normal dose hardly affect the respiratory and the cardiovascular systems, and virtually all the effects of these drugs result from their actions on the central nervous system. These include sedation, anxiolysis, hypnotic effects, muscle relaxation, and anticonvulsant effect. The benzodiazepines are normally assumed to be devoid of antidepressant or analgesic effects. Unlike the barbiturates, alcohol, and other sedative drugs, the benzodiazepines are not general neuronal depressants. Thus, with increasing dosage sedation merges into sleep and stupor, but no true general anesthesia occurs. It is not clear whether the antianxiety effects of the benzodiazepines are separate from their sedative and hypnotic effects or an intrinsic part of this action.

The depressant effects of a single dose of benzodiazepine can be detected in normal subjects using objective intellectual, cognitive and psychomotor tests. At low doses, subjective changes such as drowsiness or torpor may be undetectable despite objective impairment (McNair, 1973). However, in the clinical context with anxious patients and with repeated dosing, impairment of functioning is much more difficult to detect. This often reflects a lessening of anxiety, but tolerance may also develop.

Despite the extensive long-term usage of the benzodiazepines, few studies have evaluated the chronic effects of these drugs. It is not clear whether therapeutic effects are maintained for longer than a few weeks nor whether any changes in psychological functioning can be detected. Research in this area is urgently required.

INDICATIONS AND EFFICACY

The main decision to be taken by the physician is whether to use a drug at all. Most anxiety attacks or bouts of insomnia are self-limiting as the stress recedes, or the person adapts and copes, or remission occurs naturally. Only if the symptoms are so severe as to interfere with everyday, interpersonal, social or occupational activities, or are intolerable subjectively should drugs be used, and then only on a short-term basis.

Anxiety

The main use of the benzodiazepines is in the symptomatic management of anxiety and stress-related conditions (Greenblatt and Shader, 1974a,b,c). The indications are wide but the common factor is the symptom of anxiety (Blackwell, 1973; Lasagna, 1977). Many controlled trials have shown the therapeutic superiority of the benzodiazepines over placebo and many others have shown that benzodiazepines are generally better than the barbiturates with respect to both the quality and the quantity of improvement in anxiety and stress-related symptoms. There seems little to choose among the benzodiazepines in terms of effectiveness. Hundreds of trials have compared one benzodiazepine with another, the earlier ones generally using chlordiazepoxide as the standard treatment, the more recent ones diazepam. Differences have been marginal, providing administration was flexible to avoid inappropriate dosages.

The initial choice of benzodiazepine should take into account the temporal pattern of the anxiety state. A benzodiazepine with a long half-life, such as diazepam or clorazepate, is appropriate if the anxiety levels are high and sustained. For episodic anxiety, shorter-acting compounds such as lorazepam can be used, taken 30 minutes or so before entering the anxiety-provoking situation.

Some patients are reassured by carrying some lorazepam or similar compounds for such an eventuality, which might be dubbed a "talismanic" use.

Many patients report increases in anxiety on the background of an already raised anxiety level. Here, the most appropriate drug pharmacokinetically is diazepam. A half or more of the daily dose can be given before the patient goes to bed. This acts as an hypnotic because of its rapid absorption and transient peak levels. During the day, the long half-life of diazepam and its major metabolite, N-desmethyldiazepam, ensures a background anti-anxiety effect. Superimposed on this, small doses of diazepam can be given during the day as required.

Some patients take their antianxiety medication regularly but many take their medicines only when feeling particularly anxious or when they fear they will encounter a particularly anxiety-provoking situation. Most such patients can be trusted to keep to a small dose of benzodiazepine (e.g., 5 mg of diazepam), but if there is any sign of escalation of dosage or frequency of administration, the patient's case should be urgently reviewed.

A major therapeutic difficulty concerns patients with chronic disabling anxiety. Their symptoms are usually alleviated by tranquilizers but as the anxiety recrudesces on stopping medication, long-term usage becomes inevitable with the risk of dependence. This risk is worth taking if: (a) the patient is handicapped by his anxiety, and (b) if response to medication is unequivocal. However, we know little about the longterm outcome of patients with mild, chronic anxiety, most studies confining themselves to hospital inpatients or outpatients.

Insomnia

The largest use for short-acting benzodiazepines is in managing insomnia, especially that related to stress and anxiety. The essential criterion for a hypnotic where daytime sedation is not required is that it should not cumulate on repeated dosage during the course of treatment. To this end its average half-life should not exceed 8 to 10 hours. Triazolam has a very short half-life, that of temazepam is about this duration but those of nitrazepam and flurazepam (and metabolites) are too long to meet this criterion.

Other Indications

Other uses for which the short-acting benzodiazepines are appropriate are as preoperative medication and as deep sedation for minor operative procedures such as in dentistry. The drugs render the patient calm, conscious and cooperative, yet anterograde amnesia may be total for the operation or procedure. Benzodiazepines are also in great vogue as skeletal muscle relaxants in the management of acute conditions such as tetanus and trauma and chronic conditions such as the relief of spasticity and athetosis in patients with neurological illnesses.

Benzodiazepines can be used as adjuncts to various types of relaxation therapy especially where the patient is very tense and anxious and is unable even to commence relaxation. Benzodiazepines have also been advocated in the management of alcohol withdrawal, but the dependence may be transferred from alcohol to the benzodiazepine.

UNWANTED EFFECTS

All antianxiety drugs have adverse effects upon the central nervous system and higher cerebral functions, the main problem being oversedation (Edwards, 1981). Relatively innocuous side-effects frequently occur during short-term benzodiazepine treatment. In contrast, little is known about potentially adverse, longterm effects such as chronic psychological impairment.

Acute Toxicity

Overdosage with the benzodiazepines occurs frequently but fortunately deaths as a result of benzodiazepines *alone* are rare (Greenblatt et al., 1978). Typically, other drugs or alcohol have been taken. Only in children and the physically frail, especially those with respiratory problems, are the benzodiazepines hazardous.

Side-Effects During Therapy

The commonest unwanted side-effects are tiredness, drowsiness, and torpor, most marked within the first two hours after large doses. Drowsiness is complained of most frequently during the first week of treatment and then wanes and disappears, suggesting that the tolerance effect outweighs any cumulation. Accordingly, patients should be warned of the potential side-effects of any prescribed benzodiazepine. The dosage should initially be cautious until the effects of the drug can be gauged. In particular, patients should be advised not to drive a vehicle during the initial adjustment of dosage. Once the optimal dosage has been determined, danger of interference with mechanical skills such as driving or operating dangerous machinery recedes.

As with most depressant drugs the effects of alcohol can be markedly potentiated (Linnoila et al., 1979). Patients must be warned not to drink alcohol when taking benzodiazepines, whether chronically or intermittently. In particular, the combination of alcohol and a benzodiazepine may profoundly impair ability to drive, even when the patient has been taking the benzodiazepine for some time (Linnoila and Häkkinen, 1974). Generally speaking, the benzodiazepines can be given safely in combination with other drugs. As with other tranquilizers, however, they may enhance the sedative effects of phenothiazines, antidepressants, narcotic analgesics and antihistamines. Cimetidine, by virtue of its liver microsomal enzyme competitive effect, may potentiate some benzodiazepines.

Other Adverse Reactions

Patients taking benzodiazepines may show paradoxical behavioral responses. Such phenomena include increased aggression and hostility (Gaind and Jacoby, 1978), uncharacteristic criminal activities such as shop-lifting, sexual improprieties or offenses such as importuning or self-exposure, and excessive emotional responses such as uncontrollable giggling or weeping.

Administration of benzodiazepines can cause respiratory depression in patients with respiratory problems such as chronic bronchitis and emphysema. Other side-effects include excessive weight gain, skin rash, impairment of sexual function, menstrual irregularities, and (rarely), blood abnormalities. Benzodiazepines should be avoided during pregnancy, especially during the first three months. Benzodiazepines pass readily into the fetus and have been suspected of causing respiratory depression in the newborn. Benzodiazepines also pass into the mother's milk and can oversedate the baby so breast feeding should be discontinued if a benzodiazepine is prescribed for the mother.

Very recently, CT-scan abnormalities have been reported in longterm benzodiazepine users (Lader et al., 1983). The abnormalities resemble those in alcoholics. The relationship between the cortical abnormalities and ventricular enlargement in the patients and benzodiazepine usage is quite unclear.

TOLERANCE AND DEPENDENCE

Although benzodiazepines are reputed to cause only a low rate of abuse and dependence, the possibility of this adverse effect on chronic use is currently a subject of much concern. Tolerance develops to some of the effects of anti-anxiety drugs, but dosage escalation is uncommon. Metabolic tolerance is probably of little clinical importance, but experimental evidence shows that receptor site tolerance occurs (Greenblatt and Shader, 1978). Tolerance to benzodiazepines confers cross-tolerance to methaqualone, barbiturates, and, to some extent, alcohol.

Although numerous reports describe human abuse and dependence, the number of case reports with convincing evidence of dependence is small in relation to the extensive and widespread use of benzodiazepines (Marks, 1978). Furthermore, a few patients escalate their dosage to levels so high that the prescriber suspects that dependence has supervened.

A definite withdrawal syndrome has been described in patients who have escalated their dose of benzodiazepine and have been on a *high* dose for a long time. The mildest symptoms are anxiety, tension, apprehension, dizziness, insomnia, and anorexia. More severe physical dependence is manifested by withdrawal symptoms of nausea and vomiting, tremor, muscle weakness, and postural hypotension. Occasionally, hyperthermia, muscle twitches, convulsions, and confusional psychoses may occur (Fruensgaard, 1976).

Tolerance and dependence in patients who take therapeutic doses of benzodiazepines for long periods of time is less easy to establish (Covi et al., 1973). On withdrawal of medication, symptoms appear often resembling those for which the benzodiazepine was originally prescribed, for example, anxiety, tension, insomnia, trembling, palpitations, and sweating. This is sometimes taken as evidence that the anxiety has continued, merely being kept under control by the drug, and that the symptoms have reemerged when the drug was withdrawn, rather than a true withdrawal syndrome ensuing (Rickels et al., 1978). Recently, evidence has been adduced to suggest that patients on normal therapeutic doses (e.g., up to 30 mg per day of diazepam or equivalent), who report difficulty in discontinuing their drugs, develop a fullblown withdrawal syndrome if their drug is stopped. On withdrawal, affective and perceptual changes occur identical in nature, extent and severity to those experienced in patients discontinuing high doses. Many patients may be reluctant to have their medication withdrawn because of previous unpleasant experiences when attempting themselves to lower the dose. This was apparent in a study by Tyrer et al. (1981) in which only 40 out of 86 suitable patients consented to withdrawal.

The management of benzodiazepine withdrawal is to lower the dose over 2 to 4 weeks and to rely on supportive psychotherapy to help the patient over the worst of the withdrawal period which is usually about 2 weeks. Substitution of an antipsychotic drug such as chlorpromazine is not advisable because the convulsive threshold is lowered. Propranolol, the beta-adrenoceptor antagonist, may help especially if tremor is extreme.

CONCLUSIONS

Of the recommendations of the American Medical Association (1974) concerning sedatives the following are the most cogent.

Reserve anxiolytics for the relief of severe symptoms, not for minor ephemeral complaints.

Keep doses modest so that psychological impairment does not supervene.

Be familiar with need for gradual withdrawal with much support and encouragement when abuse does occur or when discontinuing after longterm use.

Monitor the possibility of dependence when patients are on long courses of treatment. Four to six months seems the crucial time when the risk of dependence becomes appreciable.

REFERENCES

American Medication Association (1974). Committee on alcoholism and drug dependence: Barbiturates and barbiturate-like drugs; considerations in their medical use. *J. Am. Med. Assoc.* 230:1140–1141.

Berger, F.M. (1963). The similarities and differences between meprobamate and barbiturates. *Clin. Pharmacol. Ther.* 4:209–231.

Blackwell, B. (1973). The role of diazepam in medical practice. *J. Am. Med. Assoc.* 225:1637–1641.

Covi, L., Lipman, R.S., Pattison, J.H., Derogatis, L.R., and Uhlenhuth, E.H. (1973). Length of treatment with anxiolytic sedatives and response to their sudden withdrawal. *Acta Psychiatr. Scand.* 49:51–64.

Edwards, J.G. (1981). Adverse effects of antianxiety drugs. *Drugs* 22:495–514.

Fruensgaard, K. (1976). Withdrawal psychosis: A study of 30 consecutive cases. *Acta Psychiatr. Scand.* 53:105–118.

Gaind, R.N. and Jacoby, R. (1978). Benzodiazepines causing aggression. In: Gaind, Hudson, ed., *Current Themes in Psychiatry*, London: McMillan, p. 371-379.

Greenblatt, D.J. and Shader, R.I. (1974a). *Benzodiazepines in Clinical Practice.* New York: Raven Press, p. 68-69.

Greenblatt, D.J. and Shader, R.I. (1974b). Benzodiazepines. Part I. *N. Engl. J. Med.* 291:1011–1015.

Greenblatt, D.J. and Shader, R.I. (1974c). Benzodiazepines. Part II. *N. Engl. J. Med.* 291:1239–1243.

Greenblatt, D.J. and Shader, R.I. (1978). Dependence, tolerance and addiction to benzodiazepines: clinical and pharmacokinetic considerations. *Drug Metabolism Rev.* 8(1):12–28.

Greenblatt, D.J., Shader, R.I. and Koch-Weser, J. (1975). Flurazepam hydrochloride. *Clin. Pharmacol. Ther.* 17:1–14.

Greenblatt, D.J., Allen, M.D., Noel, B.J. and Shader, R.I. (1978). Acute overdosage with benzodiazepine derivatives. *Clin. Pharmacol. Ther.* 21:497–514.

Lader, M. (1974). The peripheral and central role of the catecholamines in the mechanisms of anxiety. *Int. Pharmacopsychiat.* 9:125–137.

Lader, M., Ron, M. and Petursson, H. (1983). CT-scan brain abnormalities in longterm benzodiazepine users. *Psychol. Med.* in press.

Lasagna, L. (1977). The role of benzodiazepines in non-psychiatric medical practice. *Am. J. Psychiatry* 134:656–658.

Linnoila, M. and Häkkinen, S. (1974). Effects of diazepam and codeine, alone and in combination with alcohol, on simulated driving. *Clin. Pharmacol. Ther.* 15:368-373.

Linnoila, M., Mattila, M.J. and Kitchell, B.S. (1979). Drug interactions with alcohol. *Drugs* 18:299-311.

Marks, J. (1978). *The Benzodiazepines. Use, Overuse, Misuse, Abuse.* Lancaster: MTP Press.

McNair, D.M. (1973). Antianxiety drugs and human performance. *Arch. Gen. Psychiatry* 29:609–617.

Mendelli, M., Tognoni, G. and Garattini, S. (1978). Clinical pharmacokinetics of diazepam. *Clin. Pharmacokin.* 3:72–91.

Rickels, K. (1978). Use of antianxiety agents in anxious outpatients. *Psychopharmacol.* 58:1–17.

Rickels, K., Downing, R.W. and Winokur, A. (1978). Antianxiety drugs: clinical use in psychiatry. In Iversen, Iversen and Snyder, *Handbook of Psychopharmacology*, New York: Plenum, p. 395–430.

Shader, R.I. and Greenblatt, D.J. (1977). Clinical implications of benzodiazepine pharmacokinetics. *Am. J. Psychiatry* 134:652–656.

Tyrer, P. (1980). Use of blocking drugs in psychiatry and neurology. *Drugs* 20: 300–308.

Tyrer, P., Rutherford, D. and Huggett, T. (1981). Benzodiazepine withdrawal symptoms and propranolol. *Lancet* i:520–522.

21

Clinical Trial Methodology: Issues for the Psychopharmacologic Treatment of the Anxiety Disorders

ALLEN RASKIN

INTRODUCTION

A number of years ago a Food and Drug Administration task force was established to develop guidelines for the conduct of psychoactive drug trials with geriatric patients. After three days of sometimes heated discussion one of the panel members volunteered to write a first draft of these guidelines for the next meeting. Other panel members were very impressed by this individual's willingness to take on this formidable task. In due time a draft of the guidelines arrived and read very well until one came to a sentence that contained the word "children." It then became apparent that these were the guidelines that had been developed for pediatric drug trials and what our volunteer had done was to substitute the word elderly for the word children in the pediatric guidelines. This true story is a dramatic example of the fact that, in general, methodological issues in the conduct of drug trials transcend age, sex, or psychiatric diagnosis. Small sample size is a problem whether you are conducting a drug trial with children, the elderly, men, schizophrenics or patients with panic disorders.

With this caveat in mind it is also fair to say that there are some methodologic issues that are especially relevant to the conduct of drug trials with anxiety disorder patients. The focus in this chapter will be on these issues:

(a) diagnosis as an entry criterion, (b) sample size, (c) quasi-experimental designs and (d) distinguishing anxiety and depression.

DIAGNOSIS AS AN ENTRY CRITERION

Although it is felt by many that the latest, or Third Edition of the Diagnostic and Statistical Manual (*DSM-III; American Psychiatric Association*, 1980) provides better diagnostic criteria and a more meaningful classification of the anxiety disorders than its predecessor, there are problems in applying these diagnoses to specific criteria for patient inclusion in drug trials. These problems can be illustrated by reference to the diagnosis of panic disorder. Although DSM-III lays out in very specific terms certain criteria for this diagnosis, such as the presence of at least four specified symptoms during each panic attack, the investigator is left with the task of documenting the presence of these attacks in patients admitted to his or her study. The problem with documenting these attacks is that they generally tend to occur in situations and circumstances when the rater or researcher is not likely to be present. Some patients have also learned to mask the outward expressions of their panic attack so that even a keen observer cannot always tell when a ptient is having an attack.

Unfortunately, there is no simple solution to this problem. A 17-item self-report rating scale has been developed to assess signs of a panic attack (Klein, 1982). This scale has shown good correspondence with physiological measures taken when phobic patients with spontaneous panic attacks are administered sodium lactate. Sodium lactate only induces panic attacks in patients with histories of spontaneous panic attacks. However, sodium lactate does not induce a panic attack in all patients with histories of spontaneous panic attacks and investigators may be understandably reluctant to administer sodium lactate to their patients to document the presence of these attacks. Other approaches that have been tried include attaching a Holter monitor to patients to monitor heart rate and other cardiac functions when the patient is engaged in normal activities on the outside and to relate changes in these measures to patient reports of having experienced panic attacks. Efforts are also currently underway to develop an electronic method of measuring respiration that is also portable and can be worn by a panic disorder patient during the day (Klein, 1982).

Another diagnostic issue of considerable importance today is the relationship of depression to a number of the anxiety disorders, most notably to agoraphobia with panic attacks, panic disorder, and obsessive-compulsive disorder. There is ample evidence that these disorders show a good response to anti-depressant drug therapy. However, there are two divergent views on why these drugs work in these disorders. One view holds that the drugs only work in anxiety disorder patients with significant depression in addition to their other symptoms and the benefits derived are primarily in alleviating the symptoms of depression (Marks, 1982). Another school believes that the antidepressants have a direct effect on spontaneous panic attacks and obsessive-compulsive symptoms and see the presence of depression in these patients as an extraneous and possibly a contaminating influence (Klein, 1981). Hence, investigators holding this latter view exclude patients with significant depressive symptoms from their studies. It should be noted that the presence of significant amounts of depression is not an exclusionary factor per se in DSM-III diagnoses of agoraphobia with panic attacks, panic disorder, or obsessive-compulsive disorder.

Although both of the above schools have been able to marshall evidence to support their respective points of view, the definitive study in this area has not been performed. An adequate test of the various hypotheses surrounding the role of the antidepressants in the treatment of these disorders would require sufficient numbers of these patients with both high and low initial levels of depression. The results one would expect of a hypothetical study of antidepressant drug treatment on agoraphobic symptoms, based on the views of these two schools, are illustrated in Figure 1. School "A" reflects the view that the antidepressants work primarily on the symptoms of depression and School "B" that there is a direct effect of the antidepressants on the spontaneous panic attacks. The major discrepancy between these schools would be for the patients with low initial levels of depression. School "B" would predict significant reduction in agoraphobic symptoms for these patients whereas School "A" would not.

Other methodological issues are also illustrated in this figure. The first is that when there is little or no pathology to start with, as in the case with the low depression group, then you cannot expect much of a treatment effect. What we are dealing with here is a phenomenon known as the floor effect. A good example of this effect would be a study of the use of aspirin to treat headaches in subjects who do not have headaches. The table also illustrates the fact that recovery or improvement in symptom reduction is seldom complete and that even a 40 or 50 percent improvement rate over pretreatment levels is considered quite good. This point was recently illustrated by Karl Rickels (1982) who reviewed a number of his early studies of drug treatment with generalized anxiety disorders. Although there were quite a few statistically significant drug-placebo differences on subscales of the Hopkins Symptom Checklist (Derogatis, et al., 1974) mean levels of improvement seldom exceeded one point on a four point scale of severity.

SAMPLE SIZE

It was earlier noted that sample size is a problem that transcends the anxiety disorders. However, sample size is also a special problem for some of these disorders because of the low incidence of patients with diagnoses such as

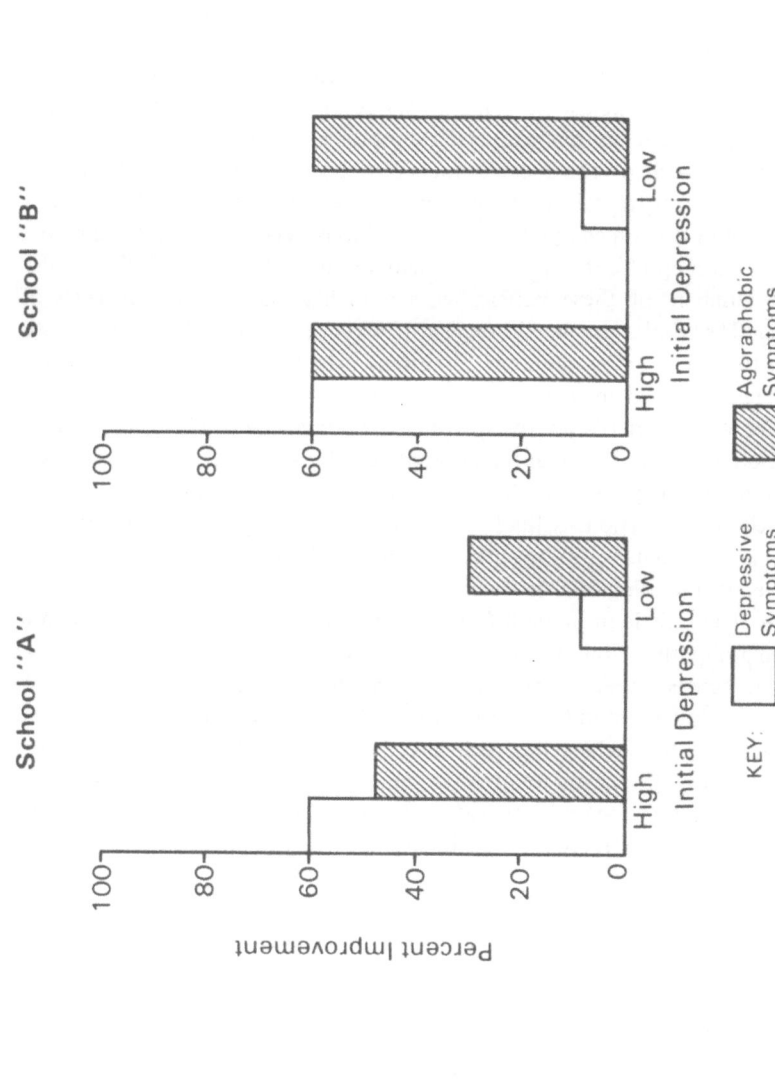

Figure 1. Predicted percent of improvement for School "A" and School "B" on symptoms of depression and agoraphobia with antidepressant treatment.

agoraphobia with panic features or obsessive-compulsive disorders. This problem is heightened if one has to further subdivide these groups into high and low initial levels of depression or if one is interested in a mixed modality study comparing the effects of drugs and/or psychotherapy.

Power analysis tests are available to estimate the sample size necessary to show clinically meaningful treatment differences. Two reviews done some time ago of the sensitivity to treatment effects of rating scales such as the Brief Psychiatric Rating Scale (Overall, et al., 1967) and the Inpatient Multidimensional Psychiatric Scale (Derogatis, et al., 1968) indicated that sample sizes of 40 to 60 subjects per treatment group would be required in most studies to show psychotropic drug effects. Fortunately sample size is not the only factor one can manipulate to reduce or account for variation within treatment groups. For example, an adequate placebo washout period (Ainslie et al., 1965), or the matching of patients on relevant characteristics (McNair et al., 1970), increases sensitivity to treatment effects and reduces the need for large sample sizes.

There are also some statistical approaches one can use to maximize cell sizes. For example, to demonstrate differential treatment effects as a function of initial level of depression, it may not be necessary to subdivide the population under study into high, moderate, or low levels of depression. If frequency distributions indicate that the relationship between initial level of depression and the outcome measures are essentially linear and normally distributed, then one could test for treatment effects with the initial severity of depression score entered as the covariate in an analysis of covariance. The tests for homogeneity of regression in these analyses will indicate whether there are significantly different treatment effects on the criterion variables as a function of initial level of depression. Generally, the test for homogeneity of regression is performed only for the purpose of determining whether one of the major assumptions of covariance analysis is met (i.e., that the slopes or regressions of the covariates on the outcome measure are not significantly different from each other). If these differences are significant then one is not justified in using covariance analysis. However the presence of significant heterogeneity of regression can be an important finding in its own right in treatment assessment studies. Figure 2 illustrates significant heterogeneity of regression in a fictitious study examining the effects of six weeks of treatment with imipramine or diazepam on spontaneous panic attacks. The ordinate is the covariate mean on initial depression and the abscicca is the six-week score on number of spontaneous panic attacks. The figure indicates that imipramine is very effective in reducing panic attacks for patients with high initial levels of depression but a poor choice for patients with low initial levels. Diazepam, on the other hand, is a good treatment for reducing symptoms of agoraphobia for patients with low initial levels of depression but is ineffective if patients have high initial levels of depression. As stated earlier, the advantage of this statistical approach is that it utilizes all of the subjects in a particular

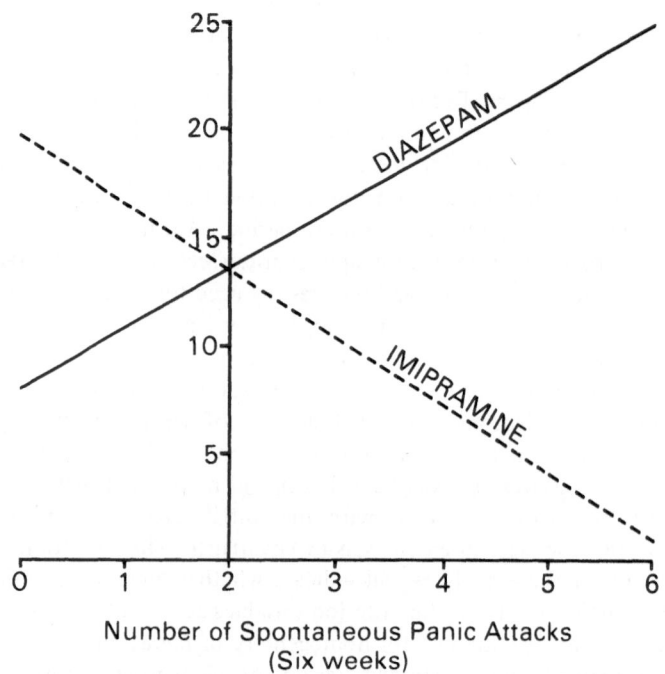

Initial Level of Depression
(Covariate mean)

Figure 2.   An example of significant heterogeneity of regression.

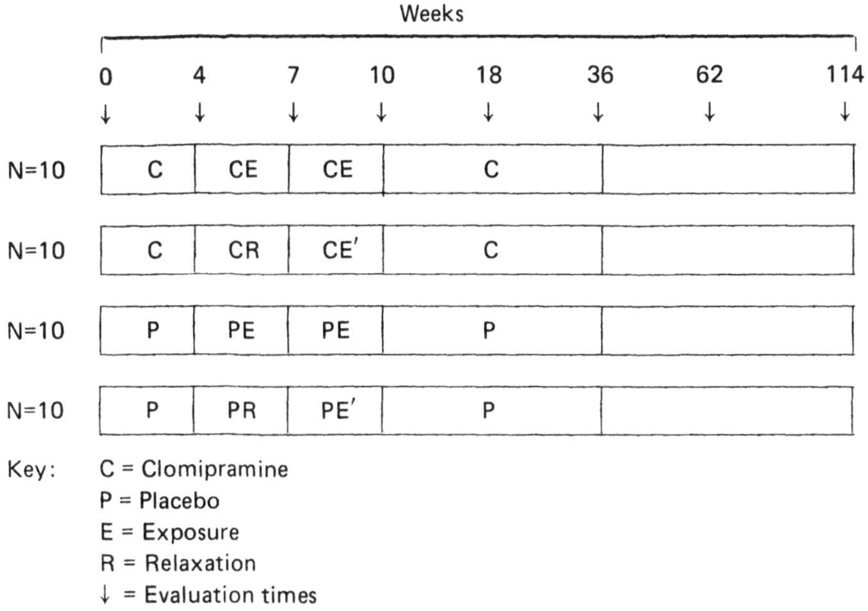

Figure 3 Study design. Reprinted with permission from Marks, I.M., Stern, R.S., Mawson, D., Cobb, J. and McDonald, R. (1980) Clomipramine and exposure for obsessive-compulsive rituals: I. *Br. J. Psychiatry* 136:1–25.

treatment group instead of dividing them into subgroups on the basis of initial level of depression.

Designs utilizing subjects as their own controls have also been used by investigators in this field to contend with small sample size. This approach can be illustrated by a recent study by Marks and associates (1980) comparing the effects of clomipramine, placebo, exposure therapy and relaxation therapy in 40 obsessive-compulsive patients. The design of this study is outlined in Figure 3. This study design can perhaps best be characterized as an incomplete cross-over study. In a complete cross-over study all patients receive one of the two treatments and then are crossed-over to the alternate treatment after a suitable trial on the initial treatment. In the Marks et al., (1980) study two groups of patients received clomipramine and two groups placebo for four weeks. At that time exposure therapy was added to one of the clomipramine groups and one of the placebo groups and relaxation therapy was added to the other clomipramine group and placebo group. At seven weeks, patients who received relaxation therapy were crossed over to exposure therapy. At 10 weeks exposure therapy was terminated for all patients and at 36 weeks patients were taken off all medications. Final evaluations were performed at 114 weeks. This design is a compromise between a simple random assignment to treatment design and the more traditional cross-over design previously described. The drugs are the constant factor in this design with all patients receiving either clomipramine or placebo for 36 weeks.

With a total pool of 40 subjects Marks et al. (1980) were able to examine simple drug effects unconfounded with behavior therapy effects, the differential effects of exposure and relaxation therapy when combined with either an active drug or placebo, the effects of switching from relaxation therapy to the more potent exposure therapy and finally long-term effects following discontinuation of first behavior therapy and then chemotherapy. The design is also rational in the sense that it follows accepted clinical practice which is to start these patients on an antidepressant and then add behavior therapy.

This is a powerful research design that is unfortunately flawed in one important respect (i.e., it is not possible to partial out the effects of time and of prior treatments on the later treatments). This is the classic problem with all cross-over designs. In this case one needs to assume that there is sufficient residual psychopathology after four weeks treatment with either clomipramine or placebo to show behavior therapy effects. Marks et al. (1980) tried to minimize this problem by the addition of a placebo group and by limiting the initial drug trial to four weeks. Four weeks represented a compromise on their part but it is somewhat brief to show major drug effects. On the other hand, drug effects could be dissipating or masking behavior therapy effects in the four to seven-week period. There are also data to show a high spontaneous recovery rate with some of the anxiety disorders after entry into a study and placement on either a placebo or into a waiting group (Frank et al., 1963). However, this appears to be a particular problem with generalized anxiety disorders.

The major problem with the Marks et al. (1980) design is that it leaves proponents of behavior therapy wondering what the effects of exposure therapy would have been if there had been a separate exposure therapy group from the start of the study and this treatment, and this treatment alone, had been continued for 10 weeks or longer.

QUASI-EXPERIMENTAL DESIGNS

Because of increased public awareness of patient rights and human subject concerns, investigators have become wary of utilizing traditional drug treatment designs containing features such as random assignment of patients to treatment, use of placebo controls and a drug "wash-out" period or waiting phase prior to instigating active drug treatment. Quasi-experimental designs (Campbell and Stanley, 1963) have been proposed as an alternative to the more traditional designs because they do not impose any restrictions on usual or customary treatment practices. Quasi-experimental designs have been used in studies with schizophrenics (Gillis, 1979) and depressed patients (Gillis and Moran, 1980) and may be of special value for drug trials of anxiety disorder patients who are mainly treated as outpatients where it is more difficult to impose restrictions or controls than in a hospital.

One form of quasi-experimental design is known as an *in situ* study (Gillis, in press). This type of study involves (1) surveying the drug regimes being used in a given facility; (2) identifying those agents given with sufficient frequency that the number of patients receiving each is large enough to constitute a separate treatment group; (3) specifying each treatment group, within previously defined limits of dose levels and time; (4) evaluating patients in these groups on the dependent measures of interest; and (5) comparing the groups' results on these measures.

Treatment conditions can be established for specific diagnostic categories with limits set on dosage and time of use for each drug. For example, an imipramine group can be established for panic disorder patients who received between 100 and 150 mg/day of imipramine for at least four weeks. Once these groups have been assembled it is possible to immediately test the patients on critical measures of outcome. No waiting period is required in this design and it is not necessary to titrate dose level to the maximally effective dose for each patient as one assumes this has already been done by the prescribing physician. The design can be tightened by building into the patient selection procedures independent criteria for assuring that a "stable" and maximally effective dose has been attained, based on clinical status, time on the drug and blood level of the drug.

Although the quasi-experimental design has obvious appeal to proponents of naturalistic research there are some serious shortcomings with this approach. Most of these shortcomings stem from the fact that patients were not randomly assigned to the various treatments and no systematic effort was made to initially match patients in each of the treatment groups on presenting symptoms or on background variables such as age, sex, severity of illness and level of chronicity. If these are systematic biases operating at a treatment setting such that patients with certain symptoms or diagnoses are routinely given a particular drug this could confound and make uninterpretable any differences that may later emerge among the drug groups.

Surveys of prescribing practices within treatment settings indicate that the major bias that occurs in these settings is the assignment of certain kinds of patients to specific classes of drugs, for example, psychotics to major tranquilizers and depressed patient to antidepressants (Gillis and Moran, 1981). There is considerably less agreement among physicians on the choice of drugs within a class. This finding suggests that *in situ* studies examining treatment effects among drugs within a class stand a reasonable chance of ending up with groups fairly evenly matched on presenting symptoms and other critical control variables.

DIFFERENTIATING DEPRESSION AND ANXIETY

A variety of parameters have been explored to differentiate anxiety and depression. These include biological differences such as cortisol secretion, sleep differences such as total time awake (Akiskal, 1982) differences in cognitive schemata (Beck, 1981) and differences on scales rating psychopathology (Lipman, 1982). The focus in this chapter will be on the use of symptom rating scales to differentiate anxiety and depression.

Before launching into a discussion of rating scales it is important to recognize that the presence of mixed symptoms of both depression and anxiety in the same patient is the rule rather than the exception. For example, two-thirds of the patients in a large collaborative study of drug treatment in hospitalized depressed patients fell into Overall's (Raskin, et al., 1970) anxious-depression subtype.

The admixture of symptoms of anxiety and depression also spills over into the rating scales themselves so that the Hamilton Depression Scale (Hamilton, 1960), for example, includes items sampling agitation, psychic anxiety, somatic anxiety, and somatic symptoms—items more often associated with anxiety than depression. Snaith and associates (1971) also argued that the Wakefield Inventory provided a better measure of depression than the Beck or Zung Scales because the latter scales failed to include items dealing specifically with anxiety.

The extent to which anxiety and depression symptoms commingle is also related to the source of the ratings. Psychiatrists and psychologists are better able to separate out symptoms of anxiety and depression than patients. Hence when one factor analyzes rating scales completed by psychiatrists and psychologists, one is more likely to get distinct factors reflecting depression and anxiety than when one factor analyzes comparable scales completed by patients (Raskin et al., 1967). These findings may merely reflect the fact that mental health professionals have certain biases regarding the symptoms they associate with anxiety and depression which are not shared by the patients.

Rating scales, including self-report scales, are available that have well defined anxiety and depression clusters or factors. One scale in this category is the Hopkins Symptom Checklist (HSCL; Derogatis et al., 1974). The HSCL has been used in a number of collaborative studies of drug treatment in both anxious and depressed patients. Prusoff and Klerman (1974) performed a discriminant function analysis to determine if the five original factors from the HSCL would reliably differentiate their anxious and depressed samples. These were patients initially diagnosed as anxious or depressed by DSM-II criteria. The five HSCL subscales successfully differentiated 66% of the patients in these two groups. Although this is significantly better than chance it still indicates considerable overlap between the diagnostic groups. The HSCL factor that contributed most to this discrimination was Somatization which was higher in the anxious sample despite the generally higher level of distress in the depressed group.

Another large collaborative study used initial cut-off scores on HSCL clusters of anxiety or depression to assign patients to primarily anxious or primarily depressed groups. These assignments were compared with independent judgments by psychiatrists. There was 87% agreement between initial rating scale assignment and psychiatrist assignment for patients classified as depressed and 75% agreement for patients classified as anxious (Lipman, 1982).

Other rating scales such as the Raskin-Covi Three-Area Scales for Depression and Anxiety, the ACNP Anxiety and Depression Checklist and the Hamilton Anxiety and Depression Scales also significantly differentiated these two groups (Lipman, 1982). However, what was most striking in this study was the similarity in symptom profiles on the HSCL clusters for the primarily anxious and primarily depressed groups. Anxiety and depression were dominant clusters for both groups although the anxiety cluster was higher for the anxious patients and the depression cluster higher for the depressed patients.

What these findings indicate is that there is considerable overlap of symptomatology with mainly quantitative rather than qualitative differences between patients assigned to primarily anxious or primarily depressed groups. However, symptom differences do emerge when finer distinctions are made within these broad categories. For example, single items on the Newcastle Scale did discriminate patients who could be characterized as panic anxiety from others characterized as endogenous depression (McNair and Fisher, 1978).

This is obviously an area in which additional research is needed. Normative data on existing rating scales is sorely lacking for patients falling into the different anxiety disorder diagnostic groups.

REFERENCES

Ainslie, J.D., Jones, M.B. and Stiefel, J.R. (1965). Practical drug evaluation method: Imipramine in depressed outpatients. *Arch. Gen. Psychiatry* 12: 368-373.

Akiskal, H.S. (1982). Biochemical and psychopharmacological strategies in the study of anxiety disorders and their phenomenology. Presented at Anxiety Disorders Workshop sponsored by the Clinical Research Branch, NIMH, Bethesda, MD, May 6-7.

American Psychiatric Association (1980). *Diagnostic and Statistical Manual of Mental Disorders (Third Edition).* Washington, D.C.: American Psychiatric Association.

Beck, A.T. (1971). Cognition, affect, and psychopathology. *Arch. Gen. Psychiatry* 24:495-500.

Campbell, D.T., and Stanley, J.C. (1963). *Experimental and Quasi-Experimental Designs for Research.* Chicago: Rand McNally and Co.

Derogatis, L.R., Lipman, R.S., Rickels, K., Uhlenhuth, E.H. and Covi, L. (1974). The Hopkins symptom checklist (HSCL): A self-report symptom inventory. *Behav. Sci.* 19:1-15.

Derogatis, L.R., Bonato, R.R. and Yang, K.C. (1968). The power of IMPS in psychiatric drug research: As a function of sample size, number of raters, and choice of treatment. *Arch. Gen. Psychiatry* 19:689-699.

Frank, J.D., Nash, E.H., Stone, A.R., and Imber, S.D. (1963). Immediate and long-term symptomatic course of psychiatric outpatients. *Am. J. Psychiatry* 120:429-439.

Gillis, J.S. (1979). The effects of trifluoperazine and fluphenazine injection on conflict resolution and interpersonal learning with schizophrenics. *Curr. Ther. Res.* 26:547-556.

Gillis, J.S. and Moran, T.J. (1980). The effects of amitriptyline and imipramine on interpersonal learning with depressed patients. *Res. Commun. Psychol., Psychiatry, Behav.* 5:157-176.

Gillis, J.S. (in press). Applications of a quasi-experimental design to research in psychopharmacology. *Psychol. Rep.*

Gillis, J.S. and Moran, T.J. (1981). An analysis of drug decisions in a state psychiatric hospital. *J. Clin. Psychol.* 37:32-42.

Hamilton, M. (1960). A rating scale for depression. *J. Neurol. Neurosurg. Psychiatry,* 23:56-62.

Klein, D.F. (1982). Personal communication, May 8.

Klein, D.F. (1981). Anxiety reconceptualized. In: Klein, D.F., and Rabkin, J.G. (eds.), *Anxiety, New Research, and Changing Concepts.* New York: Raven Press.

Lipman, R.S. (1982). Differentiating anxiety and depression in anxiety disorders: Use of rating scales. *Psychopharmacol. Bull.* 18:69-77.

Marks, I. (1982). Are there anticompulsive or antiphobic drugs? Review of the evidence. *Psychopharmacol. Bull.* 18:78-84.

Marks, I.M., Stern, R.S., Mawson, D., Cobb, J. and McDonald, R. (1980). Clomipramine and exposure for obsessive-compulsive vituals: I. *Br. J. Psychiatry* 136:1-25.

McNair, D.M., Fisher, S., Kahn, R.J. and Droppleman, L.F. (1970). A drug-personality interaction in intensive outpatient treatment. *Arch. Gen. Psychiatry* 22:128-135.

McNair, D.M. and Fisher, S. (1978). Separating anxiety from depression. In: Lipton, M.A., DeMascio, A. and Killam, K.F. (eds.), *Psychopharmacology: A Generation of Progress.* New York: Raven Press.

Overall, J.E., Hollister, L.E. and Dalal, S.M. (1967). Psychiatric drug research: Sample size requirements for one vs. two raters. *Arch. Gen. Psychiatry* 16:152-161.

Prusoff, B. and Klerman, G.L. (1974). Differentiating depressed from anxious neurotic outpatients: Use of discriminant function analysis for separation of neurotic affective states. *Arch. Gen. Psychiatry* 30:302-309.

Raskin, A., Schulterbrandt, J., Reatig, N. and Rice, C.E. (1967). Factors of psychopathology in interview, ward behavior, and self-report ratings of hospitalized depressives. *J. Consult. Psychol.* 31:270-278.

Raskin, A., Schulterbrandt, J.G., Reatig, N. and McKeon, J.J. (1970). Differential response to chlorpromazine, imipramine, and placebo: A study of subgroups of hospitalized depressed patients. *Arch. Gen. Psychiatry* 23:164–173.

Rickels, K. (1982). Benzodiazepines in the treatment of anxiety. Paper presented at the Pharmacology of Benzodiazepines Workshop sponsored by the National Institutes of Health, Bethesda, MD, April 12–14.

Snaith, R.P., Ahmed, S.N., Mehta, S. and Hamilton, M. (1971). Assessment of the severity of primary depressive illness: Wakefield Self-Assessment Depression Inventory. *Psychol. Med.* 1:143–149.

22

Pharmacokinetics and Drug Concentrations Measurement: Relevance to Treatment of Anxiety Disorders

MARKKU LINNOILA

DIAGNOSTIC CONSIDERATIONS

Anxiety is a mood state accompanied by psychophysiological changes (such as rapid heart rate, increased perspiration, tremor, and often by feelings of tingling of extremities, going crazy, choking or dying) associated with fear, but occurring in the absence of generally threatening stimuli. However, it is a symptom rather than a diagnostic entity. There is a group of mental disorders with anxiety as a primary symptom in the absence of major affective symptomatology and/or thought disorder. In the DSM-III, most of these have been classified under the titles of anxiety disorders, or anxiety states (Table 1). Moreover, in psychiatric outpatients anxiety commonly coexists with mild to moderate depressive symptoms in the cyclothymic and dysthymic disorders (DSM-III #300.13 and 300.40, respectively).

A series of clinical studies started in the early 1960s have provided data consistent with the view that successful pharmacotherapy requires a differential diagnosis of anxiety disorders and states. Patients suffering from panic and/or phobic attacks respond best to antidepressants, β-blockers and possibly clonidine, whereas patients with a more generalized, relatively constant, high level anxiety or reactive anxiety have been customarily treated with benzodiazepines (Klein, 1967; Kline, 1967; Robinson et al., 1973; and 1978; Tyrer, 1976;

329

Table 1. Mental Disorders with Significant Anxiety Symptoms

Anxiety Disorders
   Agoraphobia with panic attacks (DSM-III # 300·21)
   Agoraphobia without panic attacks (DSM-III # 300·22)
   Social phobia (DSM-III # 300·23)
   Simple phobia (DSM-III # 300·29)

Anxiety States
   Panic disorders (DSM-III # 300·01)
   Generalized anxiety disorder (DSM-III # 300·02)
   Obsessive compulsive disorder (DSM-III # 300·30)
   Post-traumatic stress disorders (DSM-III # 308·30 and 309·81)
   Atypical anxiety disorder (DSM-III # 300.00).

Cyclothymic Disorder (DSM-III # 301·13)
   Dysthymic disorder (DSM-III # 300·40)

Adjustment Disorders with Anxious Mood (DSM-III # 309·24)

Drug-use of drug-withdrawal related anxiety disorders are omitted.

Granville-Grossman and Turner, 1966; Kathol et al., 1980; HoehnSaric et al., 1981; Greenblatt and Shader, 1974). Furthermore, in obsessive-compulsive disorders (DSM-III # 300.30) serotonin reuptake inhibitors have recently had the best therapeutic effect (Thoren et al., 1979; Stern et al., 1980).

Some early and recent, large-scale, clinical studies, however, have produced results which suggest that a majority of patients, even those suffering from a generalized anxiety disorder, will respond better within a few weeks to treatment with antidepressants than with benzodiazepines (Bianchi and Phillips, 1972; Rickels et al., 1969; Johnstone et al., 1980; Kahn et al., 1981). Since the same seems to be true of patients suffering from a mixture of depression and anxiety, one group (Johnstone et al., 1980) raised the question, whether a differential diagnosis between a generalized anxiety disorder and a dysthymic disorder with anxiety is warranted. At least it does not predict differential response to drugs which have relatively specific and very different mechanisms of action (tricyclics vs. benzodiazepines). Consequently, the somewhat different clinical syndromes may not be indicative of differential pathophysiology.

The pertinent question then becomes: when would the benzodiazepines, presently the most widely prescribed anxiolytics, be indicated in psychiatric practice? They are indicated in adjustment disorders with anxious mood and/or somatic symptoms and in acute post-traumatic stress disorders. Obviously, the benzodiazepines have therapeutic efficacy in generalized anxiety disorder as well, even though it may not rival that of the tricyclics for this indication. Moreover, in anxious outpatients with suicide potential their low toxicity following overdose is an asset (Greenblatt and Shader, 1974).

Table 2. Clinical Usefulness of Plasma Level Measurements

1. Drug shows large interindividual variation in kinetics.
2. Drug causes significant acute or chronic toxicity which is related to its kinetics.
3. There is known relationship between plasma levels of the drug and therapeutic outcome in a disorder.
4. There is a group of patients with altered endorgan sensitivity.
5. Suspicion of patient noncompliance.

PHARMACOKINETIC CONSIDERATIONS

The basic tenet of clinical pharmacokinetics is that during steady state the free plasma concentration of a drug is the same as that at the relevant receptor. Because total rather than free plasma concentrations are generally measured, an implicit assumption is made that the interindividual variations in total plasma concentrations provide a reasonable estimate of the variation in free concentrations. Thus, within a diagnostically uniform group of patients, presumed to represent relatively similar pathophysiology, determination of the total drug concentration is useful under certain circumstances (Table 2).

In the field of clinical psychopharmacology, measurement of lithium concentrations is of indisputable value in guiding both the treatment of acute exacerbations of primary, major, bipolar, and unipolar affective disorders and the maintenance of a remission (Cooper and Simpson, 1978). In "endogenous" or primary, major depressions with prominent vegetative symptoms, quantitation of imipramine and nortriptyline and their metabolite levels has been convincingly proved to be of value. Adjusting the dose of these tricyclics to produce "therapeutic" plasma levels increases the incidence of favorable therapeutic outcomes from around 60 to between 80 and 90% of patients (Table 3). The data concerning "therapeutic" plasma levels of other tricyclics in primary, major depressions are controversial (for review see Linnoila, 1981).

Table 3. "Therapeutic" Plasma Levels of Tricyclic Antidepressants in Primary, Major Depressions with Vegetative Symptoms

Imipramine + desipramine (90% favorable therapeutic outcome)	> 220 ng/ml (Glassman et al., 1977; Perel et al., 1978)
Nortriptyline (80% favorable therapeutic outcome)	> 50 but < 150 ng/ml (Asberg, 1973; Kragh-Sorensen et al., 1976; Ziegler et al., 1978)

The active hydroxymetabolites were not quantified in these studies.

DRUG CONCENTRATION MEASUREMENTS IN
PANIC AND PHOBIC DISORDERS

Monoamine oxidase inhibitors (MAOIs) currently on the market are nonspecific in the sense that they inhibit both MAO type A and B, and their action is irreversible. Thus, the duration of the effect of these drugs is dependent on the rate of synthesis of the MAO protein itself. There are no data concerning the relationship between plasma levels and therapeutic response to MAOIs in anxiety disorders. Because of the irreversible action of these drugs, measurement of their plasma levels, once a minimum has been exceeded, should not yield information useful for titrating the dose. Such a minimum therapeutic dose for phenelzine seems to be 60 mg/24 hours for most patients (Robinson et al., 1978). Conceivably, side effects of these drugs could be unrelated to their MAO inhibiting potency and positively correlated with their kinetics. If this were the case, then quantifying these drugs could prove to be useful.

Tricyclic antidepressants, particularly desipramine and imipramine, and probably others, as well (Gloger et al. 1981) have a potent antipanic and antiphobic effect, but they do not reduce the anticipatory anxiety experienced by these patients (Sheehan et al., 1980; Zitrin et al., 1980). The tricyclics work in patients with or without mitral valve prolapse (Gorman et al., 1981) which is common in this disorder (Venkatesh et al., 1980), and they probably block panic attacks produced by lactate infusions as well (Rifkin et al., 1981).

Because the tricyclic antidepressants are "high extraction" drugs and show large, interindividual variability in their kinetics, they are good candidates for plasma concentration measurements (Wilkinson and Shand, 1975).

The only studies concerning plasma tricyclic levels in panic attack and phobic patients have been on a small scale and have not shown any correlation between plasma tricyclic levels and therapeutic response (Jobson et al., 1979; Davidson et al., 1981). In these studies the patients responded to tricyclic plasma levels which were significantly below those necessary for response in patients with "endogenous" depressions. Interestingly, Davidson et al. found that there was a modest positive correlation between the degree of platelet MAO inhibition produced by amitriptyline and relief of phobic symptoms (r > .05). This preliminary finding is intriguing because of the similarity of the effects of MAOIs and tricyclic in these patients and because of the rapid onset of the therapeutic action of these drugs in phobic patients (days instead of weeks).

Thus, even though measurements of tricyclic concentrations may not be useful in the management of phobic patients, pharmacokinetic analysis is helpful in elucidating the mechanisms of action of these drugs in this disorder.

β-Blockers seem to act in phobic-anxious patients by blocking peripheral B_1 receptors. This conclusion is derived from studies demonstrating that practolol which is a relatively specific B_1 receptor blocker, and sotalol, which is mainly active in the periphery, are as active as D-L and D propranolol in relieving anxiety (Bonn and Turner, 1971; Bonn et al., 1972; Tyrer and Lader, 1973). The usefulness of β-blocker plasma concentration measurements, however, has not been evaluated in phobic patients. Because propranolol like the tricyclic antidepressants is a "high extraction" drug and consequently shows large inter-individual variability in its kinetics, measuring its plasma levels could be of value. Some patients respond to clonidine but the side effects of this drug prohibit its use in these disorders (Hoehn-Saric et al., 1981). However, its similarity to the β-blockers reduces the effects of adrenergic nervous system stimulation. This common action may provide a clue to the pathophysiology of panic and phobic disorders.

DRUG CONCENTRATION MEASUREMENTS IN GENERALIZED ANXIETY DISORDER, ADJUSTMENT DISORDER WITH ANXIOUS MOOD AND/OR DYSTHYMIC DISORDER

Benzodiazepines There are two short-term studies, one on clordiaze-poxide and another on diazepam, which found a positive correlation between drug concentrations and anxiolytic response (Linn and Friedel, 1979; Dasberg et al., 1974). In the chlordiazepoxide study, the subjects were 15 mildly anxious patients who were followed for a week on placebo and then for another week on chlordiazepoxide (60 mg/24 hours). The treatments were administered in a random order. Chlordiazepoxide was a more effective anxiolytic than placebo and the efficacy correlated positively with the plasma levels of two of its active metabolites (Table 4).

Table 4. "Therapeutic" Benzodiazepine Levels in Anxious Patients
Short-Term Studies (< 3 weeks duration)

Chlordiazepoxide's anxiolytic efficacy on day 7 correlated with the levels of desmethylchlordiazepoxide and demoxepam (r = .6; Lin and Friedel, 1979)

Diazepam plasma levels > 400 ng/ml are associated with a favorable therapeutic outcome in severely anxious patients on day 5 (Dasberg et al., 1974)

Diazepam levels > 400 ng/ml prior to the next dose are associated with reduced anxiety following a 10 mg dose in severely anxious patients on day 14 (Linnoila et al., unpublished)

N-desmethyldiazepam plasma levels correlated negatively with duration of sleep (r = -.6) in anxious insomniacs on day 7 (Tansella et al., 1975).

In the diazepam study, 15 acutely anxious inpatients of a crisis intervention center received 20 mg/24 hours of diazepam. They were followed for five days. Diazepam was slightly better than placebo, and highly anxious patients with plasma diazepam levels in excess of 400 ng/ml improved more than patients having plasma levels below this "threshold" (Dasberg et al., 1974; Table 4). High plasma N-desmethyldiazepam levels were interpreted to be antagonistic to diazepam's anxiolytic efficacy. A common feature of these two studies was that the severity of anxiety was rated within a few hours after the previous dose of the benzodiazepines such that steady state conditions were not present. This may be of significance, because both objectively and subjectively measurable mood effects of these drugs seem to be strongest during the absorption phase (Bliding, 1974).

We recently conducted a study investigating efficacy, psychomotor side effects and pharmacokinetics of diazepam in 30 nonpsychotic, nondepressed and chronically anxious patients. All of them had Hamilton anxiety ratings in excess of 25 at the time of admission (Linnoila et al., unpublished). After a 3 week withdrawal from previous treatments and a week on placebo, equal numbers of patients received double-blind diazepam 10 mg t.i.d., diazepam 5 mg t.i.d. or placebo for three weeks. All groups improved significantly according to psychiatrist's ratings obtained prior to ingesting a dose but there were only marginal differences between the treatments (Figure 1). Subjective ratings conducted during the absorption phase of the drug on day 14, however, showed diazepam 10 mg t.i.d. to be more efficacious than placebo. Interestingly, the rate of absorption of diazepam is significantly higher after a 10 mg dose than after a 5 mg dose (Ellinwood et al., 1981). There were no significant correlations between the steady state plasma levels and reduction of anxiety. But those patients who had steady state levels in excess of 400 ng/ml of diazepam on day 14 responded best, similar to the Dasberg et al. study (Table 4).

In conclusion, these controlled but relatively small scale studies suggest that chlordiazepoxide and diazepam are somewhat more effective than placebo in the short term treatment of generalized anxiety. At least in the case of diazepam, the anxiolytic effect may be associated with the absorption phase of the drug. Furthermore, a minimum predose plasma level of 400 ng/ml of diazepam may be necessary for a therapeutic response to appear during the initial two weeks of treatment. Importantly, psychomotor side effects of diazepam are associated with its absorption phase as well (Ellinwood et al., 1981).

In an Italian inpatient study, 60 anxious patients suffering from insomnia were treated, double-blind, with placebo, amylobarbital 200 mg, or N-desmethyldiazepam 10 or 20 mg q.h.s. (Tansella et al., 1975). On day 7, the high dose N-desmethyldiazepam group who had higher plasma drug levels than the low dose group was reported to sleep significantly better than the placebo group. However, a significant difference in anxiety levels was not found between the

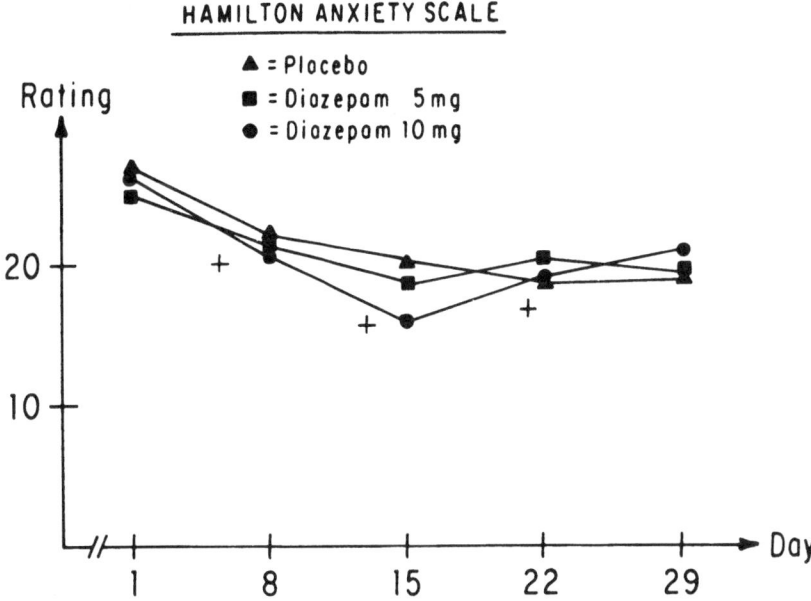

Figure 1. Hamilton Anxiety Scale ratings in 30 anxious patients. All patients received placebo from day one to day eight. Thereafter, equal numbers of patients were randomly allocated to the placebo, diazepam 5 mg and 10 mg t.i.d. groups. There were no differences in the ratings between the groups, but all groups were less anxious on days 8, 15, and 22 than at the baseline (non-parametric anova; method of at least differences; + = p<.05, two-tailed probability).

groups. There was a negative correlation (r = -0.55) between the plasma levels of N-desmethyldiazepam and self-rated duration of sleep in the high dose group.

In a recent, large scale, British experiment (Johnstone et al., 1980 and 1981) 240 neurotically depressed or anxious outpatients were treated double-blind with a maintenance dose of placebo, amitriptyline 150 mg/24 hours, diazepam 20 mg/24 hours or a combination of the two drugs for four weeks. Plasma "levels" of the drugs were measured with radioimmuno and radioreceptor assays. These assays are of questionable value in evaluating plasma levels. Moreover, the time of blood sampling relative to the last dose was not reported. Because of these flaws, the finding of no significant relationship between drug "concentrations" and therapeutic response cannot be evaluated, even though the observation tallies with other investigators' results in intermediate duration studies (see below). This study remains, however, as a valuable contribution in elucidating the drug of choice for these patients, as reviewed above.

In chronic use, diazepam apparently induces its own metabolism, even though this conclusion may be partially confounded by outpatient noncompliance, and no relationship can be found between it and its active metabolites' plasma levels and therapeutic efficacy (Kanto et al., 1974). Yet, in spite of presumably decreasing plasma levels in chronically anxious patients continuous treatment with diazepam can reduce the reappearance of symptoms from 45% to 22% compared to placebo (Rickels et al., 1982). Furthermore, an early response at 1 week (which can be speculated to be related to diazepam plasma levels above 400 ng/ml in treatment responsive patients) is a good predictor of a chronic response.

Monoamine oxidase inhibitors are probably the most effective treatment for dysthymic disorder (Ravaris et al., 1980). The above discussion concerning their use in panic/phobic patients pertains to the dysthymic disorder as well, except that the onset of the therapeutic effect may be slow in generalized anxiety and dysthymic disorders.

Tricyclic Antidepressants Despite the efficacy of tricyclic antidepressants in the treatment of generalized anxiety and dysthymic disorders, all studies concerning "therapeutic" plasma levels of these drugs in these disorders have been negative (Norman et al., 1980; for review, Linnoila, 1981). Generally, doses needed for a therapeutic response are lower than those used in the treatment of "endogenous" depressions, but the onset of the therapeutic effect is slow (1 to 4 weeks) in the depressive and generalized anxiety disorders similar to "endogenous" depressions.

Obsessive-Compulsive Disorder Chlorimipramine is an effective treatment of this previously very difficult to treat anxiety disorder. According to two well recognized groups of investigators it has a curvilinear dose response curve (Table 5). Therefore, plasma level monitoring of chlorimipramine and its active metabolites could be important in treating obsessive-compulsive patients.

Regrettably, the "therapeutic" plasma level ranges for chlorimipramine reported by the two groups of investigators do not overlap. Thus, more studies are needed to solve this discrepancy before using chlorimipramine levels in clinical practice.

Table 5. Chlorimipramine Plasma Levels and Therapeutic Response in Obsessive-Compulsive Patients

Patients with plasma chlorimipramine levels < 93 ng/ml were most likely to respond (Thoren et al., 1979)

Patients with plasma chlorimipramine levels > 100 but < 250 and N-desmethyl chlorimipramine levels > 230 but < 550 ng/ml were most likely to respond (Stern et al., 1980).

General Conclusions In anxiety disorders other than obsessive compulsive disorder, plasma level monitoring of the commonly used drugs is of questionable therapeutic value. In the obsessive-compulsive disorder, monitoring plasma chlorimipramine and active metabolite levels can probably increase the incidence of favorable therapeutic outcome once a "therapeutic" plasma level range has been defined. The only anxiolytic drug for which a case has been made to measure plasma levels is diazepam during the first and second weeks of treatment. However, since the clinical titration of diazepam dose is generally not limited by toxicity the dose can be rationally adjusted without knowing the plasma levels in most patients.

REFERENCES

Asberg, M. (1973). Plasma nortriptyline levels: Relationship to clinical effects. *Clin. Pharmacol. Ther.* 16:215–229.

Bianchi, G.N. and Phillips, J. (1972). A comparative trial of doxepin and diazepam in anxiety states. *Psychopharmacol.* 25:86–95.

Bliding, A. (1974). Effects of different rates of absorption of two benzodiazepines on subjective and objective parameters. *Eur. J. Clin. Pharmacol.* 7: 201–211.

Bonn, J.A. and Turner, P. (1971). D-propranolol and anxiety. *Lancet* 1:1355–1356.

Bonn, J.A., Turner, P. and Hicks, D.C. (1972). Beta-adrenergic-receptor blockade with practolol in treatment of anxiety. *Lancet* 1:814–815.

Cooper, T.B. and Simpson, G.M. (1978). Kinetics of lithium and clinical response. In: M.A. Lipton, A. DiMascio and K.F. Killam, eds., *Psychopharmacology: A Generation of Progress,* New York, Raven Press, pp. 923–931.

Dasberg, H.H., van der Kleijn, E., Guelen, P.J.R. and van Praag, H.M. (1974). Plasma concentrations of diazepam and its metabolite N-desmethyldiazepam in relation to anxiolytic effect. *Clin. Pharmacol. Ther.* 15:473–483.

Davidson, J., Linnoila, M., Raft, D. and Turnbull, C.D. (1981). MAO inhibition and control of anxiety following amitryptyline therapy. *Acta. Psychiatr. Scand.* 63:147–152.

Ellinwood, E.H., Linnoila, M., Easler, M.E. and Molter, D.W. (1981). Onset of peak impairment after diazepam and after alcohol. *Clin. Pharmacol. Ther.* 30:534–538.

Glassman, A.H., Perel, J.M., Shostak, M., Kantor, S.J. and Feiss, J.L. (1977). Clinical implications of imipramine plasma levels for depressive illness. *Arch. Gen. Psychiatry* 34:197–204.

Gloger, G., Grunnhaus, L., Birmacher, B. and Tuondart, T. (1981). Treatment of spontaneous panic attacks with chlorimipramine. *Am. J. Psychiatry* 138: 1215–1271.

Gorman, J.M., Fyer, A.F., Glicklich, J., King, D. and Klein, D.F. (1981). Effect of imipramine on prolapsed mitral valves of patients with panic disorder. *Am. J. Psychiatry* 138:977–978.

Granville-Grossman, K.L. and Turner, P. (1966). *The Effect of Propranolol in Clinical Practice.* New York, Raven Press.

Hoehn-Saric, R., Merchant, A.F., Keyser, M.L. and Smith, V.K. (1981). Effects of clonidine on anxiety disorders. *Arch. Gen. Psychiatry* 38:1278-1282.

Jobson, K., Linnoila, M., Gillam, J. and Sullivan, J.L. (1978). Successful treatment of severe anxiety attacks with tricyclic antidepressants: a potential mechanism of action. *Am. J. Psychiatry* 135:863-864.

Johnstone, E.C., Owens, D.G.C., Frith, C.D., McPherson, K., Dowie, C., Riley, G. and Gold, A. (1980). Neurotic illness and its response to anxiolytic and antidepressant treatment. *Psychol. Med.* 10:321-328.

Johnstone, E.C., Bourne, R.C., Crow, T.J., Frith, C.D., Gamble, S., Lofthouse, R., Owen, F., Owens, D.G.C., Robinson, J. and Stevens, M. (1981). The relationships between clinical response, psychophysiological variables and plasma levels of amitriptyline and diazepam in neurotic outpatients. *Psychopharmacol.* 72:233-240.

Kanto, J., Iisalo, E., Lehtinen, V., Salminen, J. (1974). The concentrations of diazepam and its metabolites in the plasma after an acute and chronic administration. *Psychopharmacologia* 36:123-131.

Kathol, R.G., Noyes, R., Slymen, D.J., Crowe, R.R., Clancy, J. and Kerber, R.E. (1980). Propranolol in chronic anxiety disorders. *Arch. Gen. Psychiatry* 37:1361-1365.

Kahn, R.J., McNair, D.M., Covi, L., Downing, R.W., Fisher, S., Lipman, R.S., Rickels, K. and Smith, V.K. (1981). Effects of psychotropic agents in high anxiety subjects. *Psychopharmacol. Bull.* 17(3):97-100.

Kelly, D., Guirguis, W., Frommer, E., Mitchell-Heggs, N. and Sargant, W. (1970). Treatment of phobic states with antidepressants. *Br. J. Psychiatry* 116: 387-398.

Klein, D.F. (1967). Importance of psychiatric diagnosis in prediction of clinical drug effects. *Arch. Gen. Psychiatry* 16:118-126.

Kline, N.S. (1967). Drug treatment of phobic disorders. *Am. J. Psychiatry* 123: 1447-1450.

Kragh-Sorensen, P., Eggert-Hansen, C., Baastrup, C. and Hvidberg, E.F. (1976). Self-inhibiting action of nortriptyline's antidepressive effect at high plasma levels. *Psychopharmacology* 45:305-312.

Lin, K.-M. and Friedel, R.O. (1979). Relationship of plasma levels of chlordiazepoxide and metabolites to clinical response. *Am. J. Psychiatry* 136:18-23.

Linnoila, M. (1981). Relationship between plasma levels of antidepressants and therapeutic response. In T.A. Ban, R. Gonzales, A.S. Jablensky, N.A. Sartorius and F. E. Vartanian, eds., *Prevention and Treatment of Depression,* Baltimore, University Park Press, pp. 219-232.

Norman, T.R., Burrows, G.D., Bianchi, G.N., Maguire, K.P. and Wurm, J.M.E. (1980). Doxepin plasma levels and anxiolytic response. *Int. Pharmacopsychiat.* 15:247-252.

Perel, J.M., Stiller, R.L. and Glassman, A.H. (1978). Studies on plasma level/effect relationships in imipramine therapy. *Comm. Psychopharmacol.* 2:429-439.

Ravaris, C.L., Robinson, D.S., Ives, J.O., Nies, A. and Bartlett, D. (1980). Phenelzine and amitriptyline in the treatment of depression. *Arch. Gen. Psychiatry* 37:1075-1080.

Rifkin, A., Klein, D.F., Dillon, D. and Levitt, M. (1981). Blockade by imipramine or desipramine of panic induced by sodium lactate. *Am. J. Psychiatry* 138:676-677.

Rickels, K., Perloff, M., Stepansky, W., Dion, H.S., Case, W.G. and Sapra, R.K. (1969). Doxepin and diazepam in general practice and hospital clinic neurotic patients: a collaborative controlled study. *Psychopharmacologia* 15:265-279.

Robinson, D.S., Nies, A., Ravaris, C.L. and Lamborn, K.R. (1973). The mono-amine inhibitor, phenelzine, in the treatment of depressive-anxiety states. *Arch. Gen. Psychiatry* 29:407-413.

Robinson, D.S., Nies, A., Ravaris, L., Ives, J.O. and Bartlett, K. (1978). Clinical pharmacology of phenelzine. *Arch. Gen. Psychiatry* 35:629-635.

Sheehan, D.V., Ballenger, J. and Jacobsen, G. (1980). Treatment of endogenous anxiety with phobic, hysterical, and hypochondriacal symptoms. *Arch. Gen. Psychiatry* 37:51-59.

Stern, R.S., Marks, I.M., Mawson, D. and Luscombe, D.K. (1980). Clomipramine and exposure for compulsive rituals: II: Plasma levels, side effects and out-come. *Br. J. Psychiatry* 136:161-166.

Tansella, M., Sicilliani, O., Burti, L., Schiavon, M., Zimmerman-Tansella Ch., Genna, M., Tognoni, G. and Morselli, P.L. (1974). N-desmethyl-diazepam and amylobarbitone sodium as hypnotics in anxious patients. Plasma levels, clinical efficacy and residual effects. *Psychopharmacologia* 41: 81-85.

Thoren, P., Asberg, M., Bertilsson, L., Mellstrom, B., Sjogvist, F., and Traskman, L. (1979). Clomipramine treatment of obsessive compulsive disorder. II. *Arch. Gen. Psychiatry* 37:1289-1294.

Tyrer, P.J. and Lader, M. (1973). Effects of beta adrenergic blockade with sotalol in chronic anxiety. *Clin. Pharmacol. Ther.* 14:418-425.

Tyrer, P. (1976). Towards rational therapy with monoamine oxidase inhibitors. *Br. J. Psychiatry* 128:354-360.

Venkatesh, A., Pauls, D.L., Crowe, R., Noyes, R., van Valkenburg, C., Martins, J.B. and Kerber, R.E. (1980). Mitral valve prolapse in anxiety neurosis (panic disorder) *Am. Heart J.* 100:302-305.

Wilkinson, G.R. and Shand, D.G. (1975). A physiological approach to hepatic drug clearance. *Clin. Pharmacol. Ther.* 18:377-390.

Ziegler, V.E., Clayton, P.J., Taylor, J.R., Co, B.T. and Biggs, J.T. (1976). Nor-triptyline plasma levels and therapeutic response. *Clin. Pharmacol. Ther.* 20:458-463.

Zitrin, C.M., Klein, D.F. and Woerner, M.G. (1980). Treatment of agoraphobia with group exposure in vivo and imipramine. *Arch. Gen. Psychiatry* 37: 63-72.

SECTION IV

Emergency Psychiatry

Hints for Clinicians

DEFINITION OF RAPID NEUROLEPTIZATION

A definition of rapid neuroleptization should include proper evaluation and establishment of a diagnosis, specific monitoring procedures and a recognizable end-point. The term has been used to describe both short-term use for initial control, to augmentation of an ongoing program during a period of agitation, restlessness, combativeness, or increased psychotic symptoms. Moreover it has also been used to describe rapid treatment over several days in increasing amounts to reach high-dose oral regimens which may continue for an indefinite time.

METHOD OF TREATMENT

When one embarks on rapid neuroleptization, it must be in a setting with close medical supervision and staff trained in the management of hypotension, acute dystonias and other serious side effects. The most serious diagnostic risk is the fact that once this treatment has been started, critical re-assessment of diagnosis may be ignored. If it is effective, there is rapid symptom-reduction and the pressure to make an accurate diagnosis is lessened. In particular, the critical examination of the diagnosis of schizophrenia, so frequently made, is rendered difficult.

341

High or rapidly increasing oral doses are not always an advantage. Focal control of severe psychotic symptoms may be achieved by repeated parenteral administration of high potency neuroleptics using 2 to 10 mg of haloperidol or similar doses of other high potency drugs. Two to four injections at hourly intervals are usually adequate. Low potency drugs are not recommended because of the possible development of hypotension and local irritation. Administration should be repeated at intervals of one hour, up to a maximum dose of 100 mg of haloperidol in 24 hours or the equivalent of other high potency drugs.

Following the parenteral control, the oral medication required for continuing control will be equal to or as much as twice the amount administered in the preceding 24 hours parenterally. This may be begun six to twelve hours after the last intramuscular dose. Parenteral medication should be stopped as soon as the patient is sleeping, sedated, or cooperative enough for oral medication to be instituted. Individualized dose is the most essential principle in *all* phases of treatment. Non-response or partial-response requires reevaluation, not increased dosage; some patients get worse on high doses.

UNWANTED EFFECTS

While there is yet no direct evidence suggesting that rapid neuroleptization is more likely to lead to rare important side effects than other forms of high dose neuroleptic administration, it is important to be aware of their existence. These side effects include behavioral toxicity, malignant neuroleptic syndrome, and drug-induced catatonia. Behavioral toxicity is typified by a drug-induced psychosis with dysphoria and worsening mental status which may resemble the original symptoms. It is a consequence of anticholinergic effects of the drugs; or an unusual extrapyramidal side effect with akathisia. Malignant neuroleptic syndrome may lead to death. Catatonia may be mistaken for worsening of the clinical picture and should be recognized so that medication can be interrupted.

A dose of 60 to 100 mg of haloperidol or its equivalent of other acceptable high potency drugs may be given in the initial 24-hour period. Should such an initial regimen not be effective, then selection of a second high-potency drug is indicated. Studies suggest that 2 to 5 mg of fluphenazine, trifluoperazine, haloperidol, and thiothixene, may all have a potency equal to 100 mg of chlorpromazine.

Some patients do not calm down even with very large doses of neuroleptics. As the main concern is to reduce disturbed or aggressive behavior, judicious use of conventional sedatives may be required. An intramuscular dose of 130 mg sodium phenobarbitol often calms a patient not yet tranquilized by neuroleptics. It is important to remember that electroconvulsive therapy is still a useful modality for treating a disturbed patient, even though it is rarely used today. The reported interaction between haloperidol and lithium, with severe neurologic sequelae, does not seem to have much substance.

Thioridazine has at least three disadvantages, namely, strong adrenergic blocking effects that can lead to postural hypotension; strong anticholinergic effects that might aggravate the mental disorder, and possible cardiotoxicity. Hallucinogens like LSD, mescaline, and psilocybin produce "bad trips" that are best managed by simple sedative-hypnotic drugs, such as an oral dose of 10 to 20 mg diazepam. Phencyclidine (PCP) may induce a state closely resembling schizophrenia. Antipsychotic drugs are useful in acute treatment of these disorders. Continual gastric suction and acidification of the urine with ammonium chloride in doses of 1 to 2 g 4 times daily are effective ways to hasten the disappearance of PCP. The drug is secreted into the stomach from the blood and then reabsorbed through the enteric tract; gastric suction interferes with this gastroenteric recycling. Because PCP is a basic drug that remains ionized in an acid urine and thus is not reabsorbed by the kidney, its excretion is hastened by urine acidification.

PHARMACOKINETIC CONSIDERATIONS

Intravenous doses lead to initial high concentration in plasma. As intramuscular doses lead to lower initial concentrations, they are more likely to give a prolonged elevated level. Oral doses lead to a growth and decay pattern of drug concentration like intramuscular doses, but because of the first pass effect, the area under the curve, after an oral dose, does not have to be the same as that after the injected doses. The first pass effect reflects the chemical change or metabolism of the drug, with conversion of products not detected in assays of the parent drug. It occurs during the transfer from the gastrointestinal tract through the gut mucosa, portal circulation and liver, before the drug reaches the general circulation in which measurements are conventionally made. Over 90% of the steady state plateau is reached after approximately 5 drug half-lives have elapsed, regardless of the frequency and magnitude of dosing. If the initial dose of the multiple dosing regimen is higher than the ensuing doses, and if the relationship between the levels of the two doses is properly chosen, then the steady state of concentration is reduced by the initial loading dose and maintained by the later doses.

Chlorpromazine is the most extensively studied drug. After single or multiple doses enzyme induction occurs and the plasma level is reduced. There is wide variation between patients. Intramuscular doses induce detectable concentrations rapidly, but absorption is prolonged. Plasma levels and CSF levels are correlated but the distribution ratio varies between patients.

For haloperidol: approximately 30% is lost as the result of the first-pass effect after oral administration. There is wide variation in plasma levels. Enzyme induction plays no part, either alone or in interactions with antiparkinson drugs.

Butaperazine and thioridazine levels vary widely. Use of thioridazine is complicated since it has metabolites which have been proved to possess clinical activity, and there is no injectible form of the drug. There is also a wide range in the non-protein bound fraction, similar to that known to occur with chlorpromazine.

Trifluoperazine concentrations are proportional to dose and its half-life is in the general region of 7 to 20 hours after single doses.

23

Summary of the Guidelines for the Use of Psychotropic Drugs in Emergency Psychiatry

GEORGE VOINESKOS

INTRODUCTION

In the years since World War II, the emergency department has grown from a single room where accident cases were taken for first aid into one of the busiest, most complex, labor intensive and sophisticated hospital departments. The reason for this growth has been the unplanned, phenomenal increase in the use of the emergency department, in both Canada and the U.S., documented as being greater than that of any of the other measures of hospital utilization, and well beyond that which could be explained by the population growth (Voineskos, 1981; Krass, 1977; Chaiton, 1975; American Medical Association, 1966; Jenkins and Van de Leuv, 1978; Baltzan, 1972). The increasing utilization of the hospital emergency room has been accompanied by a similar and often greater increase in *the percentage of psychiatric emergency visits* (Schwartz et al., 1972; Satloff and Worby, 1970; Zonana et al., 1973; Lowy, 1971).

The reasons for the upsurge in psychiatric emergency visists are numerous and complex, unlikely to change within the foreseeable future, and can be conveniently classified (Voineskos, 1981) into two categories: (a) those related to the increase in the emergency department per se, and (b) those related to changes in the psychiatric delivery system. The emphasis on treatment outside the hospital has led to increasing numbers of patients in the community, who, in the absence of adequate after-care support systems, appear in the emergency department (Schwartz, et al., 1972). Many of these patients would formerly have been inpatients for prolonged periods of time, and suffer from chronic psychotic illness.

345

The increase in emergency visits has lead to a major shift in the practice of hospital psychiatry, and to a transformation of the patterns of referral to hospital psychiatric services. In response to the increased demand the psychiatric emergency service has been developed, which now constitutes one of the essential services that should be provided by psychiatric facilities, and occupies a pivotal position in the psychiatric care delivery system. It should be emphasized that those who practice emergency psychiatry need specialized systematic training in dealing with the distinctive population, mode of presentation, assessment techniques, and treatment methods.

Morselli and Zarifian (1980) have remarked that the correct use of drugs is one of the most urgent problems facing the medical profession today. These investigators further suggest that the development of ever more active, more potent, and more specific psychotropic agents has been accompanied by risks related to the toxic effects of these drugs. This is particularly important in the use of psychotropic drugs in psychiatric emergencies. It has recently become the practice to give large doses in quick succession often without adequate data for a diagnosis.

THE NEED FOR ACCURATE DIAGNOSIS

In his presentation, Hollister concludes that one must try to make the most accurate diagnosis and then find the most appropriate drug and dose for that patient (this volume). Anderson (this volume) and Tupin (this volume) concur on the need for accurate diagnosis and evaluation of the physical, and especially neurological, status of the patient before the administration of neuroleptics. A primary objective is to exclude certain organic conditions, particularly major life threatening illnesses (Anderson, 1980).

In addition, the clinician is warned that the use of drugs might alter the natural course of the disorder to the extent that further diagnostic evaluation may be impaired; or it might lead to ignoring the critical reassessment of diagnosis because of rapid symptom reduction (Tupin, Hollister, this volume). However, in practice in many psychiatric emergencies pharmacologic treatment may have to be instituted before it is possible to make a thorough evaluation of the patient. One must assure that the patient will not be able to harm himself or others. Anderson et al. (1976, 1980) remind us that acute psychosis is an "intensely painful state." When a complete physical assessment is not immediately possible they recommend giving a dose of a high potency neuroleptic, such as haloperidol 5-10 mg. I.M. This may help calm a psychotic patient sufficiently to allow completion of the examination. Hollister wisely advises the clinician "to document fully in the record why various agents were used." He suggests obtaining the consent of the relatives, when available (Hollister, this volume).

CHOICE OF NEUROLEPTIC AND SETTING OF ADMINISTRATION

Anderson, Hollister and Tupin are all in agreement that in the emergency treatment of acute psychosis it is preferable to use the high potency neuroleptics rather than low potency drugs. Their advice is not based on the therapeutic but on the adverse effects of the various neuroleptics, notably hypotension. Hollister (this volume) states unequivocally that chlorpromazine is now obsolete. Thioridazine is not suitable in the emergency situation. The properties of the long acting neuroleptics make them inappropriate for use in rapid neuroleptization (Tupin, this volume).

While the feasibility of rapid neuroleptization on an out-patient basis has been suggested (Anderson et al., 1976), it is definitely best to follow Dr. Tupin's recommendation that it is best done in the hospital. This is a serious medical procedure. The patient needs careful medical and nursing supervision of his condition, progress and possible side effects. Attempts at ambulatory management because of expediency or economy should be resisted.

SIDE EFFECTS

Side Effects and Antiparkinsonian Medication

Dr. Anderson, having drawn attention to the high incidence of dystonias in rapid neuroleptization with high potency neuroleptics, recommends the concurrent routine use of antiparkinsonian medication during the initial titration and for about two weeks thereafter. If antiparkinsonian medication is not used routinely, Dr. Tupin suggests that p.r.n. orders be left for the parenteral use of such drugs; he further warns about the possible appearance of respiratory distress arising from laryngeal-pharyngeal dystonia. Recently, Modestin et al. (1981) reported on the sudden death of a woman who received high doses of haloperidol, and suggested that the cause of death in such cases may be due to a neuroleptic-induced laryngeal spasm leading to cardiac arrest via vagal reflexes.

The prophylactic use of antiparkinsonian medication, nevertheless, awaits clarification. The differences in the practice of routine versus as required use of antiparkinsonian medication reflects partly the lack of agreement in the literature on the frequency of side effects in rapid neuroleptization. Some argue that, since dystonias do not always or only rarely occur, the addition of antiparkinsonian medication may bring about unnecessary side effects (Tupin, this volume).

In addition, a few reports suggest the possibility of an interaction between anticholinergic antiparkinsonian drugs and neuroleptics (Morselli and Zarifian, 1980; Gautier et al., 1977; Rivera-Calimlin et al., 1976; Yesavage et al., 1982).

Gautier et al. (1977) found that the plasma level of 4 different neuroleptics was reduced in patients when they received benztropine, triexyphenidyl or procyclidine. After withdrawal of the antiparkinsonian drug, however, the neuroleptic plasma level increased. Similarly, others have reported that trihexyphenidyl has led to a significant decrease in the plasma level of chlorpromazine (Rivera-Calimlin et al., 1976) and of haloperidol (Morselli and Zarifian, 1980). These findings are probably relevant to rapid neuroleptization even during the intramuscular phase, because the mechanism of the neuroleptic plasma level reduction is unclear. Two mechanisms have been postulated (a) an absorption effect (Gautier et al., 1977; Davis et al., 1978), and (b) an enzymatic or metabolic effect (Gautier et al., 1977).

No definite relationship has been shown between neuroleptic plasma levels and side effects. Reviewing studies for five phenothiazines, Dahl (1979) concluded that a well defined and generally valid toxic plasma level limit has not been established. Some patients have side effects but relatively low plasma levels, while others have high plasma levels and no side effects. Recently Zarifian et al. (1982) reported that no conclusions could be drawn on the incidence of extrapyramidal side effects in high dose neuroleptic treatment (plasma haloperidol levels 140 to 250 ng/ml).

Grave Rare Complications

In addition to laryngeal-pharyngeal spasm, Dr. Tupin (this volume) has drawn attention to other serious and rare complications such as behavioral toxicity, malignant neuroleptic syndrome and catatonia.

Behavioral toxicity may be a consequence of massive central anticholinergic effects (Curry, this volume). It demands reduction or discontinuation of the neuroleptic.

Tupin cautions that, while he is not aware of reports suggesting that rapid neuroleptization is more likely than other drug regimens to lead to malignant neuroleptic syndrome, it may be induced by giving rapidly increasing doses over a short period of time. Malignant neuroleptic syndrome and catatonic reactions have been described in patients who were on high doses of haloperidol, trifluoperazine, and fluphenazine (Gellenberg and Mandel, 1977; Weinberger and Kelly, 1977; Geller and Greydanus, 1979), but also they have occurred on small doses, such as haloperidol 7.5 mg or 5 mg daily (Weinberger and Kelly, 1977). Nevertheless, one cannot overemphasize the need for the physician to bear in mind the drug induced nature of catatonia and the malignant neuroleptic syndrome, particularly when the patient's condition unexpectedly worsens in the course of treatment. The neuroleptic must then be discontinued (Gellenberg and Mandel, 1977). It may be difficult to differentiate these complications on clinical grounds from the rare syndrome of lethal catatonia first described in the pre-phenothiazine era (Weinberger and Kelly, 1977).

NEUROLEPTIC DOSAGE, DOSING AND ROUTE OF ADMINISTRATION

The large dosage of neuroleptics given in rapid neuroleptization have recently been questioned (Kirkpatrick and Burnett, 1982). In this regard Hollister and Tupin suggest that regular doses may be as effective as high doses, and that mega doses seem to be less justified than was previously thought. Dr. Tupin cautions against the uncritical adoption of "routine" techniques. He also cautions the clinician to resist the pressures for early discharge of patients on high doses, whose symptoms are in incomplete remission. This can only result in poor compliance and perpetuation of the "revolving door". He suggests that 'focal neuroleptization' can be both effective and desirable as a method of controlling emergent symptoms or initiating ongoing treatment, especially when it is carefully titrated against the patient's individual needs and has a specific end point. However it should not be seen as a method of establishing high dose maintenance medication.

Tupin (this volume) recommends that up to 100 mg of haloperidol or the equivalent of other high potency neuroleptic may be given in the first 24 hours. Should such a regimen not be effective, a selection of another drug should be considered. A maximum amount is, therefore, defined. This makes good sense, particularly in the light of studies (Zarifian et al., 1982) which have reported that very high doses of haloperidol, such as 200 mg per day resulting in plasma levels of up to 250 ng/ml, failed to produce clinical improvement. There are indeed patients who are poor responders to a neuroleptic or neuroleptics. Davis et al. (1978) have pointed out that variables unrelated to plasma levels play a role in determining clinical response.

In the light of our present knowledge of the relationship of neuroleptic plasma levels and therapeutic response the upper limit of 100 mg haloperidol may be rather arbitrary. Professor Curry (this volume) outlines the therapeutically "desirable" plasma range for two high potency neuroleptics namely haloperidol and fluphenazine, but the evidence for this is by no means conclusive.

Recently Baldessarini (1979) reported that blood assays of neuroleptic drugs had little clinical usefulness and remained essentially an experimental procedure needing further guidelines for interpretation and clinical use. Included in the assay methods were gas chromatography, radioimmunoassays, and radioreceptor assays. More recently Hollister (1981) suggested that the data on neuroleptics are too sparse and contain too many possible sources of error to accept claims of a range of therapeutic plasma concentrations.

In recent years, studies on the relationship of neuroleptic plasma level and therapeutic response, while reporting conflicting results, have been encouraging (Evans, 1981; Tune et al., 1981; Magliozzi et al., 1981; Sakalis and Traficante, 1981). The issue, however, is still far from settled. Furthermore, it should be emphasized that none of the correlation studies has been conducted in relation to emergency psychiatry, and rapid neuroleptization (Curry, this volume).

Hollister (this volume) suggests that the only unequivocal advantage of parenteral administration is that the treating physician can be sure the drug enters the body. Tupin (this volume) recommends that parenteral administration should be stopped as soon as the patient is cooperative enough to take oral medication. However, in view of the difference in the absorption rate between oral and intramuscular administration these suggestions should be questioned.

The therapeutic or toxic effect, of the plasma concentration built-up by the *hourly* multiple doses during the first phase of neuroleptization should be assessed before proceeding to the next dose. These effects are more likely to be apparent within an hour with I.M. than with oral dosing. The mean lag between ingestion of haloperidol and appearance of the drug in the blood is about one and a half hours, and maximal concentrations in serum are reached after five hours (Forsman and Ohman, 1979). On the other hand, following intramuscular injection the maximum plasma level is reached within 20 minutes (Hollister, 1981).

One other question pertains to the validity of the method of determining the amount of the neuroleptic given orally during phase II of rapid neuroleptization. This amount is usually taken to be about 1.5 times the I.M. amount in view of the reduced biological availability of the oral preparation, which is reported to vary between 44% and 79% with a mean of 60% ± 11% (Forsman and Ohman, 1976). Morselli and Zarifian, however, have drawn attention to the great inter-individual variability (8-12 fold) for a given oral dose whereas after intramuscular administration it is reduced to 1-3 fold (Morselli and Zarifian, 1980). This is by no means unique to haloperidol; even higher magnitude interpatient variability for a given oral dose has been reported for thiothixene (Yesavage et al., 1982) and for fluphenazine (Dysken et al., 1981). Such large inter-individual variability with oral doses should pose questions on the practice of arrival at the amount of the dose for the oral phase of rapid neuroleptization.

FACTORS AFFECTING RESEARCH IN EMERGENCY PSYCHOPHARMACOTHERAPY

Human experimentation committees in this and other Universities are increasingly concerned with informed consent. Many acute psychotic patients may not be able to give consent or when they appear to consent this may not be truly informed consent. This is particularly true when the patient is required to make choices in a complex experimental design. But even consent for, what used to be regarded, as relatively simple matters (for instance drawing blood samples for the study of an established treatment procedure) can pose limitations on studies (Yesavage et al., 1982).

The establishment of a 2-3 week drug free period for the purposes of obtaining base-line clinical and biological measurements, highly important to research, is not attainable for many emergency patients. The clinical picture and the behavioral manifestations of the emergency patient are often of a nature and severity that treatment may have to be initiated without delay. This may preclude even a single pre-treatment measurement, an acceptable diagnosis or adherence to the methodology of a carefully designed study.

In the light of the usefulness of psychotropic drugs the use of placebo, still possible in some psychiatric research, is likely to be disallowed in studies of emergency psychotic patients. Fixed dose regimens, especially fixed total dosage, eloquently argued by Davis and associates (1978) for the purposes of establishing the therapeutic range or window, are often impractical when faced with an individual whose behavior continues to be very disturbed and disturbing. In such situations when the usual upper limit is reached many clinicians will resort to "clinical judgement", and may probably wish to increase the medication (Dysken et al., 1981).

In emergency psychiatry many patients are admitted on an involuntary basis, and they constitute a special group when it comes to research. Their involuntary status does not give permission for treatment or participation in studies, although they may be eminently suitable for participation in a given study on other grounds. The involuntary status, however, calls for the exercise of extra care by clinicians and investigators to avoid to be or appear to be exerting any pressure whatsoever in obtaining informed consent.

REASONS FOR DOING RESEARCH IN EMERGENCY PSYCHOPHARMACOTHERAPY

Research in emergency psychopharmacotherapy is of utmost importance and utmost urgency.

The emergency population has been increasing and this is unlikely to be reversed. The emergency service is the major interface between the hospital psychiatric services and the public. Thus the quality of the emergency service, which a psychiatric facility provides, is of paramount importance for its relationships with the community and its standing among the other medical disciplines of the parent hospital. High quality clinical service must be based on sound research.

The studies on emergency use of neuroleptics are inconclusive, far from perfect and it is difficult to compare them. There are differences in design, and even in the better designed studies there are shortcomings. Most studies employ a flexible dose regimen, fixed dosage schedules are lacking, and the amount of the neuroleptic given is based on clinical improvement or side effects. A frequently quoted study of haloperidol (Eriksen et al., 1978) comparing a high loading dose to a standard dose, is hardly applicable to the emergency situation, and to date it has been reported only in a preliminary form, therefore proper evaluation is not possible.

Patient selection is not uniform, the criteria used for establishing the diagnosis are frequently not stated or when they are stated they are of questionable value. Very few studies such as that of Anderson et al. (1976) have used acceptable criteria. Duration of illness or relapse, chronicity and severity of illness are usually not reported. The role that each of these has in relation to drug effect in rapid neuroleptization or other neuroleptic treatment awaits clarification. In this regard, it is interesting to note that in the study by Neborsky et al. (1981) all the patients (N=20) were under 27 years of age, and 15 suffered their first psychotic episode, making them entirely noncomparable to the patients who fail to improve on very high doses of neuroleptics. There are no reports of studies endeavoring to correlate biological and clinical measurements during the first phase of rapid neuroleptization.

In his contributions to this volume, Professor Curry concludes with very important observations: while much useful information is now available on the pharmacokinetics of neuroleptic drugs, very little of it is relevant to emergency psychiatry; there is a definite need for intensive study of neuroleptic dosing regimens in the emergency situation; the techniques for this now exist; and research should be pursued immediately.

Much of the use of psychotropic agents in emergency psychiatry, especially with the high potency neuroleptics, is under question. The optimum dose, or dose range, upper limit, frequency and route of dosing, and the relationship of clinical improvement and side effects to plasma levels in rapid neuroleptization, as well as the relationship of the clinical and biological parameters of rapid neuroleptization to those related to steady state plasma levels are but a few of the questions requiring thorough investigation.

Emergency psychiatry presents opportunities for research in the use of psychotropic drugs that are not as readily found in other areas of psychiatry. Davis et al. (1978) writing on neuroleptic plasma levels and drug response point out that it is important to be able to measure improvement in schizophrenia, and that "this requires patients who have a reasonably florid symptomatology who improve in a fairly dramatic fashion with antipsychotic medication". Patients sufficiently ill to demonstrate a drug effect are abundant in emergency psychiatry. Another fruitful area of pursuit is that of side effects. Davis and associates (1978) make the point that clinically patients develop tolerance to such side effects as extrapyramidal signs, sedation, postural hypotension, and so forth. These investigators suggest that in view of the confounding influence of tolerance the relationship between side effects and plasma levels would probably be most visible in patients treated in the acute situation.

REFERENCES

American Medical Association (1966). *Emergency Departments*. American Medical Association, Chicago.

American Hospital Association (1972). *Emergency Services*. American Hospital Association. Chicago.

Anderson, W.H. Emergency treatment of psychosis. This volume.

Anderson, W.H., Kuehnle, J.C. (1980). Treatment of psychosis by rapid neuroleptization: update 1980. In *Haloperidol Update: 1958-1980*. Edited by Ayd, F.J. Baltimore, Ayd Medical Communications, pp. 31-39.

Anderson, W.H., Kuehnle, J.C., Catanzano, D.M. (1976). Rapid treatment of acute psychosis. *Am. J. Psychiatry* 133:1076-1078.

Baldessarini, R.J. (1979). Status of psychotropic drug blood level assays and other biochemical measurements in clinical practice. *Am. J. Psychiatry* 136:1177-1180.

Baltzan, M.A. (1972). New role of the hospital emergency department. *Can. Med. Assoc. J.* 106:249-256.

Chaiton, A. (1975). Trends in emergency department utilization. *Can. Fam. Phys.* 21:115-121.

Curry, S.H. Assessment of psychotropic drugs following acute doses: II. Clinical significance of neuroleptic plasma levels. This volume.

Curry, S.H. Assessment of psychotropic drugs following acute doses: I. Pharmacodynamics and pharmacokinetics. This volume.

Dahl, S.G. (1979). Monitoring of phenothiazine plasma levels in psychiatric patients. In *Proceedings XI CINP Congress*. Oxford; Pergamon Press, pp. 567-575.

Davis, J.M., Bettis, D.B., Dekirmenjian, H., Ericsen, S.E., Garver, D.L. (1978). Plasma levels of neuroleptics and antipsychotic drug response. *Clinical Neuropharmacology*. Edited by H.L. Klawans, New York, Raven Press, pp. 85-102.

Dysken, M.W., Jaraid, J.I., Chang, S.S., Schaffer, C., Shaid, A., Davis, J.M. (1981). Fluphenazine pharmacokinetics and therapeutic response. *Psychopharmacology* 73:205-210.

Eriksen, S.E., Hurt, S.W., Chang, S. et al. (1978). Haloperidol dose, plasma levels, and clinical response: a double-blind study. *Psychopharmacol. Bull.* 14:15-16.

Evans, L. (1981). Butyrophenones plasma levels and therapeutic effect. In *Psychotropic Drugs Plasma Concentration and Clinical Response*. Edited by Burrows, G., Norman, T., New York, Dekker Publishing, pp. 319-329.

Forsman, A., Öhman, R. (1979). Pharmacokinetics and pharmacodynamics of haloperidol in man. In *Proceedings XI CINP Congress*. Oxford, Pergamon Press, pp. 559-565.

Forsman, A., Öhman, R. (1976). Pharmacokinetic studies on haloperidol in man. *Cur. Ther. Res.* 20:319-336.

Gautier, J., Jus, A., Villeneuve, A., Jus, K., Pires, P., Villeneuve, R. (1977). Influence of the antiparkinsonian drugs on the plasma level of neuroleptics. *Biol. Psychiatry* 12:389-399.

Gellenberg, A.J., Mandel, M.R. (1977). Catatonic reactions to high-potency neuroleptic drugs. *Arch. Gen. Psychiatry* 34:947-950.

Geller, B., Greydanus, D.E. (1979). Haloperidol-induced comatose state with hyperthermia and rigidity in adolescence: two case reports with a literature review. *J. Clin. Psychiatry* 40:102-103.

Hollister, L.E. (1981). Monitoring plasma concentrations of psychotherapeutic drugs. *Trends Pharmacol. Sci.* 2:89-92.

Hollister, L.E. Sedatives in the management of psychiatric emergencies. This volume.

Jenkins, A.L., Van de Leuv, J.H. (1978). *Emergency Department Organization and Management.* C.V. Mosby, St. Louis, Missouri.

Kirkpatrick, B., Burnett, G.B. (1982). Observation on neuroleptic use in acutely psychotic patients. *J. Clin. Psychopharmacology* 2:205-207.

Krass, M.E. (1977). Non-urgent use of hospital emergency department. *Ont. Med. Rev.* 44:181-184.

Lowy, F.H. (1971). Lessons from emergencies. *Can. Psychiatr. Assoc. J.* 16:103-104.

Magliozzi, J.R., Hollister, L.E., Arnold, K., Earle, G.M. (1981). Relationship of serum haloperidol levels to clinical response in schizophrenic patients. *Am. J. Psychiatry* 138:365-367.

Modestin, J., Krapf, R., Böker, W. (1981). A fatality during haloperidol treatment: mechanism of sudden death. *Am. J. Psychiatry* 138:1616-1617.

Morselli, P.L., Zarifian, E. (1980). Clinical significance of monitoring plasma levels of psychotropic drugs. In *Drug Concentrations in Neuropsychiatry.* Ciba Foundation Symposium 74. Amsterdam, Excerpta Medica, pp. 115-139.

Neborsky, R., Janowsky, D., Munson, E. Depry, D. (1981). Rapid treatment of acute psychotic symptoms with high- and low-dose haloperidol. *Arch. Gen. Psychiatry* 38:195-199.

Rivera-Calimlin, L., Nasrallah, H., Strauss, J., Lasagna, L. (1976). Clinical response and plasma levels: effects of dose, dosage, schedules and drug interactions on plasma chlorpromazine levels. *Am. J. Psychiatry* 6:646-652.

Sakalis, G., Traficante, L. (1981). Fluphenazine. In *Psychotropic Drugs Plasma Concentration and Clinical Response.* Edited by Burrows, G., Norman, T., New York, Dekker Publishing, pp. 287-301.

Satloff, A., Worby, C.M. (1970). The psychiatry emergency services: mirror of change. *Am. J. Psychiatry* 126:1628-1632.

Schwartz, D.A., Weiss, A.T., Miner, J.M. (1972). Community psychiatry and emergency service. *Am. J. Psychiatry* 129:710-715.

Tune, L.E., Creese, I., DePaulo, J.R., Slarney, P.R., Snyder, S.H. (1981). Neuroleptic serum levels measured by radioreceptor assay and clinical response in schizophrenic patients. *J. Nerv. Ment. Dis.* 169:60-63.

Tupin, J.P. Rapid neuroleptization: origins and future developments. This volume.

Voineskos, G. (1981). Psychiatric training in the emergency service: the need for change. *Univ. Tor. Med. J.* 58:36-39.

Weinberger, D.R., Kelley, M.J. (1977). Catatonia and malignant syndrome: a possible complication of neuroleptic administration. *J. Nerv. Ment. Dis.* 165:263-268.

Yesavage, J.A., Becker, J., Wermer, P.D., Mills, M.J., Holman, C.A., Cohn, R. (1982). Serum-level monitoring of thiothixene in schizophrenia: acute single-dose levels at fixed doses. *Am. J. Psychiatry* 139:174-178.

Zarifian, E., Scatton, B., Bianchetti, G., Cuche, H., Loo, H., Morselli, P.L. (1982). High doses of haloperidol in schizophrenia. *Arch. Gen. Psychiatry* 39:212–215.

Zonana, H., Henisz, J.E., Levine, M. (1973). Psychiatric emergency services a decade later. *Psych. Med.* 4:273–290.

24

Rapid Neuroleptization: Origins and Future Developments

JOE P. TUPIN

INTRODUCTION

Rapid neuroleptization has been defined as a "method of administering repeated doses of neuroleptic medication under close clinical supervision that provides rapid control of acute functional psychotic symptoms" (Donlon et al., 1979). In this definition are emphasized the acute nature of mental illness under treatment, the repeated administration over a brief period of time of neuroleptic medication, and the establishment of rapid control under careful supervision. Other elements implied in the definition include proper evaluation and establishment of a diagnosis, specific monitoring procedures, and a recognizable endpoint. A variety of oral and injectable agents have been used.

The term has been used to describe both short-term use for initial control to augmentation of an ongoing program during a period of agitation, restlessness, combativeness, or increased psychotic symptoms, as well as used over several days in increasing amounts to reach high-dose oral regimens which may continue for an indefinite time. This paper will review the history and differentiate these two applications of repeat dose of neuroleptics and establish guidelines for appropriate use.

ORIGINS AND TRENDS

The concept originated in the mid-1950s (Kinross-Wright, 1955) and was subsequently often associated with Community Mental Health programs gaining popularity in the 1970s (Polak and Laycob, 1971). Refinements and studies have continued to the present. General agreement has been achieved that inject-able, high potency neuroleptics are the drugs of choice (Mason et al., 1980) because of their safety and effectiveness.

In 1955, John Kenross Wright reported the use of large doses of chlorpro-mazine for the treatment of schizophrenia. He reported the use of rapid increas-ing oral doses with remission of symptoms within a week or two and subsequent dose reduction to maintenance levels. In the early 1960s there was another report on the use of "loading doses" as a way of initiating treatment (Mountain, 1963). That author observed that intramuscular administration could be used if the patient were uncooperative. The Fort Logan Mental Health Center Staff reported on three years experience with "rapid tranquilization". This technique used both oral and intramuscular forms depending upon the patient's coopera-tion. Generally, oral chlorpromazine was used in extremely high doses (2,400 mg achieved by 48 hours with rapid dose reduction following).

Systematic comparison studies using appropriate research design began to appear by the late 60's often comparing high potency antipsychotics with chlor-promazine. These studies focused on the comparative effectiveness and safety of the two medication types as well as on establishing a pattern or program of use (Brauser and Goldstein, 1968; Feldman et al., 1969). Supplemental medications, often barbiturates (Nilson, 1969), were used in the early studies. Medications studied were trifluoperazine, mesoridazine, (Brauser and Goldstein, 1970), per-phenazine, (Fitsgerald, 1969), thiothixene, (Levenson et al., 1976), fluphenazine HCl (Anderson et al., 1976), and haloperidol (Man and Chen, 1973).

Chlorpromazine was noted to produce a higher incidence of hypotension, local irritation at the site of injection and sedation (Klein and Davis, 1964). Thus, by the early 1970s the advantages of the high potency drugs over the low potency drugs was emerging. The high potency drugs produced less hypotension and sedation and local irritation but more extrapyramidal effects, particularly dystonia. By the mid 70's a pattern of usage emphasizing parenteral administra-tion for 1-3 days followed by high dose oral programs reduced to lower mainte-nance levels after acute symptoms remitted. Technical questions were being raised about the relationship of parenteral dosage and subsequent oral doses, fre-quency of administration of the parenteral (every ? hours, three times a day, etc.) and other details.

It was during this time that the long-acting antipsychotics were tried. Chien and Cole (1973) and Corbett (1975) advocated such drugs as fluphenazine deconate using 12.5 mg – 75 mg weekly, for noncompliant, chronic patients in an ambulatory setting.

MANAGEMENT ISSUES

Although the advantages were noted of rapid control of severe psychosis, shortened hospital stay, relief of suffering, etc., cautionary notes were sounded about excessive sedation and severe dystonias and of crucial significance laryngeal and pharyngeal spasms with breathing difficulties (Flaherty and Lahmeyer, 1978). Sudden death was reported (Modestin et al., 1981). Some authors (Klein, 1975) advocated an initial drug free period for purposes of diagnostic evaluation. However, on the other side, Anderson and Kuehnle (1976) suggested that acute psychosis was much like emergency surgery and should be dealt with promptly and with the same level of intensive supervision required in surgery. The latter point bears emphasis. The risk of untoward effects, drug interactions and medical misadventures or interactions with pre-existing physical disease are all real problems. When one embarks on rapid neuroleptization it must be in a setting with close medical supervision and staff trained for the management of hypotension, acute dystonias, and other serious side effects.

All authors have emphasized the need for accurate diagnosis and evaluation of neurologic status as soon as possible and before administration of drug, if possible. Attention should be given to the potential for the psychosis arising from illegal drugs, particularly hallucinogens. Perhaps the most serious diagnostic risk in addition to those already noted is the fact that once embarked on this treatment, critical resassessment of diagnosis may be ignored because of rapid symptom reduction and the *assumption* of schizophrenic psychosis which may or may not be true.

Mason et al. (1980), Ayd (1980) and Donlon et al. (1979) have recently reviewed rapid neuroleptization and a number of general principals result: Many of the early studies were open, non-blind and few had appropriate controls. Nebrosky et al. (1981) recently conducted a carefully controlled study. Patients were treated either on low-dose or high-dose regimen of haloperidol in a 3-phase protocol. During Phase I the patient received on an hourly basis, up to 4-hours, IM haloperidol, either 2 or 10 mg. These hourly injections continued up to 4 times or until it was judged that the patient could comply with an oral regimen. Phase II consisted of hourly doses of oral haloperidol, either 2 or 10 mg until the identified target symptoms were considered to have decreased clinically to a satisfactory degree. Phase III was a continuation of oral regimen for "maintenance." These researchers concluded that there was no difference between the two groups. There was good response in both groups, however the high dose group in Phase I tended to be better at one hour. This and other research suggests that after the first few hours there may be little difference for many patients in any reactive "loading" regimen. Individualized doses and change of medication is important. While some patients respond to high doses, elapsed time on drugs is also an important variable. High or rapidly increasing oral doses do not seem uniformly an advantage. General conclusions, derived from all studies, seem to be substantially positive.

PHASE I – PARENTERAL USE

1. Focal control of severe psychotic symptoms may be achieved by re-peated parenteral administration of high potency neuroleptics using 2-10 mg of haloperidol or similar doses of other high potency drugs. Two to four injections at hourly intervals are usually adequate. Low potency drugs are not recom-mended because of hypotension and local irritation. Dose and drug choice should be based on previous response, plans for future treatment, experience of the physician, setting (hospital or clinic), and experience and training of the nursing staff. All have a high potency per cc and have minimal life-threatening side effects with acute laryngeal dystonia and the malignant neuroleptic syn-drome being the most serious problem during the initiation of treatment. Donlon et al. (1978) studied the EKG and blood pressure effects by using parenteral hyloperidol and found it was safe in amounts from 10-40 mg/6 hours.

2. Administration should be repeated at intervals of one hour up to a maximum dose of 100 mg in 24 hours of haloperidol or the equivalent of other high potency drugs. High potency drugs are preferred by most authorities. Halo-peridol has probably been the most studied and used by fluphenazine HCl, thio-thixene, perphenazine, and trifluoperazine have been studied and found effec-tive. However, research by Donlon et al. (1978, 1980) Naborsky et al. (1981), and Wijsendek et al. (1974) finds regular doses of high potency neuroleptics administered orally or parenterally as effective as high doses after several days. Repeated parenteral doses are effective and 5 mg of haloperidol is superior to 2 mg in the first few hours. Daily increasing oral doses do not seem to exhibit an advantage over a fixed daily dose after the first four or seven days (Donlon et al., 1978; Donlon et al., 1980). Thus, neither oral or parenteral rapidly escalating daily doses hold advantage for the patient. Moderate, repeated, parenteral administration appears useful for short-term, acute control to reduce dangerous behaviors but not as a method of achieving high dose continuing treatment. Exceptionally high doses given orally may benefit a few non-responding indi-viduals but are not routinely helpful in speeding remission (Donlon, 1976). High doses have been associated with clinical deterioration (Van Putten et al., 1974) in a few patients using both oral and IM administration.

3. Long-acting drugs are not recommended for multiple doses over a short time and the slowness with which initial appropriate blood levels are achieved.

4. Administration is best done in the hospital in a very carefully super-vised setting so that side effects can be assessed, diagnosis continuously evalu-ated, neurological status reviewed, and dose amount and route continuously reviewed.

Careful medical monitoring including repeated diagnostic assessment, toxi-cology screens as indicated, and observation for extrapyramidal side effects should be mandatory. Availability of PRN order of anti-Parkinson agent should be written and nursing staff instructed on medications so that serious dystonias, particularly laryngeal, can be treated rapidly.

PHASE II – ORAL CONTINUING USE

1.   Generally the oral medication will be equal to or as much as twice the amount administered in the preceeding 24 hours parenterally. This may be begun 6-12 hours after the last intramuscular dose. Naborsky et al. (1981) uses two oral phases – the first continuing a "loading" concept, the second a regular daily dose.

2.   Parenteral medication should be stopped as soon as the patient is sleeping well, sedated, or cooperative enough that oral medication can be instituted. Occasionally, after oral medication is begun, supplemental parenteral medication may be needed for the first 24-48 hours.

3.   Prophylactic antiparkinson agents are used by some clinicians (Anderson and Kuehnle, 1980), others wait for the emergence of symptoms (Ayd, 1980).

4.   Plasma measures are not yet established for routine use in either initial or continuing neuroleptic treatment.

5.   Individualized dose is the most essential principal in *all* phases of treatment. Non-response or partial response is only a call for evaluation of not increased dosage; some patients get worse on high doses which may account for "non-response."

In conclusion, the studies both open and double-blind, support the fact that the high potency neuroleptics (fluphenazine HcL, thiothixene, and haloperidol) are effective as a method of focal control of specific symptoms or for the initiation of continuing treatment of functional psychosis given intramuscularly in repeated doses. Surprisingly low doses can be effective.

SIDE EFFECTS AND DISADVANTAGES

Given that repeated administration of neuroleptics is effective and the general safety is clear, additional comments need to be made about safety and side effects. Altough usual side effects of sedation, hypotension and extrapyramidal problems have been adequately discussed in the literature, the focus should be shifted to some remaining serious issues. Questions have been raised as to whether or not this procedure may reduce the risk of tardive dyskinesia because of the highly controlled and ultimately quicker establishment of clinical improvement, thus reducing the patient's exposure to medication – rather than a longer initiation of treatment using low or inadequate dosage.

Unusual side effects that may be more common with this technique include behavioral toxicity, malignant neuroleptic syndrome, and drug induced catatonia. All of these are rare but extremely important side effects. Behavioral toxicity is typified by a drug induced or aggregated psychosis with dysphoria and worsening mental status. They may resemble the original symptoms, but they may be a consequence of anticholinergic effects of the drugs or an unusual extrapyramidal side effect with akathisia. Irrespective of the origin, the dose must be reduced. When symptoms increase (or fail to remit) with increasing dose, the clinician should consider this possibility.

Malignant neuroleptic syndrome which consists of rigidity, fever, hypertension, tachycardia and dyskinesia may lead to death. Although I know of no reports suggesting that rapid neuroleptization is more likely to lead to this unfortunate side effect, one must acknowledge that rapidly increasing doses over a short period of time might increase the likelihood of it happening.

Catatonia as a side effect may be mistaken for worsening of the clinical picture (Gelenberg and Mandel, 1977) and should be recognized so that medication can be interrupted. Treatment of the catatonia may require a second neuroleptic and/or administration of the dopamine agonist, amantidine.

Dystonias are often observed in the initial treatment period, and since this can occasionally effect the upper airway and pharynx leading to obstruction and respiratory distress, great care must be exercised in watching for this serious side effect. Some authors (Anderson) recommend prophylactic use of Benztropine, 1 or 2 mg bid, while others will use medications at the time of the onset of extrapyramidal symptoms. There are advantages and disadvantages to both procedures. However, if the latter model is to be followed, then the cause of the seriousness of the upper airway obstruction, a PRN order should be left for parenteral antiparkinson drugs. Disadvantages: 1) Dx blurring, 2) disinterest in total care and aftercare, 3) excess drug, 4) accelerating dose.

MANAGEMENT PROCEDURE

Ayd has reviewed the indications and the techniques and emphasizes the importance of initial diagnosis and the importance of excluding patients with organic brain disease. Generally the candidates include the following: schizophrenics, manics, psychosis characterized by agitation, aggressiveness and combative behavior, which may arise from certain drugs (amphetamines or LSD), psychotic depression and in some situations, delirium and organic brain syndrome.

Doages based on body size — but it would appear that low doses, 2-5 mg of haloperidol or its equivalent of fluphenizine, trifluoperazine, or thiothixene, is suitable for most patients. This may be repeated within 30 to 60 minutes.

However, longer intervals are appropriate and sometimes desirable. The clinician must be clear about the end-point and again, not use it as a continuing method of routine treatment, but rather to achieve a specific goal, i.e., compliance with oral medication, control of agitation, reduction of aggressiveness, etc.

Sixty to 100 mg of haloperidol or its equivalent of other acceptable high-potency drugs, may be given in the initial 24-hour period. Should such an initial regimen not be effective, then selection of a second high-potency drug would seem to be indicated.

Lastly, the clinician must be aware that any procedure, if done automatically and without individualization, is more likely to cause serious side effects than the careful individualization of dosage. The more recent studies emphasize that low doses may be quite effective in establishing initial control and in the initial phases of treatment. Thus, high dose, or megadoses, seems to be less and less justified than previously considered.

One must remember the substantial potency of the newer and high potency drugs. Often, doses under 20 mg per day of oral medication would be adequate for the majority of patients and will avoid or minimize extrapyramidal side effects. I am increasingly concerned that uncritical application of rapid neuroleptization techniques in ths hospital may lead to continuing oral high doses. The high doses are continued in the outpatient setting where they are doubly inappropriate and where side effects then develop and patient compliance suffers. High-potency drugs are relatively free of side effects when dosage is properly titrated. Studies suggest that fluphenazine, trifluoperazine, haloperidol and thiothixene, may all have a potency such that 2–5 mg of these drugs is equivalent to 100 mg of chlorpromazine.

DISCUSSION

One is tempted to speculate on how rapid neuroleptization developed. As I have already noted, it came about and was originally described and studied primarily in community based active treatment programs. A number of reasons have been given for its development. Those include alleviation of patient distress, protection of patients and others from potential hazards of unrestrained psychotic behavior, and averting hospitalization or making the duration of hospitalization as brief as possible. All of these reasons are laudable and promote the early return of the patient to the community. Other reasons, particularly in some of the community programs, have included the pressure for short hospitalization so that small number of beds can service a large population. Short staffing, occasionally with inexperienced or poorly trained individuals, has probably also contributed to the introduction of these techniques. Some of these clearly reflect problems with funding, space, and the availability of trained clinicians willing to work in settings where the seriously psychotic are seen. These pressures, along with the success of rapid neuroleptization, may lead to early discharge before the patient has achieved optimal remission and the maintenance programs in poorly supervised settings, may have little chance of success. This is part of the "revolving door." We should not underestimate the advantages of proper use of this technique for focal application of repeated doses of high potency neuroleptics can be extremely effective and desirable as a way of controlling emergent symptoms or initiating ongoing treatment when carefully titrated to patient's need and the avoidance of "routine" techniques that may only serve to oversedate and over-treat patients and expose them to the risk of increased side effects.

The future in this area seems to be clearly emerging — that rapid neuroleptization will continue to be a valuable technique. Although the techniques seem both effective and generally safe, the clinician is warned to use it with a clear understanding of the procedure, the potential side effects and to grasp clearly the difference between focal neuroleptization and high dose medication, for a specific endpoint. It is not a method of establishing high-dose maintenance medication without attention to the individual patient. Furthermore, low-potency drugs and long acting injectables should not be used for these purposes. The term rapid neuroleptization should be retired since it may too often encourage inappropriate routine use of large doses of high potency drugs continued into the outpatient setting. Focal use of short-term goals then followed by usual doses is advised for most patients. Individualized doses following application of the refined concept of *focal* neuroleptization is a better, safer and more scientifically valid technique.

REFERENCES

Anderson, W.H. and Kuehnle, J.C. (1974). Strategies for the treatment of acute schizophrenics. *J.A.M.A.* 229:1884–1889.

Anderson, W.H. and Kuehnle, J.C. (1980). Treatment of psychosis by rapid neuroleptization: Update 1980. Chapter 3. In (Ed.), AYD, F.J., Jr. *Haloperidol Update: 1958-1980.* AYD Medical Communications, 1980.

Anderson, W.H., Kuehnle, J.C. and Catanzano, D.M. (1976). Rapid treatment of acute psychosis. *Am. J. Psychiatry* 133:1076–1078.

Ayd, F.J., Jr. (1980). Guidelines for using intramuscular haloperidol for rapid neuroleptization. Chapter 5. *Haloperidol Update: 1958-1980.* (Ed.) AYD, F.J., Jr. (1980).

Brauzer, B. and Goldstein, B.J. (1968). Imperative effects of intra-muscular thiothixene and trifluoperazine in psychotic patients. *J. Clin. Pharmacol.* 8: 400–403.

Brauzer, B. and Goldstein, B.J. (1970). The differential response to parenteral chlorpromazine and mesoridazine in psychotic patients. *J. Clin. Pharmacol.* 10:126–131.

Chien, C.P. and Cole, J.O. (1973). Depot phenophiazine treatment in acute psychosis: A sequential comparative clinical study. *Am. J. Psychiatry* 130: 13–17.

Corbett, L. (1975). Techniques of fluphenazine decanoate therapy in acute schizophrenic illnesses. *Dis. Nerv. Syst.* 36:573–575.

Donlon, P.T. (1976). High dosage neuroleptic therapy: A review. *Int. Pharm. Psychiatry* 11:235–245.

Donlon, P.T., Hopkin, J. and Tupin, J.P. (1979). Overview: Efficacy and safety of the rapid neuroleptization method with injectable haloperidol. *Am. J. Psychiatry* 136(3):273–278.

Donlon, P.T., Hopkin, J., Schaffer, C.B. and Amsterdam, E. (1979). Cardiovascular safety of rapid treatment with intra-muscular haloperidol. *Am. J. Psychiatry* 136:233–234.

Donlon, P.T., Hopkin, J., Tupin, J.P., Wicks, J.J., Wahba, M. and Meadow, A. (1980). Haloperidol for acute schizophrenic patients: An evaluation of three oral regimens. *Arch. Gen. Psychiatry* 37:691–695.

Donlon, P.T., Meadow, A., Tupin, J.P. and Wahba, M. (1978). High versus standard dosage fluphenazine HCl in acute schizophrenia. 39:800–804.

Feldman, P., Bay, A.P., Baser, A.N., Bhasker, K.N. and Kennedy, L.L. (1969). Parenteral haloperidol in controlling patient behavior during acute psychotic episodes. *Curr. Ther. Res.* 11:362–366.

Fitzgerald, C.H. (1969). A double-blind comparison of haloperidol with perphenazine in acute psychotic episodes. *Curr. Ther. Res.* 11:515–516.

Flaherty, J.A. and Lahmeyer, H.W. (1978). Laryngeal-pharyngeal dystonia as a possible cause of asphyxia with haloperidol treatment. *Am. J. Psychiatry* 135:1414–1415.

Gelenberg, A.J. and Mandel, M.R. (1977). Catatonic reactions to high-potency neuroleptic drugs. *Arch. Gen. Psychiatry* 34:947–950.

Kinross-Wright, J. (1955). The intensive chlorpromazine treatment of schizophrenia. *Psychiat. Res. Rep.* 1(53–62).

Klein, D.F. (1975). Who should not be treated with neuroleptics but often are. In: AYD, F.J., Jr. (Ed.). *Rational Psychopharmaco Therapy and the right to refuse treatment.* Baltimore Aid in Medical Communications, Ltd.

Klein, D.F. and Davis, J.M. (1964). *Diagnosis and Drug Treatment of Psychiatric Disorders.* Baltimore, Williams & Wilkins.

Levenson, A.J., Burnett, G.B., Nottingham, J.B., Sermas, C.E. and Thornby, J.I. (1976). Speed and rate of remission of acute schisophrenia: A comparison of the intra-muscularly administered through fluphenazine HCl with thiothixene haloperidol. *Curr. Ther. Res.* 20:695–700.

Man, P.L. and Chen, C.H. (1973). Rapid tranquilization of acutely psychotic patients with intra-muscular haloperidol and chlorpromazine. *Psychosomatics* 14:59–63.

Mason, A., Aaron, S. and Granacher, R.P. (1980). *Clinical Handbook of Antipsychotic Drug Therapy.* Chapter 3, pg. 109–141.

Modestin, J., Krapf, R. and Böker, W. (1981). A fatality during haloperidol treatment: Mechanism of sudden death. *Am. J. Psychiatry* 138:12–13.

Mountain, H.E. (1963). Crash tranquilization in a milieu therapy setting. *J. Fort Logan Mental Health Center* 11:42–44.

Naborsky, R., Janowsky, D., Munson, D. and Deprey, D. (1981). Rapid treatment of acute psychotic symptoms with high- and low-dose haloperidol. *Arch. Gen. Psychiatry* 38:195–199.

Nilson, J.A. (1969). Immediate treatment expedites hospital release. *Hosp. Com. Psychiatry* 20:36-38.
Polak, P. and Laycob, L. (1971). Rapid tranquilization. *Am. J. Psychiatry* 118: 300-307.
Van Putten, T., Mutalipiassia, L.R. and Malkin, M.D. (1974). Phenothiazine-induced decompensation. 3:102-105.
Wijsendek, H., Steiner, M. and Goldberg, S.C. (1974). Trifluoperazine: A comparison between regular and high doses. *Psychopharmacologia* 36:147-150.

25

Sedatives in the Management of Psychiatric Emergencies

Leo E. Hollister

For purposes of discussion, the term "sedative" will be used, not in the strict pharmacologic sense, but to denote any drug that may be used to calm patients. The term "emergency" will be used to denote any situation in which a person may require immediate psychiatric intervention regardless of the locale.

PRESENTATION OF PATIENTS

No two patients present with exactly the same problems, but common patterns can be discerned. Almost always the patient is brought to the attention of medical facilities by other persons: the police, family members, friends or strangers. Seldom do patients themselves seek help. Indeed, the precipitating factor is often not so much the absolute degree of emotional disorder as its social, economic or legal consequences.

Aggressive or excited behavior is a common presentation. Patients may have become threatening to their spouses, children, other family members or neighbors. Or they may disturb the peace, by excited responses to hallucinations or persecutory delusions. Such behavior is likely to come to the attention of the police, who may be called because the patient is brandishing a weapon or making threatening remarks or gestures.

Acute anxiety or panic occurs when patients are suddenly overwhelmed with anxiety or panic to the extent that they can no longer function, but are "frozen". They may show abnormal behavior in trying to deal with the panic, such as locking themselves in a room or climbing to the rooftop. Panic attacks are often associated with known phobias, but some occur without any known precipitant.

Strange or inappropriate behavior calls attention to itself. When it becomes intolerable to those about, the patient may be brought to psychiatric attention. We have all seen people on the street who talk loudly and disjointedly to an unseen audience. They are often ignored, but if the behavior becomes bothersome, the police may be called. The "bag ladies" of major cities show another sort of relatively harmless behavior that is more a manifestation of society's neglect of their problem than anything else.

A suicidal attempt that has been foiled is usually secondary to an acute episode of depresson. When suicide has not been attempted, the prevailing anxiety or agitation may mask the seriousness of the underlying depression. Depressive episodes, whether they be part of endogenous depression or manic-depressive disorder, often begin abruptly. The apparent need for emergency care is largely determined by the reaction of others to the patient's mood or behavior.

States of abnormal consciousness, such as stupor, or impaired memory, such as amnesia, clearly disrupt the patient's ability to function normally. The ability of the patient to continue to function seems to be the critical determinant in determining the perceived need for medical attention for many of these conditions we have been discussing.

Various complications of drug use, such as drug-induced abnormal behavior or drug withdrawal syndromes, create psychiatric emergencies. Hysterical manifestations, especially amnesia, seem to be less frequent than formerly but still occur.

The common characteristics of the psychiatric emergency are that people other than the patient are almost always involved and that the presentation occurs when other support systems have proven not to be adequate.

INITIAL MANAGEMENT

As with medical and surgical emergencies, diagnosis and treatment must often proceed simultaneously (Bridges, 1971). One should try as quickly as possible to assess the problem at hand and to decide what needs to be done immediately and what can best be deferred. Any immediate action that may be required should be done, such as the use of drugs, physical restraint, or suicidal precautions. Physical and laboratory evaluations, as well as the collection of additional historical data from as many sources as can be mustered, should follow. Finally, when one has established a working diagnosis, emergency treatment can be initiated and long-term management planned.

When planning on the use of drugs, one must realize that one will alter the natural course of the disorder to the extent that further clinical diagnostic evaluation may be impaired. On the other hand, one must assure that the patient will not be able to harm himself or others. Although the use of drugs in emergency conditions is not so controversial, one would be well advised to document fully in the record why various agents were used. The assent of the patient's relatives who may be available would also be desirable.

SPECIFIC PROBLEMS

The Excited Schizophrenic

An episode of schizophrenia-like psychosis in a patient not previously diagnosed may represent the initial stages of a chronic, debilitating life-long infirmity, or may be a transient psychosis in someone vulnerable to schizophrenic decompensation under severe life stresses. In any case, the initial treatment of the episode is the same. Antipsychotic drug treatment is well founded in acute schizophrenia even though some patients may improve spontaneously (Casey et al., 1960; National Institute of Mental Health-Psychopharmacology Service Center, 1964). Good premorbid function, acute onset of the disturbance, and strong social support may indicate the "reactive" or "good prognosis" form of schizophrenia. Subsequent clinical course is the best measure of the situation, however.

A rapid treatment course might be initiated with oral or parenteral doses of 5 to 10 mg of haloperidol or thiothixene repeated at intervals of one to two hours until adequate symptomatic control is achieved. When the parenteral drug is used the subsequent daily dose of the less bioavailable oral form may have to be somewhat higher, but usually it remains the same as the parenteral dose. There is very little evidence to suggest that the parenteral route produces more satisfactory or expeditious outcomes than the oral. The only unequivocal advantage of parenteral dosage lies in the fact that acutely psychotic patients may not take oral drugs reliably, and, with injection, the treating physician can be sure the drug enters the body. Although daily doses of 80 mg or more seem to achieve the desired aims, further experience by the original proponents of high dosage has led to the conclusion that 80 mg of fluphenazine a day is no better than the standard 20 mg since both produce equivalent benefits and adverse effects (Donlon and Tupin, 1974; Donlon et al., 1978).

Some patients do not calm down, even with very large doses of neuroleptics. As the main concern is to reduce disturbed or aggressive behavior, judicious use of conventional sedatives may be required. An intramuscular dose of 130 mg of sodium phenobaribital often calms a patient still not tranquilized by neuroleptics. Oral doses of 10 mg of diazepam, if the patient will accept oral medication, can be given every hour until the patient is calm. The management of the severely disturbed psychotic is still a difficult and not completely solved problem. In older times, one might have used electroconvulsive therapy, but recourse to this modality of treatment is rare today. Experience with carbamazepine or propanolol in this situation is limited.

The Excited Manic

Manic psychoses may be difficult to distinguish from those of acute schizophrenia. Many are lumped in the emergency treatment of acutely agitated states with vague diagnoses. Although lithium carbonate is the preferred treatment for milder exacerbations of mania, it is inappropriate as the sole treatment of severely manic patients because of its slow onset of action (Prien et al., 1972).

Today, clinicians prefer to use a high-potency antipsychotic, despite the reputation of chlorpromazine for having greater sedative effects. The reported interaction between haloperidol and lithium, with severe neurologic sequelae, does not seem to have much substance (Baastrup et al., 1976). Nevertheless, the combined action of lithium and antipsychotics may produce more severe extrapyramidal syndromes than those associated with antipsychotics alone. Since lithium treatment should be started simultaneously with antipsychotics, the choice of drug is a matter of some concern. With careful monitoring, however, any of the high-potency drugs may be used in the same pattern as outlined for schizophrenia.

Excitements of Uncertain Cause

In many clinical situations, the exact cause for an excited psychosis is not known. Treatment must be given as an emergency measure. One study of the use of haloperidol and chlorpromazine in 58 such patients found the former to be preferable, 15 of 30 patients who received a single 5 mg injection of haloperidol were controlled and another 8 patients were improved. Results with injections of 50 mg of chlorpromazine were however less satisfactory (Gerstenzang and Krulisky, 1977).

Differences between high potency drugs are small, if indeed they exist. In a controlled comparison between haloperidol and thiothixene in 30 patients with acute psychosis, using doses of from 4 to 32 mg, findings were equally satisfactory with both drugs (Stotsky, 1977). Although the small sample — only 15 patients in each group — might have failed to detect a subtle but real difference, the results are credible in the light of clinical experience with such drugs.

Considering the many adverse reactions that are unique to chlorpromazine, some of us have argued that it is now obsolete. Thioridazine is not amenable to emergency use, both because a parenteral form is not available and because the total daily dose must be limited to 800 mg. Thus, the field has been pretty well narrowed down to the high-potency agents.

Agitated, Suicidal Depressions

Many manifestations of agitated depressions are similar to those of the schizophrenic excitements. Some years ago, a rash of reports of suicidal behavior following the use of depot fluphenazine appeared. It was a mystery why they should have been caused by a simple change in dosage form, when for years before no such association had been made with the drug. The solution became evident when the pattern of use of this preparation became known. Emergency clinics were using the depot form for the treatment of almost every excited patient, without bothering to establish a diagnosis. Clearly, some of these patients were depressed and the use of the antipsychotic drug was inappropriate. Without effective treatment, many of the patients, who had not been hospitalized in the zeal to avoid hospitalization, later committed suicide.

A place exists for the use of neuroleptics in these patients, but the patient should also be placed on treatment with tricyclic antidepressants. If hospitalization is warranted, doses of imipramine or amitriptyline of 150 mg/day should be given immediately rather than the usual incremental dosing pattern. Such immediate intensive treatment with oral doses of drug may result in the rapid recovery that has been reported from parenteral use of tricyclics (Beaumont, 1973). The augmented sedative effects of such doses may also suffice to curb the excited behavior, without use of neuroleptics. Such treatment should only be attempted in patients whose physical health is good and who can be hospitalized for several days.

Not all patients who make a suicidal attempt need to be hospitalized for psychiatric observation. If the degree of depression is not severe, and the attempt seems to have lacked conviction, such patients may be entrusted to the care of a responsible relative or friend. One might then resort to the more traditional method of initiating treatment with tricyclic antidepressants, starting with oral doses ranging from 25 to 75 mg/day and increasing gradually until a level of 150 mg/day is attained.

The Panicked Patient

Patients with true panic attacks often respond better to tricyclic antidepressants than to benzodiazepines (Klein et al., 1980). The latter drugs may be effective for alleviating the anticipatory anxiety associated with panic attacks but are often inadequate, when used alone, for allaying the acute attack. Tricyclic antidepressants are the drugs of choice for treating this situation. If, however, the panic attack is associated with a known phobia, the simplest immediate management is reassurance and removal from the negative stimulus. A combination of 10 mg of diazepam and 25 mg of amitriptyline one to three times daily may be required to treat the acute attack, with the tricyclic being continued in the usual incremental pattern until 150 to 300 mg/day is reached, depending on the control of recurrent attacks. Experience with alprazolam, a triazol benzodiazepine, in treating panic attacks has been limited.

The Hysteric Patient

Hysteria seems to be decreasing, presumably due to increasing sophistication of patients. Amnesic disorders are more common than the motor or sensory manifestations of the past. As hysteria may represent an escape from some threat, one should not be too eager for a rapid resolution. One should allow time for the patient to resolve the conflict.

A sedative dose of a benzodiazepine, say 10 to 20 mg of diazepam, may allow the patient to "sleep it off". If the manifestation is refractory to simple measures such as this and to passage of time, one may wish to conduct an interview under sedation, using either intravenous thiopental sodium or diazepam. The doses should be only enough to make the patient relaxed, not anesthetic. Resuscitation should be available if needed.

The Confused Elderly Patient

Patients with senile brain disease (Alzheimer's disease) run a variable course. For reasons that are not always clear, these patients occasionally become acutely disturbed. This may be associated with some major life change, such as moving, or with an illness or operation. One must be especially alert to physical causes of agitation, such as pain, e.g., when a previously quiet, demented patient becomes agitated, when paranoid delusions and visual or auditory hallucinations become evident, or when behavior is bizarre and sleep-wake cycles are profoundly disturbed.

Antipsychotic drugs do not remedy the specific illness but may be useful for symptom control, which is usually necessary since these patients are disruptive.

Thioridazine, which is highly sedative but has little tendency to evoke extrapyramidal reactions, has been the favored drug for treating these patients. This drug has at least three disadvantages: strong adrenergic blocking effects that can lead to postural hypotension; strong anticholinergic effects that might aggravate the mental disorder; and possible cardiotoxicity. Recent studies have shown that high-potency neuroleptics, such as fluphenazine, haloperidol, and thiothixene, are equally effective and well tolerated (Branchey et al., 1978). Most patients will respond to relatively low doses, which should always be used initially; a few will ultimately require fairly high doses before full symptomatic control is reached.

One drug combination used successfully to control "wild wanderers" is haloperidol, 3 mg, combined with lorazepam, 1 mg, three times daily. Antiparkinson drugs are added as needed. Control is rapid and any extrapyramidal syndromes are rapidly reversible (Fine and Walker, 1977). For long-term maintenance treatment, it may be advisable to try a depot preparation such as fluphenazine decanoate. Doses of 12.5 mg IM every two weeks have been reported to be safe and effective (Green, 1977).

The Drugged Patient

Alcohol The social drug most likely to be associated with emotional disturbance is alcohol, because of its widespread use. Some patients may become aggressive and abusive when acutely intoxicated, whereas others may have this response to relatively small amounts of alcohol; a form of pathological intoxication. Sedation is desirable but conventional sedative-hypnotics are usually not very effective — patients may be as tolerant of these drugs as they have become to alcohol. Further, the respiratory depressant effects of these drugs and alcohol, to which tolerance does not develop, may be additive.

When such patients require sedation, a parenteral dose of a high-potency antipsychotic is generally effective — haloperidol, 5 mg IM, every 30 to 60 minutes until control is achieved. Usually no further treatment is needed once the effects of alcohol have passed.

The most common form of alcohol withdrawal syndrome is delirium tremens (DT). A patient with the full-blown syndrome does not seem to respond specifically to any drug treatment, but in those with incipient DT the conventional sedative-hypnotic drugs often stop its progression. Diazepam, given repeatedly in intravenous boluses of 10 mg followed by 5 mg every five minutes, can be titrated to produce the exact level of sedation desired. Once that level has been attained, the patient can be maintained with oral doses of this drug or some other (Thompson et al., 1975). Milder cases of alcohol withdrawal may be treated with oral doses of sedative-hypnotics. During withdrawal from alcohol, some patients retain a clear sensorium but have marked hallucinations, the so-called alcoholic hallucinosis. Many authorities believe that this occurs in patients vulnerable to schizophrenia who become psychotic under the stress of alcohol withdrawal or heavy drinking. Treatment with conventional sedative-hypnotic drugs is not highly effective. Good responses are obtained with high-potency neuroleptics, however. The treatment program might be the same as that for acute alcholic intoxication. Most patients require drug therapy only temporarily.

Stimulants Prolonged use of amphetamines or cocaine may produce a paranoid psychosis that closely resembles paranoid schizophrenia. Usually, simple withdrawal of the drug will remedy the situation. If the psychosis is severe, however, antipsychotic drug treatment is warranted. Haloperidol is preferred over chlorpromazine since it does not interfere with the clearance of amphetamines from the brain.

Hallucinogens Hallucinogens like LSD, mescaline, and psilocybin produce "bad trips" that are best managed by simple sedative-hypnotic drugs, such as an oral dose of 10 to 20 mg of diazepam. When the sedated patient awakens, the effects of the hallucinogen have disappeared. Long-lasting psychoses associated with this class of hallucinogens are uncommon, and the general feeling is that their occurrence probably reflects incipient schizophrenia provoked by the drug. Thus, treatment would be the same as for any other type of schizophrenia.

Phencyclidine (PCP), currently the favored hallucinogen, is much more likely to produce a state closely resembling schizophrenia. Such patients are difficult to control (Burns et al., 1975). Antipsychotic drugs are useful in the acute treatment of these disorders and may have to be maintained if the psychosis does not remit promptly after the effects of PCP have waned.

Continual gastric suction and acidification of the urine with ammonium chloride in doses of 1 to 2 g four times daily, are effective ways to hasten the disappearance of PCP (Domino and Wilson, 1977). The drug is secreted into the stomach from the blood and then reabsorbed through the enteric tract; gastric suction interferes with this gastroenteric recycling. Because PCP is a basic drug that remains ionized in an acid urine and thus is not reabsorbed by the kidney, its excretion is hastened by urine acidification.

CONCLUSIONS

Not all possible psychiatric emergencies have been covered, but those discussed are those most often treated with drugs. As is the case with any treatment involving drugs, each case is individual. One must try to make the most accurate diagnosis and then find the most appropriate drug and dose for that patient. Guidelines are not cookbooks.

REFERENCES

Baastrup, P.C., Hollnagel, P. and Schou, M. (1976). Adverse reactions in treatment with lithium carbonate and haloperidol. *J.A.M.A.* 236:2645-2646.
Beaumont, G. (1973). Oral and intravenous clomipramine in depression. *J. Intern. Med. Res.* 1:361-364.

Branchey, M.H., Lee, J.H., Amin, R. and Simpson, G.M. (1978). High- and low-potency neuroleptics in elderly psychiatric patients. *J.A.M.A.* 239:1860–1862.

Bridges, P.K. (1971). *Psychiatric Emergencies. Diagnosis and Management.* C.C. Thomas, Springfield, Ill., pp. 195.

Burns, R.S., Lerner, S.E., Corrado, R., James, S.H. and Schnoll, S.H. (1975). Phencyclidine – states of acute intoxication and fatalities. *West. J. Med.* 123:345–349.

Casey, J.F., Bennett, I.F., Lindley, C.J., Hollister, L.E., Gordon, M. and Springer, M.N. (1960). Drug therapy in schizophrenia: A controlled study of the relative effectiveness of chlorpromazine, promazine, phenobarbital and placebo. *Arch. Gen. Psychiatry* 2:210–217.

Domino, E.F. and Wilson, A.E. (1977). Effects of urine acidification in plasma and urine phencyclidine levels in overdose. *Clin. Pharmacol. Ther.* 22: 421–424.

Donlon, P.T., Meadow, A., Tupin, J.P. and Wahba, M. (1978). High vs. standard dosage fluphenazine HCl in acute schizophrenia. *J. Clin. Psychiatry* 39: 19–23.

Donlon, P.T. and Tupin, J.P. (1974). Rapid "digitalization" of decompensated schizophrenic patients with antipsychotic agents. *Am. J. Psychiatry* 131: 310–312.

Fine, W. and Walker, D.J. (1977). Management of the elderly agitated demented patient. *Br. Med. J.* 2:580.

Gerstenzang, M.L. and Krulisky, T.V. (1977). Parenteral haloperidol in psychiatric emergencies; double-blind comparison with chlorpromazine. *Dis. Nerv. Syst.* 38:581–583.

Green, M.F. (1977). Depot tranquilizers for disturbed behavior. *Br. Med. J.* 2: 1027.

Klein, D.F., Gittelman, R., Quitkin, F. and Rifkin, A. (1980). *Diagnosis and Drug Treatment of Psychiatric Disorders: Adults and Children,* Second Edition. Williams and Wilkins, Baltimore, pp. 561–565.

National Institute of Mental Health-Psychopharmacology Service Center, Collaborative Study Group. (1964). Phenothiazine treatment in acute schizophrenia. *Arch. Gen. Psychiatry* 10:246.

Prien, R.F., Caffey, E.M. Jr., and Klett, C.J. (1972). Comparison of lithium carbonate and chlorpromazine in the treatment of mania. *Arch. Gen. Psychiatry* 26:146–153.

Stotsky, B.A. (1977). Relative efficacy of parenteral haloperidol and thiothixene for the emergency treatment of acutely excited and agitated patients. *Dis. Nerv. Syst.* 38:967–973.

Thompson, W.L., Johnson, A.D., Maddrey, W.L. and the Osler Medical House-staff. (1975). Diazepam and paraldehyde for treatment of severe delirium tremens. *Ann. Intern. Med.* 82:175–180.

26

Rapid Treatment of Psychosis

William H. Anderson

Although the cause of psychosis may be unknown, there is a generally effective acute treatment for this idiopathic condition. Typically it involves administration of antipsychotic drugs, all of which have in common the characteristic of post-synaptic dopamine blockade. Upon administration of the appropriate dosage of such a drug, hallucinations disappear, delusional activity subsides, thought disorder abates, and affective disturbance becomes normal. This much is generally beyond dispute. The focus of the current debate on these clinical issues concerns the optimal strategy of drug dosage and duration and the methods by which these can be determined.

One view is that this optimal treatment is best approximated by beginning with a relatively small oral dose and gradually increasing it by small oral increments every few days or weeks until satisfactory remission occurs. This may be called the "standard" method. In contrast, others identify a "rapid" method which utilizes only antipsychotic drugs of the high potency type, administered intramuscularly by hourly serial titration to an individually adjusted optimum dose on the first day. The "rapid" treatment method requires the use of high potency antipsychotics because only these have a satisfactory high ratio of antipsychotic to sedative activity. Intramuscular injection is required in order to insure that adequate absorption will occur between hourly doses. Those who tend to use the standard treatment generally believe that no advantage is to be gained by the rapid method, since, they think, the psychosis "itself" takes weeks to resolve, and one only accomplishes sedation by a more rapid method.

In contrast, the advocates of the rapid method believe that there is no fixed time required for resolution of psychotic symptoms, and that the early effects of high potency drugs may be truly antipsychotic and not merely sedative.

Partisans of each side of this debate claim to base their assumptions on observation and clinical experience. This curiosity would appear to illustrate that our "empirical" observations tend to be influenced by the context of the phenomenon under observation and the belief system which we embrace. One problem in resolving the issue is that we have no thoroughly adequate instrument for determining the presence and severity of psychosis. Thus, the "standard" treatment advocates technically may be correct that the psychosis is not completely in remission after one day if rigorous mental status examination can still find traces of it. The "rapid" treatment advocates may be similarly correct in saying that *for practical purposes,* the psychosis is in remission after one day if and when the cardinal features of delusion, hallucination, thought disorder and affect disturbance are greatly improved. This may at bottom be an argument about whether a glass of water is half full or half empty.

CONDITIONS TO BE EXCLUDED

Whichever method is elected, it is first essential to determine that the illness to be treated is a primary idiopathic psychosis and not the result of some identified abnormal physiology of a toxic, metabolic, vascular, or space occupying type. Generally it is sufficient to take a careful history, and perform physical and neurological examination, augmented as necessary with laboratory studies. It is especially important to be sure that the psychotic symptoms are not the result of an acute, life-threatening medical condition such as meningitis, intracranial hemorrhage, anticholinergic poisoning, hypoglycemia or sedative withdrawal (Anderson, 1980).

Having excluded these "organic entities, it is important to recognize that it is not essential to determine at once whether the psychotic entity is better described as schizophrenia or mania. Since this determination depends to a large extent on detailed personal and family history, it is seldom possible to make a confident determination at the outset of treatment. Both illnesses are treated at the outset with antipsychotic drugs. Lithium carbonate is begun after a few days when the history is suggestive of affective illness and the main psychotic features are under control.

WHEN SHOULD RAPID TREATMENT BE CONSIDERED?

The advantage of rapid treatment is that the major behavioral features of psychosis abate quickly even though the "underlying" psychiatric process may persist. This is useful because psychosis is very often painful and dangerous (Anderson and Kuehnle, 1981). The psychic pain is generally obvious except those cases which are most insidious and indolent. It is curious how often compassionate professionals seem to forget this very plain truth. Perhaps it would be more clear if we were to be psychotic ourselves. Would we then wish to have the most rapid relief available, or would we wish to have a period of, say, seven days observation without treatment or other hardly useful delay?

Advocates of standard treatments or observation periods generally do so on the assumption that they may protect the patient from exposure to antipsychotic medication which is excessive in dose or duration. It may be that they forget that rapid treatment in no way implies high dosage, and that such treatment may also be rapidly reduced or stopped.

It is also important to remember that acute psychosis is embarrassing to the patient and his family, expensive in terms of loss of income and cost of eventual treatment, and dangerous in terms of the possibility of acting on the basis of grossly distorted judgment (Anderson and Kuehnle, 1974; Anderson, Kuehnle and Catanzano, 1976).

METHOD OF RAPID TREATMENT

The essential features of rapid treatment are (1) high potency antipsychotic drugs, (2) intramuscular administration, and (3) serial titration of dosage. Investigators disagree concerning the incremental dosage to be used, with 2-10 mg hourly of haloperidol or equivalent being used. There is no concensus among investigators as to an average effective dose. The usual observation is that a wide individual difference is noted; optimal improvement usually occurs after 8 to 30 mg on the first day. The differences in observation may result from different perceptions of endpoint or because of different populations (Donlon, Hopkin and Tupin, 1979; Naborsky, Janowsky, Munson and Depry, 1981).

Following attempt at optimal improvement by intramuscular medications on the first day, it is then necessary to continue treatment with oral medication. Generally the oral dosage on day two is the same as the intramuscular dose on day one. Factors which suggest increased oral dose are resurgence of symptoms and development of agitation or insomnia. Factors which suggest decrease are sedation and extrapyramidal symptoms.

COMPLICATIONS

The most frequent complication will be the development of an acute dystonic reaction. This may be seen in 30 to 50 percent of the cases with usually effective doses. By the prophylactic use of benztropine 1-2 mg b.i.d. from the onset of treatment, the incidence of such reactions may be reduced very markedly (Stern and Anderson, 1979). This prophylaxis need be continued only a matter of two or three weeks in most cases. Dystonia should be thus prevented if possible, since, like psychosis, it is frightening and painful. On occasion actual respiratory compromise may develop. Hence to avoid the complication is desirable. Benztropine in such doses for such a short period seldom provides unacceptable side effects in the usual population of young patients.

CONCLUSION

Rapid treatment of psychosis is a safe, effective, humane, and practical method of therapeutic intervention in a painful, dangerous and common medical disorder.

REFERENCES

Anderson, W.H. (1980). The physical examination in office practice. *Am. J. Psychiatry* 137:1188–1192.

Anderson, W.H. and Kuehnle, J.C. (1981). Diagnosis and early management of acute psychosis. *N. Engl. J. Med.* 305:1128–1130.

Anderson, W.H. and Kuehnle, J.C. (1974). Strategies for the treatment of acute psychosis. *J.A.M.A.* 229:1884–1889.

Anderson, W.H., Kuehnle, J.C., and Catanzano, D.M. (1976). Rapid treatment of acute psychosis. *Am. J. Psychiatry* 133:1076–1078.

Donlon, P.T., Hopkin, J. and Tupin, J.P. (1979). Overview: Efficacy and safety of rapid neuroleptization method with injectable haloperidol: behavioral considerations. *Am. J. Psychiatry* 136:273–278.

Naborsky, R., Janowsky, D., Munson, E. and Depry, D. (1981). Rapid treatment of acute psychotic symptoms with high-dose and low-dose haloperidol. *Arch. Gen. Psychiatry* 38:195–196.

Stern, T.A. and Anderson, W.H. (1979). Benztropine prophylaxis of dystonic reactions. *Psychopharmacol.* 61:261–262.

27

Assessment of Psychotropic Drugs Following Acute Doses: Pharmacodynamics and Pharmacokinetics

STEPHEN H. CURRY

INTRODUCTION

This chapter is principally concerned with the Clinical Pharmacokinetics of the drugs useful in emergency psychiatry, when given in single doses or as a short course of frequent doses prior to stabilization for longer term treatment. However, consideration of a few general principles is appropriate by way of introduction.

In assessing the suitability of a particular drug for use in psychiatric emergencies, attention will be focused on both the clinical pharmacology and the pharmacokinetic features of the compound in question. The clinical pharmacological considerations include differential pharmacological effects of the various candidate compounds (both desired and undesired effects), routes of administration, dose dependency of effects, duration of effects, scale of variation between individuals, and factors affecting the drug effects, such as disease states, physiological variables including genetics, interacting drugs and pharmaceutical formulation. The clinical pharmacokinetic considerations include basic information on half-life and other measurements, relevant pharmacokinetic models including compartment models, route of administration comparisons, dose dependency of kinetics, the scale of variation between patients, and factors affecting kinetics, such as diseases, physiological variables, other drugs and pharmaceutical formulation. There is obviously considerable overlap between the clinical pharmacological group and the clinical pharmacokinetic group. The relationship between the two groups is a major field of study.

MODELS

Pharmacokineticists like to draw diagrams with boxes representing compartments and arrows representing transfer between the compartments. Pharmacokineticists also like equations. This is desirable but it need not become a burden. It is important however, to differentiate between the one and two compartment models shown in Fig. 1. In the one compartment case, the drug is considered to be distributed homogeneously throughout the body. Input into the single compartment is generally at a constant rate (k_o) by intravenous infusion, or by exponential absorption processes from doses placed in the gastrointestinal tract by swallowing, or from intramuscular injection sites. Exponential absorption processes are generally assessed by means of k_a values (absorption rate constants). The single homogeneous compartment has a volume (V) obtained by multiplying the concentration in plasma by the total body content, and the removal from the compartment is by elimination, an exponential process comprising metabolism and excretion of the unchanged drug, assessed by k_{el}, the first order rate constant of elimination. The half-life of the drug (T½) is given by:

$$T½ = \frac{0.693}{k_{el}}$$

In the two compartment case, the drug is distributed unevenly, but to equilibrium, between two "spaces" or areas of the body. These compartments have volumes V_1 and V_2. Input is again by infusion or absorption, generally into the "central" compartment (1) and output is by exponential elimination from the central compartment. The rate constant of elimination is given the symbol k_{10} in this case. The transfer rate constants between the two compartments are k_{12} and k_{21}.

After an intravenous bolus dose into a single compartment, the drug concentration declines exponentially with the same rate constant at all times and concentrations. Decline of the concentration in plasma within a two compartment case is biphasic, fast at first, and slower later, with a transition point between the two parts of the decay curve being approximately identifiable. During the initial rapid phase, the drug decay is dominated by transfer of the drug from the central compartment, which includes plasma, into the peripheral compartment. The slower phase indicates decay of drug concentrations in the body as a whole.

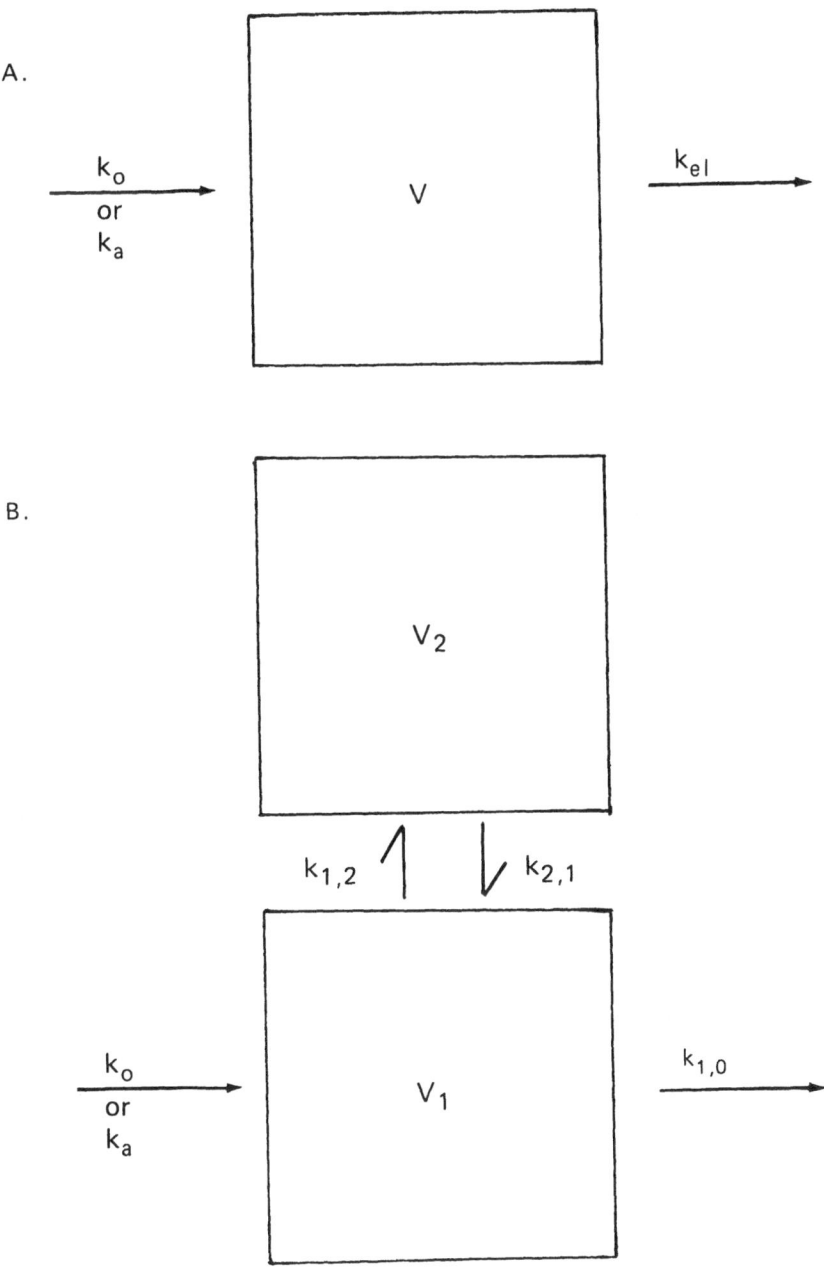

Figure 1. The one (A) and two-compartment (B) models.

Comparisons between drug concentrations in plasma after intravenous, oral, and intramuscular doses lead to the realization that intravenous doses are unique in leading to an initial high concentration in the single compartment system, or in the central compartment of the two-compartment system. Intramuscular doses generally lead to an area under the curve of a drug concentration diagram the same as that after a corresponding intravenous dose. A consequence of this is the poorly appreciated fact that, because intramuscular doses lead to lower initial concentrations, they are more likely to give a prolonged elevated level. Oral doses, like intramuscular doses, lead to a growth and decay pattern of drug concentration, but the area under the curve does not have to be the same as that after the injected doses because of the first-pass effect — chemical change or metabolism of the drug with conversion to products not detected in assays for the parent drug, during transfer from the gastrointestinal tract through the gut mucosa, portal circulation, and liver, before reaching the general circulation in which measurements are conventionally made.

When second and later doses follow an innitial dose, the doses build successively on the residues left from the previous doses. There is an overall rise in the mean concentration, but the rate of rise gradually decreases, so that the mean concentration tends to reach a plateau. It can be shown that, while the true plateau can only be reached if dosing continues for an infinite time, ninety percent of the plateau is reached after approximately four drug half-lives have elapsed, regardless of the frequency and magnitude of dosing. It is here that the concept of a steady state applies. True steady state is reached only at infinity, but the ninety percent point is a reasonable approximation. However, it must be noted that the pulsed nature of oral and intramuscular dosing causes a considerable fluctuation in the concentration both during the rise towards steady state and at the steady state.

An interesting pharmacokinetic question which is of importance in emergency psychiatry, and which appears to have been ignored by both pharmacokineticists and clinical pharmacologists, concerns concentrations of drugs in peripheral compartments during frequent multiple dosing. This issue obviously does not arise if a one compartment model is applicable. If a two compartment model is applicable, then the concentration in the peripheral compartment rises during the phase of rapid fall of concentration in the central compartment (the α-phase), and falls during the phase of slower fall of concentration in the central compartment (the β-phase). An important consequence of this is the fact that, if second and later doses are given during the α-phase following earlier doses, the drug concentration in the peripheral compartment will show a gradual rise towards its steady state, without fluctuation. If the second and later doses are given during the β-phase following earlier doses, the drug concentration in the peripheral compartment will still show a rise towards a steady state, but there will be fluctuation in the concentration in the peripheral compartment both during the rise, and at the steady state.

The last model to be considered relates to loading doses. If the initial dose of a multiple dosing regimen is higher than the ensuing doses, and if the relationship between the levels of the two doses is properly chosen, then the steady state concentration is induced by the initial loading dose and maintained by the later doses. Generally speaking, if the dosage interval is equal to the half-life of the drug, the drug concentration will double after each dose, and fall by fifty percent from the peak by the time the next dose is due. More frequent dosing will lead to less fluctuation and less frequent dosing will lead to more fluctuation. This will be made more complex if doses are given on the α-phase of the biexponential decay in two-compartment cases when dosing is frequent and on the β-phase when dosing is less frequent.

SPECIFIC EXAMPLES

It is clearly desirable in all circumstances, but especially in emergency psychiatry, to know the details of the drugs under study in regard to their many pharmacokinetic variables (Donlon et al., 1979; Menuck and Voineskos, 1981). These include whether a one or two compartment model is applicable, and if the latter, whether the receptors, in the brain are in the central or the peripheral compartment. Also, we need to know k_a values, especially as a rapid effect is sought. Whether or not a first-pass effect is prominent is also important, as is the activity of any metabolites. Also, the possibilities for enzyme induction, interpatient variation, dose relationships, and a host of other influences become important. The second half of this paper considers the state of our knowledge in relation to particular drugs.

In considering specific examples, it is appropriate to stress, as in the past, the fact that pharmacokinetic studies of neuroleptic drugs by means of plasma level research became possible more than fifteen years ago. Progress has been remarkably slow, so slow in fact that, bearing in mind the tendency of investigators to rediscover the wheel from time to time, and to be aware only of literature published during the ten years previous to the time of their own interest in a particular problem, there is now a problem with investigators merely repeating earlier work. The kinetics of neuroleptic drugs were extensively reviewed two to three years ago in several books, and the remarks which follow are largely designed to update these reviews (Curry, 1981).

Chlorpromazine is the most extensively studied drug (Alfredsson and Sedvall, 1981; Hershey et al., 1981; Loo et al., 1980; Midha et al., 1981; Wode-Helgodt and Alfredsson, 1981). Prior to 1966, it had been studied extensively for its metabolic properties, but it had resisted plasma level studies. Gas-chromatography with electron capture detection revolutionized that. The first-pass effect was demonstrated. The bi-exponential decay of intravenous doses was observed, with the α-phase lasting six to eight hours. The time course of effects and concentrations after single doses and during longer term treatment was studied, and the fact that enzyme induction occurred, reducing the plasma level induced per unit of dose was recognized as an important factor (Harmon et al., 1980). Interaction studies followed. More recently, the double exponential decay has been reemphasized, and multiple dosing clearly occurs on the α-phase. There is wide variation between patients. There are two important controversial metabolites. Intramuscular doses induce detectable concentrations rapidly, but absorption is still prolonged. Plasma levels and CSF levels are correlated but the distribution ratio varies between patients. Variation of single doses within individuals leads to a linear relationship of levels and dose, but when patients on different doses are studied, the increase per unit of dose is relatively small.

Fluphenazine also has a massive first-pass effect, with wide variations between individuals (Goldstein and Van Vunakis, 1981; Heyes et al., 1980; Midha et al., 1980). There is little or no enzyme induction with this drug. Seven hydroxy fluphenazine is a controversial metabolite. The half-life of fluphenazine is approximately sixteen hours. The depot intramuscular preparations are different. The enanthate leads to increasing plasma fluphenazine up to two to three days after the dose, after which it declines. The decanoate causes an initial sharp rise in plasma fluphenazine in the first eight hours, after which the concentration drops to a level which persists almost unchanged for almost two weeks or perhaps longer. Fluphenazine levels are not changed by antiparkinsonian drugs.

Haloperidol shows approximately thirty percent loss as the result of the first-pass effect (Romon et al., 1981). There is wide variation in levels. Enzyme induction plays no part, either with haloperidol or in interactions antiparkinsonian drugs. The conventional view for a long time has been that there are no active metabolites. There is a positive correlation between plasma and CSF levels.

Butaperazine shows immense variation in levels, as does thioridazine which has much higher levels than the other drugs. Thioridazine is complicated by having metabolites which have been proved to possess clinical activity, and by there being no injectable form of the drug (Nyberg et al., 1981; Skinner et al., 1980). There is also a wide range in the non-protein bound fraction, which is also known to occur with chlorpromazine (Curry et al., 1982).

Trifluoperazine is one of the oldest of the drugs but one of the most recently studied (Gillespie and Sipes, 1981; Javaid et al., 1982; Whelpton et al., 1982). Its concentrations are proportional to dose, and its half-life is in the general region of seven to twenty hours after single doses. However, in one study, virtually no within dose fluction was observed in a patient treated long-term.

Finally, thiothixene has been observed to have levels at steady state correlated with those after single doses, and to have these levels correlated with the age of the patient (Yesavage et al., 1981).

CONCLUSION

One of the purposes of the Toronto meeting was identification of new research frontiers. The message from this review is clear. While much useful information on the kinetics of neuroleptic drugs is now available, very little of it is relevant to the special situation of emergency psychiatry, and the need to devise specialized dosage regimens. There is definite need for intensive pharmacokinetic study of possible dosing regimens for neuroleptic drugs in this application (Cooper and Lapierre, 1981; Curry, 1982; Schley et al., 1981).

REFERENCES

Alfredsson, G. and Sedvall, G. (1981). Protein binding of chlorpromazine in cerebrospinal fluid and serum. *Int. Pharmacopsychiatry* 73:55–62.

Cooper, S.F. and Lapierre, T.D. (1981). Gas liquid chromatographic determination of pipotiazine in plasma of psychiatric patients. *J. Chromatography* 223:95–102.

Curry, S.H. (1981). Binding of psychotropic drugs to plasma protein and its influence on drug distribution. In: *Clinical Pharmacology in Psychiatry* (ed. E. Usdin). New York, Elsevier, pp. 213–223.

Curry, S.H. (1982). Assessment of Psychotropic Drugs Following Acute Doses: II. Clinical Significance of Neuroleptic Plasma Levels. This volume.

Curry, S.H., Brown, E.A., Hu, O. Y-P. and Perrin, J.H. (1982). LC assay of phenothiazine, thiothixene, and butyrophene neuroleptics and antihistamines in biological fluids with conventional and radial compression columns and UV and electrochemical detection. *J. Chromatography* 231: 361–376.

Donlon, P.T., Hopkin, J. and Tupin, J.P. (1979). Overview: efficacy and safety of the rapid neuroleptization method with injectable haloperidol. *Am. J. Psychiatry* 136:273–278.

Gillespie, T.J. and Sipes, I.G. (1981). Sensitive gas chromatrographic determination of trifluoperazine in human plasma. *J. Chromatography* 223:95–102.

Goldstein, S.A. and Van Vunakis, H. (1981). Determination of fluphenazine, related phenothiazine drugs and metabolites by combined high-performance liquid chromatography and radioimmunoassay. *J. Pharmacol. and Exp. Ther.* 217:36–43.

Harmon, A.W., Frewin, D.B. and Priestly, B.G. (1980). Comparative enzyme-inducing effects of chlorpromazine and fluphenazine therapies in psychotic patients. *Psychopharmacol.* 69:35–37.

Hershey, L.A., Gift, T., Atkins, R.W. and Rivera-Calimlin, L. (1981). Effects of a drug holiday on plasma chlorpromazine levels in chronic schizophrenic patients. *Psychopharmacol.* 73:355–358.

Heyes, W.F., Salmon, J.R. and Marlow, W. (1980). High performance liquid chromatographic separation of the N- and S- oxides of fluphenazine decanoate. *J. Chromatography* 194:416–420.

Javaid, J.I., Dekirmenjian, H. and Davis, J.M. (1982). GLC analysis of trifluoperazine in human plasma. *J. Pharm. Sci.* 71:63–66.

Loo, J.C.K., Midha, K.K. and McGilveray, I.J. (1980). Pharmacokinetics of chlorpromazine in normal volunteers. *Comm. Psychopharmacol.* 4:121–129.

Menuck, M. and Voineskos, G. (1981). Rapid parenteral treatment of acute psychosis. *Compr. Psychiatry* 22:351–361.

Midha, K.K., Cooper, J.K., McGilveray, I.J., Butterfield, A.G. and Hubbard, J.W. (1981). High-performance liquid chromatographic assay for nanogram determination of chlorpromazine and its comparison with radioimmunoassay. *J. Pharm. Sci.* 70:1043–1046.

Midha, K.K., Cooper, J.K. and Hubbard, J.W. (1982). Radioimmunoassay for fluphenazine in plasma. *Commun. Psychopharmacol.* 4:107–114.

Nyberg, G.L., Axelsson, R. and Martensson, E. (1981). Cerebrospinal fluid concentrations of thioridazine and its main metabolites in psychiatric patients. *Eur. J. Clin. Pharmacol.* 19:139–148.

Romon, R., Averbuch, I., Rozick, P., Fijman-Danilovich, L., Kara, T., Dasberg, H., Ebstein, R.P. and Belmaker, R.H. (1981). Serum and CSF levels of haloperidol by radioimmunoassay and radioreceptor assay during high-dose therapy of resistant schizophrenic patients. *Psychopharmacology* 73:197–199.

Schley, J., Riedel, E. and Muller-Oerlinghausen, B. (1981). Metabolism and excretion of the neuroleptic drug perazine in healthy volunteers. *Int. Pharmacopsychiatry* 16:201–205.

Skinner, T., Gochnauer, R. and Linnoila, M. (1980). Liquid chromatographic method to measure thioridazine and its active metabolites in plasma. *Acta Pharmacol. Toxicol.* 48:416–420.

Whelpton, R., Curry, S.H. and Watkins, G.M. (1982). Analysis of Plasma trifluoperazine by gas chromatography and selected ion monitoring. *J. Chromatography* 228:321–326.

Wode-Helgodt, B. and Alfredsson, G. (1981). Concentration of chlorpromazine and two of its active metabolites in plasma and cerebrospinal fluid of psychotic patients treated with fixed drug doses. *Psychopharmacology* 73:55–62.

Yesavage, J.A., Holman, C.A. and Cohn, R. (1982). Correlation of thiothixene serum levels with age. *Psychopharmacology* 74:170–172.

SECTION V

Forensic Psychiatry

Hints for Clinicians

PHARMACOTHERAPY OF SEXUAL DEVIATION

Drug treatments that seek to suppress sexual libido are available; some of these have been opposed on ethical grounds. The two major groups of drugs are the neuroleptics and hormones. In practice the study of drugs in the treatment of sexual deviance has been restricted to sexual offenders.

Tranquilizing drugs have an effect on sexual performance. Thioridazine has been reported to produce a diminution of sexual function in several studies. Benperidol is a neuroleptic drug belonging to the butyrophenone series and is somewhat similar in chemical structure to haloperidol. It has also been reported to reduce sexual drive.

With regard to the hormones, not surprisingly the group of patients who desire treatment for sexual deviations and who have good motivation, reasonable personality and some positive factors on which to base psychotherapy seem to do best. Stilboestrol given in repeated doses has been used to decrease libido and is a reported effective method of control. This substance has been used as implants as well as orally. In some studies its use has been limited by nausea and vomiting. A further rare but grave complication of carcinoma of the breast probably restricts it to very short term use. The use of the antiandrogen cyproterone acetate, largely results from it being a selective competitor with testosterone at organ receptor sites. Thus, its antigonadotrophic effect actually results from blocking the secretion of pituitary gonadotrophin. However, the proper chemical base of these drugs has yet to be clarified and at the present they should be used with caution and only in those cases where there is obvious clinical need to reduce sexual arousability per se.

PHARMACOTHERAPY OF AGGRESSIVE BEHAVIOR

Violence is by no means necessarily symptomatic of psychological disturbance. Two important factors need to be balanced in each case; the desire of any identified participant in a violent episode to receive psychiatric help, and the degree of psychiatric illness which is present. This is important ethically because of the pressure and temptation to intervene psychiatrically, especially with drugs, is quite considerable when violence has occurred and is likely to recur. With regard to the prevention of violent behavior by means of drugs, the benzodiazepines have been used to deal with hostility and aggressive behavior in epileptic patients. It is suggested that the addition of a benzodiazepine to the standard anticonvulsive medication may lead to a decrease in the number of convulsions and an improvement in the aggression and hostility in epileptics.

Several controlled studies with neuroleptics have shown that hostility and aggression are reduced in schizophrenics. However, there are only a few studies in which the effects of phenothiazines have been examined on hostility and aggression in non-psychotic patients.

Carbamazepine has also been used to control mood and behavior in patients with epilepsy including those with epileptic psychoses. There are some impulsive adolescents and possibly some adults who were hyperactive in childhood who have persisting psychiatric symptoms, including impulsivity and aggression who have essentially the same pathology as they had in childhood. These patients may benefit from treatment with stimulants such as methylphenidate or amphetamines.

The maintenance treatment with lithium in patients who commit unpremeditated acts of violence is said to be a promising development. Patients who are explosive, impulsive, and tend to respond with anger and aggression to small provocations tend to benefit. Unfortunately many of these patients lack the self-discipline to take lithium regularly, the side effects of the drug are poorly tolerated by impulsive patients with poor motivation and many are likely to discontinue the drug.

28

Summary of the Guidelines for the Use of Psychotropic Drugs in Forensic Psychiatry

STEPHEN J. HUCKER

The forensic psychiatrist may expect to encounter the full range of psychiatric disorders in the course of his work and in these cases he will employ psychotropic medications where indicated, following guidelines such as those suggested elsewhere in this volume. There are, however, certain types of mental aberration which are found more commonly among the offender population and for which drug treatments are particularly controversial. Most important among these disorders are the sexual anomalies and the personality disorders in which the individual is prone to repeated acts of violence.

Treatment of offenders presents many ethical as well as practical problems. Large numbers of individuals are referred to psychiatrists by families, courts and probation officers because they are seen as "sick" or "crazy." A proportion of these patients not only genuinely desire whatever help can be offered but have definable psychiatric conditions for which treatments are available. However, it is probably fair to state that the majority of offenders referred to the psychiatrist attend simply because someone else has sent them and would never have considered it of their own accord.

The issue of voluntariness is a central one. Except in emergency situations or cases where insight or judgement is impaired by serious mental disorder, most psychiatrists would see little justification in forcing an individual to accept treatment against his will. Yet this is just what the public and many professionals within the criminal justice system seem to expect. When acceptance of treatment may determine whether or not parole is granted, the pressure upon the offender is subtle but great and the situation places the treating psychiatrist in a difficult ethical position. Such important dilemmas were not ignored by the contributors to this Symposium and are discussed in the original papers themselves.

USE OF DRUGS IN THE TREATMENT OF PARAPHILIAS (SEXUAL ANOMALIES)

Although phenothiazines such as Chlorpromazine and Thioridazine and butyrophenones such as Benperidol have been used in the treatment of sexual anomalies, the drugs which have received most attention have been sex hormones. The ones used initially such as estrogens were frequently attended by unpleasant and sometimes serious side effects and their use can no longer be recommended. In the past few years, two drugs in particular have been used. Medroxyprogesterone Acetate (Provera, Upjohn) is available in North America while Cyproterone Acetate (Androcur, Schering) is not, although it has been used clinically and studied in Europe.

Recommendations

1. *The nature of the sexual anomaly must first be clearly identified.* Although anomalous sexual behavior is far from clearly understood, new laboratory techniques have been developed which assist in the assessment of the problem. As Dr. Walker points out, sexual anomalies may coexist although the patient may admit to only one of them. This observation is of theoretical as well as practical interest (Freund, Scher and Hucker, in press). The use of penile plethysmography (phallometry) using either circumferential or volumetric methods is very helpful in identifying a complex pattern of sexual arousal (Freund and Blanchard, 1980).

2. *The patient must be well motivated to receive treatment.* Paraphilic patients are frequently disinterested in receiving treatment for their problem but guilt, shame or fear of apprehension may bring a patient to accept that he has to do something to prevent himself from acting upon his impulses again. Certainly patients who come for treatment simply because they are sent by the courts or a probation officer are unlikely to cooperate satisfactorily.

3. *Other patient characteristics which affect treatment.* Antisocial personalities or individuals who seriously abused alcohol or drugs appear to do less well with the drug treatments available.

Patients who appear to respond best to hormone treatments suffer from what are now called paraphilias (formerly sexual deviations) such as transvestism, zoophilia, pedophilia, exhibitionism, voyeurism, sado-masochism, etc. These disorders consist of sexual arousal to preferred unusual or bizarre objects either animate or inanimate. Some of these are forbidden by law, for example pedo-philia (sexual arousal to children), and others are not necessarily illegal, for example fetishistic arousal to women's underwear. The aim of drug treatment is to reduce the intensity of the urge and the ease with which the individual becomes aroused and thus assist him in keeping his impulses under control.

Individuals who deny the offense or minimize their responsibility by blaming the victim, alcohol, drugs, job stress, etc., or whose crime appears to have other than sexual motives (for example anger) are not suitable.

4. *Methods of improving compliance.* Apart from careful pre-selection of suitable cases there are some other factors which are relevant to the issue of compliance. It seems that, if possible, starting the treatment regimen as an inpatient may enhance patient/therapist rapport and thus reduce the drop out rate. Also it may be helpful to inform the patient that he might not necessarily be totally impotent and if he has a consenting sexual partner he may still be capable of erection and ejaculation.

5. *Information and Consent.* With any of the drugs concerned, the patient needs to be informed of potential side effects in order to weigh them against disadvantages of declining treatment. One way of doing this is to present the prospective patient with an information sheet and the patient is then given an opportunity to go away and read it and return to discuss it or proceed immediately to signing the form. An example of such a form used on the Forensic Service at the Clarke Institute is given on the following pages. A similar one could be designed for use with Cyproterone Acetate.

6. *Concomitant Psychotherapy.* Clearly drugs are not the "cure" for sexual anomalies although they have a definite place in management. Both Walker and Tennent see Cyproterone Acetate and Medroxyprogesterone Acetate in this light and recommend that patients treated with these drugs be offered some form of psychotherapy at the same time. One would expect that provision of concomitant therapy would increase compliance as for example was shown in the study by Langevin et al. (1979).

Future Research

As was indicated by Tennent and Walker in their reviews, drug treatments for sexual anomalies often have not been investigated by rigorous scientific methods. The use of these drugs has become widespread despite almost complete absence of double-blind controlled trials and reliance on small uncontrolled series or anecdotal reports. Some feel that the effectiveness of these drugs in reducing sex drive is as clear as that of penicillin in treating pneumococcal pneu-monia and that the necessary double-blind trials are unethical. The present author is not convinced by this argument and recommends that well designed studies in suitably assessed patients be conducted as soon as possible.

CONSENT FORM FOR TREATMENT WITH PROVERA (MEDROXYPROGESTERONE ACETATE)

Your physician _____ has recommended that you accept treatment with Provera (Medroxy-progesterone Acetate). In your case the diagnosis of _____ has been made, and this implies that you have a sexual inclination or abnormality which you have difficulty in keeping under control without help.

Provera is a hormone drug which, by a complex action, has the effect of lowering the level of male hormone (especially testosterone) in your blood.

The intention of the treatment is to reduce sexual drive, and you are likely to notice a reduced number of erections and ejaculations together with a reduced frequency of sexual thoughts and urges.

In addition to changes in your sexual feelings, your prostate gland and seminal vesicles (internal organs which are part of the reproductive system) will shrink and the production of sperm will cease. In addition, you may experience other side effects including: weight gain, tiredness, restlessness, nervousness, inability to concentrate, depressed mood, decrease in body hair and hot and cold flashes. If you do experience such symptoms, you may want to discuss continuation of treatment with your doctor and will be free to discontinue the drug if side effects are too troublesome. It is believed that these side effects are reversible on stopping the drug.

While the drug has been used for several years, the possible long-term effects are not known and you are therefore taking a risk in accepting this treatment. Having carefully weighed and considered the potential harmful effects against the advantages of Provera treatment, you may be prepared to make a written undertaking that you fully accept treatment with Provera as recommended by Dr. _____.

The actual dose will need to be calculated according to your subjective response to the drug and the results of blood estimations of testosterone level.

I have read the information given above on treatment with Provera and have understood it to my satisfaction. I have been given an opportunity to ask any questions I wish. I fully accept treatment with Provera, as recommended by Dr. _____ and reserve the right to discontinue such treatment at any time without forfeiting any rights to future care.

Signed _____   Witnessed By _____
        (Patient)
                                                   Date _____

Signed _____   Witnessed By _____
        (Parent or Guardian)
                                                   Date _____

In the future, other drugs with more specific actions can be expected to appear. For example, an antagonist of the hypothalamic luteinizing hormone releasing hormone (LHRH) which is currently being used experimentally to treat prostatic carcinoma has as its only apparent side effect lowering of the libido. The possibilities for the use of this in the treatment of paraphilias are obvious.

USE OF DRUGS TO CONTROL VIOLENT BEHAVIOR

The management of acutely violent situations is discussed in the section on Emergency Psychiatry. Probably forensic psychiatrists deal less often with these immediate episodes and rather more with the problem of long term management of individuals with aggressive tendencies.

Because drugs have a small but nevertheless significant part to play in the overall management of violent behavior, Gunn's paper on the limitations of and alternatives to the use of medication is an important reminder. Violent episodes may have many possible causes not by any means all of which are appropriately treated pharmacologically.

Guidelines and Recommendations

1. *Comprehensive assessment* The initial assessment needs to investigate the nature and causes of the violent behavior. This involves evaluation of the combination of cultural, social, psychological and biological factors in a psychiatric and neurological context. For a good clinical introduction to this, the reader is referred to Lion's concise and readable text *Evaluation and Management of the Violent Patient* (Charles C Thomas: Springfield, Illinois, 1972).

2. *Patient Cooperativeness* Many violent patients are afraid of their own capacity for uncontrolled aggression. Nevertheless they often have the personality characteristics (such as impulsivity and poor tolerance of frustration) which makes cooperation with drug treatment difficult. Similarly, patients who continue to abuse alcohol and street drugs are generally unsuitable because of possible interaction with medication. As Gunn points out, it is often an important first step in the management of the violent patient to treat their alcohol or drug abuse problem and this may involve weaning them off medication which may have been prescribed by other physicians.

3. *Use of Specific Medications* As Kellner's review demonstrates, a number of different drugs have been prescribed to help violent patients control

themselves better. Very few have been submitted to satisfactory double-blind controlled trials making it difficult for the clinician to select medications which have demonstrated effectiveness. In acute situations the phenothiazines and butyrophenones have been most often used (see section on Emergency Psychiatry) and, while these may have a part to play in long term management, the evidence is generally anecdotal. A combination of a phenothiazine and an anti-convulsant (such as Diphenylhydantoin and Thioridazine) may have more effect than either alone. Carbamazepine might also be selected if an anti-convulsant with less sedative action is desirable.

Although stimulants such as amphetamine and methylphenidate may be useful in certain specific cases as discussed in Kellner's paper, the risks of abuse and habituation make them a generally unsafe recommendation.

Of all the drugs used in long term management of violence Lithium Carbonate has been subjected to the most satisfactory scientific scrutiny. Provided the patient can tolerate the inconvenience of regular blood tests and can cooperate adequately it is probably the drug of first choice at the present time. Its administration, side effects, etc., are discussed in the section on Affective Disorders.

4. *Limitations of Drug Treatment of Aggressive Tendencies* Where aggression is symptomatic of failure of psychological coping mechanisms the use of drugs which raise the violence threshold may simply be counter productive in the long run. A prescription of medication is certainly quicker, easier and less stressful to the therapist than skilled counselling, but no substitute for it. As Gunn points out in his paper, very satisfying and satisfactory control of habitually aggressive individuals has been demonstrated by means other than medication.

FUTURE RESEARCH

Medications aimed at reducing aggressiveness are likely to continue to appear. Kellner's survey shows, however, that continued reports of inadequate, uncontrolled trials are ultimately unhelpful. Promising leads, however, need to be followed up. In this context, it is unfortunate that SCH 12679 (also known as Trimopam) discussed by Kellner proved toxic during animal studies and it is not likely to be produced commercially.

The complex interaction of social, psychological and biological factors which results in aggression make the evaluation of the relative merits of pharmacological and other treatments difficult, but nevertheless challenging.

REFERENCES

Freund, K. and Blanchard, R. (1980). Assessment of anomalous erotic prefer-
    ences and coital dysfunctions. In: *Behavioral Assessment: A Practical
    Handbook* (Second ed.) M. Hersen and A.S. Bellack (Eds.). New York:
    Pergamon Press.
Freund, K., Scher, H. and Hucker, S.J. "The Courtship Disorders" *Arch. Sex.
    Behav.* (1983, in press).
Langevin, R. et al. (1979). The Effect of Assertiveness Training, Provera and Sex
    of Therapist in the Treatment of Genital Exhibitionism. *J. Behav. Ther.
    Exp. Psychiatr.* 10:275-282.

29

Review of Research on the Use of Drugs to Control Violent Behavior

ROBERT KELLNER

There is decidely less published research on the drug treatment of violent behavior than on several other topics in psychopharmacology, such as drug treatment of schizophrenia, affective disorders and anxiety. The purpose of this chapter is to review the main research on the use of drugs to control violent behavior. The chapter does not deal with the treatment of violence when this is a symptom of a psychiatric disorder for which there is effective drug treatment, such as schizophrenia or mania, because in these disorders the appropriate treatment is that of the disorder causing it; it deals only briefly with the management of the acute episode of violence and concentrates on the far more difficult topic, that of the prevention of violent behavior by the means of drugs.

THE MANAGEMENT OF THE ACUTE VIOLENT EPISODE

There have been several reports in the literature in which the treatment strategies to control acute violent episodes are discussed. For example, Tupin (1975) recommends as one of the alternatives diazepam 5-10 mg/IV given slowly, or a combination of haloperidol 20 to 40 mg daily with chlordiazepoxide up to 200 to 500 mg/i.m. in divided doses over 24 hours which was initially described by Shader and Salzman. The techniqe of rapid neuroleptization is described in the chapter on emergency psychiatry. In recent years droperidol, a derivative of haloperidol which has been used as pre-medication and an adjunct in anesthesia, has been used in the management of acute agitation and violence (van Leeuwen et al., 1977). The literature on the uses of droperidol in acutely disturbed behavior has been reviewed by Ayd (1980). My colleagues and I carried out a placebo controlled study of droperidol 5 mg/i.m. and repeated if necessary after 30 minutes in acute agitation and aggression and found droperidol to be rapidly effective. However, there are at present no controlled studies which compare droperidol to other drugs in acute agitation and aggression and it is not certain whether it is more effective than other neuroleptics in these situations.

DRUG TREATMENTS IN THE PREVENTION OF VIOLENT BEHAVIOR

The etiology of conditions in which violent behavior occurs differ widely; for example, it can be the consequence of an explosive personality, sociopathy, other inadequate socialization with poor self control, culturally acquired habitual display of courage, masculinity and daring, habitual violence to achieve a purpose such as dominance, or deliberate violence in the pursuit of crime (Tupin, 1975 op cit., Kellner, 1982a). In drug trials with violent patients different pathologies are being treated and the findings in controlled studies merely give an estimate on the effect of the drug on the majority in the sample. A conventional between subjects parallel controlled trial may hide the specific effects of a drug on a certain pathology. To choose a simple analogy let's assume that a controlled trial had been carried out in anemia at a time when the etiology of anemia was not known. The substances compared were iron and vitamin B-12 and patients with iron deficiency anemia and patients with Addisonian anemia were found in each group. The outcome of this trial would have depended on the proportion of patients in each group with the two different pathologies; the result may have shown that iron was more effective than vitamin B-12 in the treatment of anemia, merely because more patients with iron deficiency anemia were in each group. The trial would have concealed the fact that each substance had a specific effect on one of the pathologies.

In the present survey this kind of information is probably concealed although the drugs which are available for the treatment of violence are not anywhere as specific as the replacement treatment in deficiency diseases. If evidence exists that the response to a certain drug is more effective for a subgroup this will be commented upon, otherwise merely the results of the study will be reported. The emphasis is on controlled studies; uncontrolled studies will be mentioned either if no controlled studies are available or if the uncontrolled study suggests that the information may be important. Several of the earlier studies have been summarized and discussed elsewhere (Kellner, 1978).

The studies of hostility, impulsiveness and aggression will be considered together; in part because in many studies with psychotropic drugs the patients had more than one of these traits and in part, there is some evidence to suggest that decrease in hostility or in impulsiveness can decrease violent acts.

Benzodiazepines and Minor Tranquilizers

There is complex interaction of the effects of minor tranquilizers on anxiety, depression, hostility and personality. In a placebo controlled double blind study chlordiazepoxide was found to reduce hostility and irritability in neurotic oupatients and perhaps increase a healthy assertiveness. (Rickels and Clyde, 1967; Rickels and Downing, 1974). Diazepam was found to increase hostile mood in depressed female outpatients but did not appear to increase overt aggressive impulses (Covi et al., 1977). In anxious and depressed neurotic patients chlordiazepoxide was also found to increase slightly hostile feelings, whereas they remained largely unchanged with placebo and decreased significantly with imipramine (Covi et al., 1981). Paradoxical rage reactions with benzodiazepines are rare. There is some evidence to suggest that oxazepam does not increase hostility (Gardos et al., 1968; DiMascio et al., 1969; Salzman et al., 1974) and in psychiatric patients on the average there is a decrease of hostility with oxazepam (Feldman, 1967; Kochansky et al., 1975; Salzman et al., 1975). Halazepam does not appear to affect hostility (Zisook, 1978). The effects on hostility may depend in part on personality factors. For example, the effects may be more pronounced in "action oriented" than in "non-action oriented" subjects but this has been reported only in one study with normal subjects after a single dose of diazepam (McDonald, 1967).

There have been only open studies with benzodiazepines in hostility and aggressive behavior in epileptic patients. These studies suggest that the addition of a benzodiazepine to the standard anticonvulsant medication leads to a decrease in the number of convulsions and an improvement in the rating of aggression and hostility. Since benzodiazepines have anticonvulsant effects and fewer toxic side effects than sedatives and anticonvulsants, the addition of a benzodiazepine to the antiepileptic drugs has a logical appeal until controlled studies become available.

Patients with explosive outburst and personality disorders appear to need far larger doses of benzodiazepines than those used in the treatment of anxiety (Solomon, 1975; Kellner, 1982b). Lion (1979), in a double blind trial used chlordiazepoxide in doses 200 mg/daily and oxazepam in doses up to 240 mg in patients who had temper outburst and assaultive behavior and hostility. Oxazepam was somewhat more effective in the reduction of anxiety and hostility. We have treated patients with dangerous explosive outburst with oxazepam in doses up to 240 mg daily for several months; there were a few side effects and the patients reported a substantial decrease in explosive outbursts (awaiting publication). However, the long-term effects of these large doses is unknown and this treatment appears to be justified only when the consequences of the untreated condition are dangerous or incapacitating or when attempts are made to use this time period to teach the patient anger control or other strategies to control his explosive outbursts which are discussed in another chapter.

The Control of Aggression and Violence with SCH 12679

SCH 12679 is a benzazepine derivative that differs in structure from other psychotropic drugs; it shows similarities to chlordiazepoxide and perphenazine but has different effects on agitated and aggressive behavior in animals. It inhibits aggression without producing sedation and has only weak neuroleptic properties. Barnett et al. (1973), and Itil and Wadud (1975) suggested there may be a final common path for the neurophysiology of aggression and this may be sensitive to specific drug effects in humans. In early open studies in mentally retarded patients who were aggressive it appeared to have a calming effect (Itil and Wadud, op cit). In a controlled study with 20 retarded female patients it reduced violence, destructiveness and anger significantly more than placebo (Albert et al., 1977). Elie et al. (1980) in a large double blind controlled study with aggressive mentally retarded patients found SCH 12679 significantly superior to thioridazine and to placebo.

The history of this drug illustrates the extent to which the forces of the market affect research priorities. Since SCH 12679 was synthesized and its anti-aggressive properties were suggested, a large number of new antianxiety drugs and antidepressants have been developed and marketed which has entailed great effort and expense; a drug which is perhaps unique in its specific effect on aggression has been used only in a small number of studies.

Neuroleptics

Several controlled studies with neuroleptics have shown that hostility and aggression are reduced in schizophrenics. There are only a few studies in which the effects on hostility and aggression have been examined in nonpsychotic patients. From the published studies, it is difficult to evaluate the effects of neuroleptics because many of the studies have methodological shortcomings; most were uncontrolled and in some of the studies other psychotropic drugs were given concurrently.

Molling et al. (1962), in a double blind placebo controlled study of perphenazine up to 60 mg/daily with 28 institutionalized delinquent boys, found that there were no significant differences between drug and placebo on aggressivity or hostility. Barnes et al. (1977) in a small parallel six weeks double blind placebo controlled study of teenagers with personality disorders found mesorida-zine more effective than placebo on several symptoms and behaviors including frustration tolerance but the effect on aggression did not reach a significant level. Propericyazine (PPC) has been advocated for the treatment of impulsive behavior and aggression but the published studies are either uncontrolled or PPC was used in conjunction with other drugs (Kellner, 1978 op cit).

A few studies are summarized in the section of anticonvulsants which suggest that there are differences between individuals in their response to neuro-leptics and there are perhaps differences between neuroleptics in their effects on aggression and impulsive behavior. Neuroleptics (particularly low potency phenothiazines which are usually prescribed in large doses) tend to lower the convulsive threshold, may precipitate seizures and sometimes precipitate or aggravate behavior disorders (Fabish, 1957; Jonas, 1965; Itil and Myers, 1973). In aggressive mental retardates thioridazine was associated with an increase in aggression (Elie et al. op cit) yet thioridazine has been used in combination with anticonvulsants in the treatment of behavior disorders and appeared to have beneficial effects in some patients (Itil and Rizzo, 1967; Boelhouwer et al., 1968).

In several early published uncontrolled studies the authors expressed the opinion that neuroleptics exerted a beneficial effect on hostility, aggression and impulsiveness. Many clinicians use neuroleptics in the treatment of personality disorders including in patients who are violent. (Tardiff and Maurice, 1977); neuroleptics appear to be useful in the treatment of some violent patients but the evidence at present is inconclusive.

Anticonvulsants

Diphenylhydantoin (DPH) was found to decrease feelings of irritability and hostility in *neurotic* patients (Stephens and Shaffer, 1970). There are several open studies with DPH in which apparently DPH reduced aggression but this has not been confirmed in double blind placebo controlled studies.

Several writers have claimed beneficial changes in mood and behavior with carbamezapine in uncontrolled studies with epileptics including patients with epileptic psychoses; the authors reported a decrease in irritability, hostility, im-pulsiveness and a substantial improvement in social adjustment. In a few patients, irritability increased and explosiveness was aggravated, particularly in patients with brain atrophy and dementia. There are several controlled studies in which carbamezapine was compared with other anticonvulsants in epileptics and in which the psychotropic effects of the drug have been evaluated; generally the results tended to favor carbamezapine. In two placebo controlled studies the results were somewhat conflicting. These studies have been reviewed by Dalby (1975).

In uncontrolled studies carbamezapine appeared to be effective in the treatment of patients with the emotional dyscontrol syndrome and in the treatment of aggression. However, there are no controlled studies of carbamezapine in the treatment of these conditions and there is no evidence at present that carbamezapine is more effective than other anticonvulsants in the treatment of aggression or violent oubursts.

Combination of Anticonvulsants with Other Drugs

Itil and Rizzo op cit. (1967) treated adolescents who had explosive and aggressive traits with a combination of DPH and thioridazine. The authors reported that psychopathology improved and this improvement was highly correlated with a decrease of slow activity and a reduction of an epilepticlike pattern on the EEG and an increase of alpha index. Boelhouwer et al. (op cit) compared the effects of DPH, thioridazine, a combination of the two and placebo in young adults who had uncontrollable impulsive and antisocial behavior. Patients who showed 14 and 6 per second positive spiking of the EEG showed a better response to the combination of drugs than to either drug alone, whereas patients without positive spiking showed the best response to DPH alone. These studies suggest that at least in some patients a combination of an anticonvulsant drug with a psychotropic drug may be superior to the individual constituents alone. At present it is not possible to make a prediction which of the patients will respond this way and these studies require replications.

Stimulants

The findings of two uncontrolled studies with adult sociopaths suggest that some of the patients had benefited from amphetamines at least temporarily (Hill, 1947; Shovron, 1947). There are three published controlled studies in which either amphetamine or methylphenidate was used in the treatment of delinquent boys who were aggressive and impulsive. Korey (1944) in the early 1940s, found in a single blind study that about half of the teenage boys who were impulsive and aggressive had improved with amphetamine; their conduct and their school performance improved. Conners et al. (1971) found in younger delinquent boys no benefit from methylphenidate; however, this study had lasted only for two weeks. Eisenberg et al. (1963), in a four month controlled study with amphetamine, found a significant improvement in behavior in that the boys became easier to manage and less destructive. Wood et al. (1976) compared the effect of methylphenidate and placebo in adults who had persistent psychiatric abnormalities including impulsivity and emotional instability (but were not violent) who had been diagnosed in childhood as having had minimal brain dysfunction (MBD). In a short double blind part of the study, the patient appeared to benefit from methylphenidate and in an open study from pemoline or a tricyclic antidepressant. The findings tend to support the authors' conclusion that in some adults who had been diagnosed as having MBD in childhood this abnormality persists into adult life and it is concealed by other psychiatric symptoms and other diagnostic labels.

There are some impulsive adolescents and possibly some adults who were hyperactive in childhood, who have persisting psychiatric symptoms including impulsivity and aggression which have changed with the passage of years but perhaps still have essentially the same pathology as they had in childhood; these patients may benefit from treatment with stimulants. However, long-term outpatient treatment carries the obvious risks of habituation and of abuse of the drug.

Lithium

There have been several case reports and uncontrolled studies on the treatment of aggressive patients who were not manic with lithium. These studies have been listed by Dale (1980). Sheard (1971) conducted a single blind multiple crossover study of lithium; he found that in young male delinquents who were frequently aggressive and impulsive that serious aggressive episodes decreased when lithium level was high as compared at times when lithium level was below 0.6 mEq/liter. The author also found that serious aggressive incidents decreased more than total antisocial incidents without aggression. Tupin et al. (1973), in one of the early open studies, examined the effects of lithium on prisoners with explosive personalities and others who were violent and had diagnoses of schizophrenia or "possible schizophrenia;" many had either a history of brain injury or nonspecific abnormal EEGs. During treatment with lithium there was a significant decrease in the number of disciplinary actions for violent behavior. The prisoners reported a greater ability to reflect on the consequences of their actions and a greater ability to control anger when provoked. In this study also violent and aggressive behavior decreased more than nonviolent sociopathic acts. Worral et al. (1975) in a double blind crossover study of lithium and placebo with female aggressive mental defectives found significantly less aggression while on lithium.

Sheard et al. (1976) found in a double blind study with young delinquents who had committed serious aggressive crimes that lithium was significantly superior to placebo. At the end of three months treatment, the incidents of major infractions had gradually decreased until they had reached zero. The number of infractions increased again in the lithium group after medication was withdrawn.

The maintenance treatment with lithium in patients who commit unpremeditated acts of violence is a promising development. Patients who are explosive, impulsive and tend to respond with anger and aggression to small provocations tend to benefit. Unfortunately many of these patients lack the self discipline to take lithium regularly, side effects of the drug are poorly tolerated by impulsive patients with poor motivation and many are likely to discontinue the drug.

The findings in the study on the effects of lithium in epileptics are conflicting. There are at present no adequately controlled double blind studies; the evidence suggests that in some patients both epilepsy and behavior disturbance can be aggravated by the administration of lithium, whereas in other patients there is a decrease of aggressive behavior. The findings suggest that a history of brain damage or an abnormal EEG are not an absolute contraindication for treatment with lithium.

INTERMITTENT EXPLOSIVE DISORDER

This syndrome has also been described as the "emotional dyscontrol syndrome" and "the episodic behavioral disorder." Guidelines for the treatment of these conditions have been described by Elliott (1976), Monroe (1970), and Kellner (1982b op cit). At present there are no adequate controlled studies to suggest that one treatment is superior to another and the most effective treatment is probably not the same for all patients. Benzodiazepines, (preferably oxazepam or perhaps halazepam) because of their safety, may be tried first in larger doses than those prescribed for anxiety states and if this is ineffective an anticonvulsant in increasing doses can be tried alone and later in combination. The other drugs which have been used for the control of violent behavior which are listed above should be tried if the response to previous treatments is inadequate. Propranolol has been used in uncontrolled studies by Elliott (1977) in doses up to 240 mg daily and by Yudowsky-Stuart et al., (1981) in doses up to 520 mg daily with apparently good results.

FUTURE RESEARCH

There are large gaps in our knowledge on the control of aggression and violent behavior. Several of the observations from uncontrolled studies have not been tested or not been confirmed in double blind studies. For example, the long-term effects of oxazepam in large doses in seriously violent behavior is not known. There have been too few controlled studies with SCH 12679 which appears to have specific antiaggressive properties. There are no controlled studies with propranolol in aggression. There are too few studies in which the effects of combination of drugs were compared with the individual constituents; these studies are difficult to carry out and the results are difficult to interpret but they might yield valuable knowledge. In many patients the use of drugs should be the first treatment until psychotherapy, impulse control and anger control have been adequately tried. The psychotherapeutic strategies are surveyed in another chapter of this volume and have been summarized elsewhere (Kellner, 1982a,b op cit). The proportion of patients which will ultimately benefit more from psychological treatments and the proportion which will have to be treated predominantly with drugs is at present not known. It is also unknown the extent to which drug treatment and psychotherapy interact. Research in drug treatment and in the psychological management of anger and impulsiveness has shown promising leads. It will take many years to evaluate the usefulness and the limitations of the existing treatments.

REFERENCES

Albert, Jean-Marie, Elie, R., Cooper, S.F., et al. (1971). Efficacy of SCH-12679 in the management of aggressive mental retardates. *Curr. Ther. Res.* 21: (6)786-795.

Ayd, F.J. (1980). Parenteral (IM/IV) droperidol for acutely disturbed behavior in psychotic and non-psychotic individuals. *Int. Drug Ther. Newsletter* 15: (3),13-16.

Barnes, R.J. (1977). Mesoridazine (Serentil) in personality disorders: A controlled trial in adolescent patients. *Dis. Nerv. Syst.* 38:258-264.

Barnett, A., Malick, J.B., and Taber, R.I. (1973). Chemical and electrical treatment of aggression. *Psychopharm. Bull.* 9:17.

Boelhouwer, C., Henry, C.E., Glueck, B.C., et al. (1968). Positive spiking. A double blind control study on its significance in behavior disorders, both diagnostically and therapeutically. *Am. J. Psychiatry* 125:65-73.

Cereghino, J.J., Brock, J.T., van Meter, J.C., et al. (1974). Carbamazepine for epilepsy. *Neurology* 24:401-410.

Conners, C.K., Kramer, R., Rothschild, G.H., et al. (1971). Treatment of young delinquent boys with diphenylhydantoin sodium and methylphenidate. *Arch. Gen. Psychiatry* 24:156-160.

Covi, L., Lipman, R.S., and Smith, V.K. (1977). *Diazepam Induced Hostility in Depression.* Paper presented at the Annual Meeting of the American Psychiatric Association in Toronto, Canada, May 2-6.

Covi, L., Rickels, K., Lipman, R.S., McNair, D.M., Smith, V.K., Downing, R., Kahn, R. and Fisher, S. (1981). Effects of psychotropic agents on primary depression. *Psychopharmacol. Bull.* 17:100-103.

Dalby, M.A. (1975). In: J.K. Penry and D.D. Daly, eds., *Advances in Neurology.* Vol. II, Chapter 18, New York: Raven Press.

Dale, P.G. (1980). Lithium therapy in aggressive mentally subnormal patients. *Br. J. Psychiatry* 137:469-474.

DiMascio, A., Shader, R.I. and Harmatz, J. (1969). Psychotropic drugs and induced hostility. *Psychosomatics* 10:46-47.

Eisenberg, L., Lachman, R., Molling, P.A., et al. (1963). A psychopharmacologic experiment in a training school for delinquent boys: Methods, problems, findings. *Am. J. Orthopsychiatry* 33:431-447.

Elie, R., Langlois, Y., Cooper, S.F., et al. (1980). Comparison of SCH-12679 and thioridazine in aggressive mental retardates. *Can. J. Psychiatry* 25: 484–491.

Elliott, F.A. (1976). The neurology of explosive rage: The dyscontrol syndrome. *Practioner* 217:50–60.

Elliott, F.A. (1977). Propranolol for the control of belligerent behavior following acute brain damage. *Ann. Neurol.* 1:489–491.

Fabish, W. (1957). The effect of chlorpromazine on the EEG of epileptics. *J. Neurol. Neurosurg. Psychiatry* 20:185.

Feldman, P.E. (1967). *Current Views on Antianxiety Agents.* Pamphlet from a scientific exhibit presented at the Annual Meeting of the American Medical Association, Houston, Texas.

Gardos, G., DiMascio, A., Salzman, C., et al. (1968). Differential actions of chlordiazepoxide and oxazepam on hostility. *Arch. Gen. Psychiatry* 18: 757–760.

Hill, D. (1947). Amphetamine in psychopathic states. *Br. J. Addict.* 44:50.

Itil, T.M., Myers, J.P. (1973). Epileptic and anti-epileptic properties of psychotropic drugs. In: J. Mercier, ed., *International Encyclopedia of Pharmacology and Therapeutics* 2:(19), New York: Pergamon.

Itil, T.M., Rizzo, A.E. (1967). Behavior-disturbed adolescents. *Electroencephalogr. Clin. Neurophysiol.* 23:81.

Itil, T.M. and Wadud, A. (1975). Treatment of human aggression with major tranquilizers, antidepressants and newer psychotropic drugs. *J. Nerv. Ment. Dis.* 100:83–99.

Jonas, A.D. (1965). *Ictal and Subictal Neurosis, Diagnosis and Treatment.* Springfield, Ill., Charles C Thomas.

Kellner, R. (1978). Drug treatment of personality disorders and delinquents. In: W.H. Reid, ed., *Psychopath*, New York: Brunner/Mazel.

Kellner, R. (1982a). Treatment of personality disorders. In: J.W. Jefferson, J.H. Greist and R. Spitzer, eds., *The Treatment of Mental Disorders.* Oxford University Press (in press).

Kellner, R. (1982b). Treatment of disorders of impulse control. *Ibid.*

Kochansky, G.E., Salzman, C., Shader, R.I., et al. (1975). The differential effects of chlordiazepoxide and oxazepam on hostility in a small group setting. *Am. J. Psychiatry* 132:8.

Korey, S.R. (1944). The effects of benzedrine sulfate on the behavior of psychopathic and neurotic juvenile delinquents. *Psychiatr. Q.* 18:127–137.

Lion, John R. (1979). Benzodiazepines in the treatment of aggressive patients. *J. Clin. Psychiat.* 40:70–71.

McDonald, R.L. (1967). The effects of personality type on drug response. *Arch. Gen. Psychiatry* 17:680–686.

Molling, P.A., Lockner, A.W., Sauls, R.J. et al. (1962). Committed delinquent boys. *Arch. Gen. Psychiatry* 7:96–102.

Monroe, R.R. (1970). *Episodic Behavioral Disorders.* Cambridge, Mass., Harvard University Press.

Rickles, K. and Clyde, D.J. (1967). Clyde Mood Scale changes in anxious outpatients produced by chlordiazepoxide therapy. *J. Nerv. Ment. Dis.* 145: 154–157.

Rickles, K. and Downing, R.W. (1974). Chlordiazepoxide and hostility in anxious outpatients. *Am. J. Psychiatry* 131:442–444.

Salzman, C., Kochansky, G.E., Shader, R.I., et al. (1974). Chlordiazepoxide induced hostility in a small group setting. *Arch. Gen. Psychiatry* 31:401–405.
Salzman, C., Kochansky, G.E., Shader, R.I., et al. (1975). Is oxazepam associ-
ated with hostility? *Dis. Nerv. System* 36(2):30-32.
Sheard, M.H. (1971). Effect of lithium in human aggression. *Nature* 230:113–
114.
Sheard, M.H., Marini, J.L., Bridges, C.I., et al. (1976). The effect of lithium on
impulsive aggressive behavior in man. *Am. J. Psychiatry* 133:1409-1413.
Shovron, J.J. (1947). Benzedrine in psychopathy and behavior disorders. *Br. J.
Addiction* 44:58.
Solomon, K. (1975). High-dose benzodiazepines in the treatment of severe
neurotic anxiety. *J. Clin. Psychiatry* 39:610-613.
Stephens, J.H. and Shaffer, J.W. (1970). A controlled study of the effects of
diphenylhydantoin on anxiety, irritability, and anger in neurotic out-
patients. *Psychopharmacologia* 17:169-181.
Tardiff, M. D. and Maurice, W.L. (1977). The care of violent patients by psychi-
atrists. *Can. Psychiatr. Assoc. J.* 22:83-86.
Tupin, J.P. (1975). Management of violent patients. In: Richard I. Shader, ed.,
Manual of Psychiatric Therapeutics, Boston: Little, Brown and Company.
Tupin, J.P., Smith, D.B., Clanon, T.L., et al. (1973). The long-term use of
lithium in aggressive prisoners. *Compr. Psychiatry* 14:311-317.
Van Leeuwen, A.M.H., Molders, J., Sterkmans, P., et al. (1977). Droperidol in
acutely agitated patients: A double blind placebo controlled study. *J.
Nerv. Ment. Dis.* 164:(4)280-283.
Wood, G.R., Reimherr, F.W., Wender, P.H., et al. (1976). Diagnosis and treat-
ment of minimal brain dysfunction in adults. *Arch. Gen. Psychiatry* 33:
1453-1460.
Worral, E.P., Moody, J.P., and Naylor, G.J. (1975). Lithium in non-manic de-
pressives: Antiaggressive effect and red blood cell lithium values. *Br. J.
Psychiatry* 126:464-468.
Yudofsky, S., Williams, D., and Gorman, J. (1980). Propranolol in the treatment
of rage and violent behavior in patients with chronic brain syndromes. *Am.
J. Psychiatry* 138(2):218-220.
Zisook, S., Rogers, P.J. and Fachingbauer, T.R. (1978). Absence of hostility in
outpatients after administration of halazepam: A new benzodiazepine.
J. Clin. Psychiatry 39:(8)683-686.

30

Review of Research into the Use of Drugs and the Treatment of Sexual Deviations with Special Reference to the Use of Cyproterone Acetate (Androcur)

GAVIN TENNENT

INTRODUCTION

It has been known for centuries that drugs are capable of influencing sexual behavior. Generally, the search has been for drugs that will increase sexual potency, but apart from amphetamines (and even then this only in high doses) there are no truly sexually stimulating drugs.

Alcohol was probably the first drug recognized to reduce potency and although there is a lack of scientific data on the subject (Hastings, 1963), there is general agreement that there is a dose related association between alcohol and sexual performance if not libido. This differentiation between potency (which has been defined as the ability of the male to develop and sustain a penile erection sufficient to conclude coitus to orgasm and ejaculation) and libido is not always made in the literature, and although there are a large number of drugs that impair potency (sympatholytics, ganglion blockers, bromides, opiates, lithium), the evidence for any of these having a direct effect on libido is lacking.

Concern with the failure, or relative failure, of psychotherapy and behavioral methods to treat the serious or dangerous sexual deviant has led to the search for alternative lines of treatment. Castration (well reviewed by Heim and Hurst, 1979), apart from any ethical considerations, is not necessarily effective in that the sexual responsiveness of castrated males is much greater and more varied than has often been suggested (Eibl, 1978), and there is even dispute as to whether libido is (Brown and Courtis, 1970) or is not (Charneatel, 1977) reduced. Psychosurgery again poses serious ethical problems. Like castration, it is not only totally irreversible but also questionable in effectiveness (B.M.J., 1969; Dieckman et al., 1975).

Drug treatments that seek to suppress sexual libido also have been opposed on ethical grounds. Bancroft (1979) argues for the need "to distinguish between their proper use in a therapeutic relationship when the patient takes advantage of their effects to facilitate his own self control and their use as a method of social control imposed upon the person." Ethical problems become particularly acute when the individual to be treated is serving a prison sentence, when consent to treatment may increase his chance of getting parole, or if serving a determinate sentence being released at all. There are a number of papers on this subject (Field, 1975; Ferranti, 1976; Whitehead, 1981), but it is beyond the scope of this paper to go into this area. It is, however, a crucial area of concern for the future use of these drugs.

Ethical issues apart, there are many unresolved problems, both practical and theoretical, surrounding the use of drugs and the treatment of sexual deviation.

First, there are the issues surrounding not just the definition of sexual deviation but, having done that, for whom treatment is really necessary. Not only are there wide variations in what societies may call deviant, both between societies and within the given subgroup (e.g., pedophilia where the difference may be greater between individuals in such a subgroup than between them and those who do not share that label) (Barlow, 1976). What goes to make up sexual arousal and the factors that increase it or decrease it are not well understood, and it is inconsistent to assume that whereas normal sexual behavior is both complex and varied, deviant sexual behavior just consists of an inappropriate penile response (Crawford, 1979). Deviant arousal anyway is probably not purely a qualitative difference in sexual arousal but in many situations a quantitative one (Freund et al., 1972).

In practice the study of drugs in the treatment of sexual devaints has been restricted to sexual offenders, but even here there are problems, e.g., in the relevance of treatment. In general, sex offenders appear to have a lower rate of recidivism than other criminals and lower still if any further sex crimes are considered (Radzinowicz and Turner, 1957). Even with specific crimes like rape, re-conviction for a further offense is uncommon (Soothill, 1976). To further complicate the issue, several studies show that many habitual offenders have at least one sex offense in their record (Tennent et al., 1974). In theory then, one might expect that drug treatments for sex offenders will be reserved for only the dangerous serious sex offenders. It is, however, difficult to believe that this is so. Most treatment methods have been applied to diverse groupings of sexual offenders (often including large numbers of exhibitionists) making realistic assessment of the effectiveness of the procedure almost impossible.

This, then, brings us to the second mean problem in evaluating the use of treatments, that of methodology. The application of a rigorous scientific approach to the evaluation of treatment measures is rare in this field. The vast majority of studies have lacked objectivity and, even apart from the lack of controlled studies, the methods of assessment leave much to be desired.

The assessment of the action of drugs on sexual behavior does, indeed, pose considerable problems, particularly if, as often happens in this field, the subject population may have a vested interest in "feigning good." The problems of assessment too, concern not just an apprisal of how we measure but exactly what we are trying to re-measure. For example, the measurement of blood hormone levels presupposes that variations of these have some effect on sexual behavior. Similarly, measurements of sexual arousal (usually involving penile plethysmograph) assume that this has some relationship to sexual attitudes and libido. There are problems with the procedure itself, although in recent years fairly sophisticated techniques have been developed (Hinton et al., 1980). Ideally, therefore, assessments should reflect a combination of different measures involving self reports, ratings of both overt behavior and fantasies, measurement of sexual attitudes, and the measurement of physiological response.

THE USE OF MAJOR TRANQUILIZERS

It has been long observed that tranquilizing drugs have an effect on sexual performance. Apart from relief of anxiety and tension surrounding sexual difficulties, some observers suggest they have more specific effects. Sandison et al. (1960) described patients on 50 to 75 mg of thioridazine daily who developed erectional difficulties and reported failure to ejaculate. Freyhan (1961) and Singh (1961) reported similar problems and a reduction in libido on patients receiving 70 to 150 mg thioridazine daily.

Litkey and Feniczy (1967) treated a group of twelve patients who all had "excessive uncontrollable masturbation" with homosexual orientation.

This was a very miscellaneous group containing, as it did, drug addicts and schizophrenics. However, in all twelve a dramatic improvement (as judged by clinical assessment) was noted after three weeks, with a marked diminution of sexual preoccupation.

Tennent et al. (1974) in their comparison of benperidol, chlorpromazine, and placebo failed to show any effects of chlorpromazine on reducing any of their measures of sexual interest and activity. However, the dose of chlorpromazine was low (125 mg daily).

Bartholomew (1966) compared the effect of fluphenazine enanthanate (25 mg i.m. every two weeks for a period up to twenty-four weeks) on 26 psychotic patients with anxiety tension states but no sexual problems and 26 patients with a "considerable history of deviant sexual behavior," nineteen as a result of some Court Order. Seventeen patients in each group reported reduction in sexual interest, the majority after the first injection.

Butyrophenones

Benperidol is a neuroleptic drug belonging to the Butyrophenone series and somewhat similar in chemical structure to Haloperidol. In its range of clinical effects it is similar to Chlorpromazine except for the suggested anti-libidinal effect (Bobon, Collard, and Pritchard, 1966). Its use for reducing sexual drive has been reported by Sterkmans and Geertz (1966) who achieved satisfactory results in twenty out of thirty patients showing a variety of disorders of sexual behavior.

Field (1973) and Matthews (1975) have reported on its use with groups or prisoners, the latter in a controlled trial with cyproterone acetate. In Field's study, 14 were in prison and 14 were attending an out-patient clinic. The universal findings were abolition of sexual desire and inability to obtain an erection either as a result of fantasy or of masturbation. All the subjects were satisfied that the medication controlled their abnormal sexual drive although in two cases this loss of desire was not accompanied by any diminution of sexual fantasies. During the two-year period of the trial none of the 14 men at risk had been charged with any further sexual offense. Dosage required varied from 0.5 mg to 1 mg daily.

Tennent et al. (1974) compared the effects of chlorpromazine, benperidol, and a placebo in their effects on recidivist sex offenders in an English Special Hospital. This study was as much concerned with methodology as with drug effect and the duration of treatment was short (six weeks on each). The dosage of benperidol was 1.25 mg daily from the fourteenth day onwards and chlorpromazine 125 mg daily from the fourteenth day onwards. No significant difference between drugs was found except in measured sexual interest ratings and the sexual attitude scores where benperidol produced significantly lower scores than either placebo or chlorpromazine which did not significantly differ from each other.

How phenothiazines and butyrophenones work to produce these effects is not entirely clear. Effect on erection and ejaculation has been attributed to the anticholinergic properties of the drug (Sanderson et al., 1960). There is also, however, some evidence (Beaumont et al., 1972) of endocrine changes after chlorpromazine administration, and to a larger extent after butyrophenone treatment. These results were not confirmed in another study (Murray et al., 1975).

THE USE OF HORMONE TREATMENTS

The sex hormones can be divided into three groups: the estrogens, the androgens, and the progestogens. All three have been used in the treatment of sexual disorders but only the first two will be considered here, as the progestogens form the subject of a separate paper in this symposium.

THE USE OF ESTROGEN

Dunn (1940) treated a male sexual offender undergoing imprisonment for repeated convictions with stilboestrol 5 mg daily for sixty days and then 5 mg every other day for thirty-six days. Complete loss of libido was reported and gynecomastia and testicular degenerative changes were also reported.

Foote (1944) treated a sexual psychoapthic patient with stilboestrol 1 mg daily. After thirty days masturbation ceased and sexual preoccupation disappeared. After the treatment had been stopped, suppression of sexual interest lasted briefly and after thirty-two days there was a complete relapse which again yielded to further treatment with stilboestrol. During the treatment gynecomastia was again noted.

Golla and Hodge (1949) reported on the treatment of 12 persons "complaining of an uncontrollable sexual urge that had led to trouble." Their treatment was based on the observation made at the Burden Clinic that high doses of estrone used for the treatment of acromegalic patients produced complete loss of sexual power accompanied by softening of the testicles, and gynecomastia in patients being treated for pituitary adenomas. In all the male cases of acromegalia treated with estrogen, libido had practically vanished after fourteen days. Cessation of the treatment after various periods was followed by return of libido in about two weeks; but in observations lasting as long as six years it had been found that libido was absent so long as maintenance doses of estrone were continued. Potency could be restored by three times weekly injections of testosterone proprionate 25 mg, while the estrone treatment was continuing. They state in their paper that there was no reason to believe that even after years of estrone treatment sexual power is permanently abolished. In all of the 13 cases they treated they were successful in abolishing libido. Estrone and estradiol benzoate were equally effective. Among their conclusions, they comment that libido was rapidly removed in all cases, whereas after castration it may persist in an appreciable number for variable periods. They suggested that the effective action of estrone treatment was not confined to its direct action on the testicles.

Bierer and Someren (1950) reported the use of stilboestrol in the treatment of a schizoid young man who had a fear of his compulsive feeling to rape women (he had never done so) — here, stilboestrol therapy was used as an adjunct to other re-socialization therapies; when the stilboestrol therapy was stopped, although sexual desire and interest reappeared, the pathological mental symptoms did not.

Whitaker (1959) gave stilboestrol 5 mg daily to 26 patients presenting with a variety of psychosexual disorders (basing this treatment on observations suggesting that estrogen might inhibit male sexuality at psychological and physiological levels). Treatment was given for two weeks at a time only. In all subjects, inhibition of erections and sexual fantasies occurred for a minimum of six weeks and up to six months — in most cases there was a complete inhibition for about three months. He concluded that intermittent administration of estrogen had a very definite part to play in the overall management of psychosexual disorders in males, stressing that it was not a method of cure but an effective method of control.

Field and Williams (1970) report on the use of depot estradiol BPC 100 mg implanted subcutaneously. Their previous experience with oral stilboestrol and/or psychotherapy with imprisoned sex offenders had given disappointing results. They comment that "even those prisoners who were able to take the hormone (stilboestrol) in sufficient amounts to reduce libido without producing nausea, it was a too frequent finding that when the three weeks supply of stilboestrol that had been given to them on release had been exhausted they did not go the general practitioner who had been contacted to obtain a further supply or attend the psychiatric out-patient clinic in the area in which they had gone to live and at which an appointment had been made for them." The aim of the treatment was to produce impotence or near impotence. In all, 25 cases underwent the full course of treatment. A control group of men who reached criteria for treatment but did not have it were included in this study. Two year follow-up showed that there was a significantly lower rate of re-conviction in the treated group. It should be commented that the prisoners were all serving fixed sentences and that the question of parole was not a relevant factor. Assessment was done purely on the basis of individual reports and re-convictions.

Bancroft et al. (1974) carried out a double-blind crossover trial comparing the behavioral changes following estrogens and antiandrogens. Drugs were only given for a six-week period, the estrogen at a level of ethinylestradiol 0.01 mg b.d., measurements of change being made on self-ratings, rating scales, and penile plethysmography as well as measuring endocrine changes. When compared with no treatment, both ethinylestradiol and cyproterone acetate significantly lowered both the sexual interest score and the sexual activity score. Sexual attitudes were not significantly altered. With erectile responses only cyproterone acetate produced a weak effect in reducing erectile and subjective responses to erotic stimuli. Further work using estradiol implants and its effects on hormones and responses to strong erotic stimuli (film) showed that using higher doses of estradiol a complete suppression of penile response to erotic stimuli could be obtained and that both hormones and penile response returned to normal within 18 weeks after cessation of treatment (see Figure 1).

There seems very little doubt, therefore, that estrogens do produce a decrease in both libido and sexual arousal and that this is reversible probably after lengthy periods. However, with estrogens there are the risks of troublesome and irreversible side effects such as gynecomastia or thrombosis. In some studies their use has been limited by nausea and vomiting. A further rare but grave complication (carcinoma of the breast) Symmers (1968) probably restricts their use to very short term when it has been used as an additional factor in other forms of either psychotherapeutic or social rehabilitation treatments.

THE USE OF ANTIANDROGEN

The use of antiandrogen – cyproterone acetate for an extended review of the functions of androgens and antiandrogens and some of the problems involved in dissecting their modes of actions and their measurements, reference is made to the symposium "Androgens and Anti-Androgens" edited by Martini and Motta. From this, and from the earlier papers by Laschet and Neuman, an inadequately brief summary of the pharmacology and biological action of cyproterone acetate has been extracted. Two types of antiandrogen are recognized:

1) The "pure" antiandrogens, which have only antiandrogenic properties. Examples of these are cyproterone and flutamide. If pure antiandrogens are administered an androgen deficit is stimulated – this results in an increased release of gonadotrophines and thus enhanced synthesis of testosterone. It has no effect on libido or sexual responsiveness.

2) The second type of antiandrogens are those that have both androgenic and antigonadotrophic properties. Cyproterone acetate and chlomadinone acetate are examples. Both these substances also have potent progestogenic effects, particularly the latter, which is widely used as an oral contraceptive. Cyproterone acetate, on the other hand, has been developed mainly for its use in the treatment of hypersexuality, although it has also been used quite extensively in the treatment of female hirsutism.

Studies with radioactive C^{14} labelled cyproterone acetate in human volunteers (Kolb and Roepke, 1968) show that about 35% of the normal dose is absorbed, half of it disappears in the urine, the balance being excreted in bile.

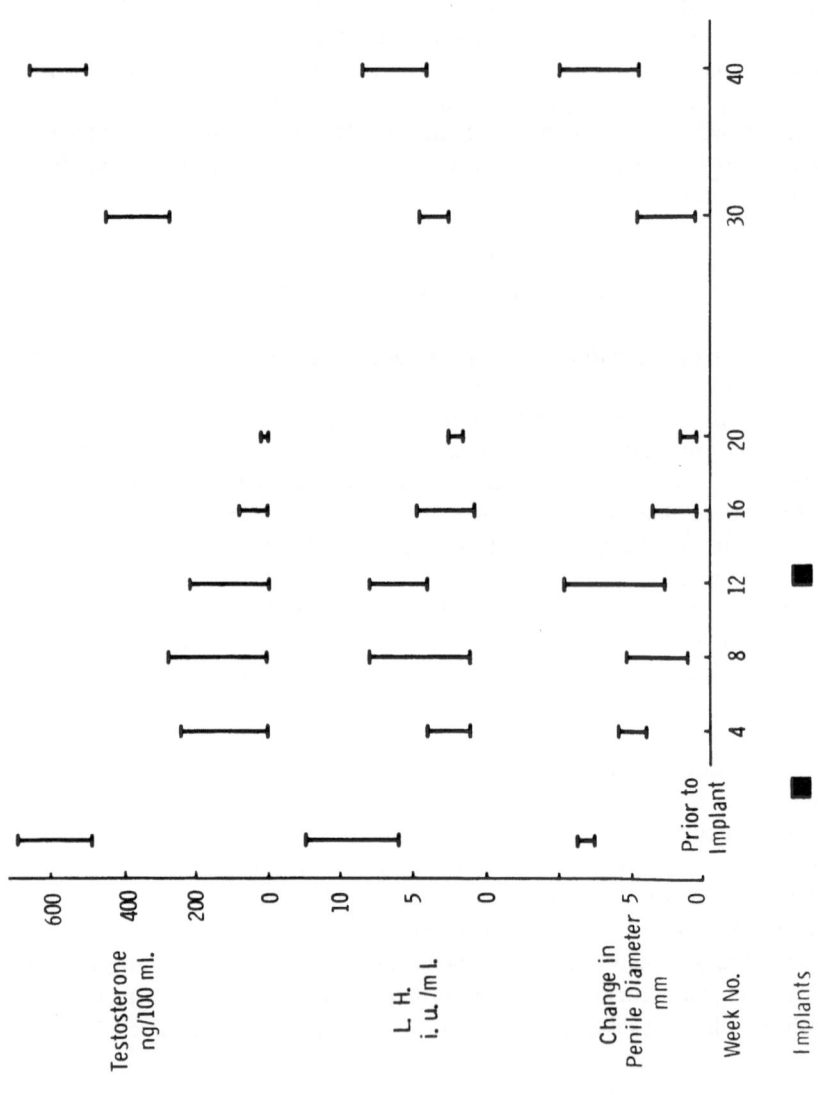

Figure 1   Testosterone LH levels and penile responsiveness before and after estrogen implants.

About 50% of the absorbed steroid is excreted within forty-eight hours of administration. Maximum blood levels seem to be reached after about 24 hours. Cyproterone acetate is available mainly in tablet form, although from Germany and New Zealand there are reports of the use of a depot preparation given by injection every ten to fourteen days.

Antiandrogens possessing antigonadotrophic properties inhibit in principle all androgen dependent functions and organ systems. The antiandrogenic action of cyproterone acetate results from it being a selective competitor with testosterone at organ receptor sites. In experimental animals, cyproterone acetate has been shown to block the stimulant effect of exogenous testosterone on seminal vesicles (Edwards, 1970), prostate gland (Neuman et al., 1968), testes (Neuman et al., 1966), and sebaceous glands (Neuman and Elgar, 1966).

Its antigonadotrophic action results in blocking the secretion of pituitary gonadotrophin (Johnson and Naqubi, 1969) and decreases the formation and excretion of testosterone and its metablites. The mode of action on the molecular level appears to involve competition between cyproterone acetate and 5 alpha dihydro-testosterone for a specific cellular androgen receptor of target tissues (Fang and Lio, 1969).

A number of studies have been made of changes in various endocrine factors during treatment. Urinary excretion of 17 oxo-steroids, 17 oxogenic steroids and total estrogens are unchanged (Laschet and Laschet, 1967; Ott and Hoffet, 1968) while urinary excretion of gonadotrophins are reduced although not completely suppressed. Murray (1975) showed that cyproterone acetate produces a reduction in plasma testosterone LH and FSH, but no change in plasma estrogen level.

Sperm counts decrease rapidly — this is not complete, however, as in Laschet studies (1978) three pregnancies have been reported. Sperm counts have been reported as returning to normal after cessation of treatment after twelve weeks and after eleven months (Ott, 1968; Petry, 1972) Hoffet (1980) and Itil (1976) have also reported an effect of cyproterone acetate on the EEG.

Side Effects

These seem to be uncommon in any of the British trials, but the more extensive German studies (Laschet, Mothes, Dein) suggest an incidence of gynecomastia of about 15-20% starting fairly late on in treatment and apparently (Mothes) disappearing after cessation of treatment. The breast enlargement is probably due to the progestational action of the drug.

Five to ten percent of patients develop a depressive reaction and during long-term treatment there tends to be a variable effect in body weight, a decrease of body hair, an increase and softening of scalp hair, and a decrease of sebum excretion. Early suggestions of alteration in nitrogen metabolism with a

Table 1. **Results of Studies using Cyproterone Acetate**

Author	Subjects	Age range	Treatment setting	Diagnosis	Type of patient/problem
Appelt (1974)	18	?	Hospital	Schizo/P.D.	Committed patients
Bancroft (1974)	12	19–34	Security Hospital	P.D.	Mixed offenses
Barron (1977)	6(10)	24–53	OP/IP	P.D. Organic factors	Persistent sex offenders
Cooper (1972)	3	40–72	OP	P.D.	Mixed offenses
Craft (1970)	6	15–31	IP	Severely subnormal	Hypersexuality with aggression
Davies (1974)	50	18–55	IP/OP	Schizo. Subnormal P.D.	Mixed offender & social problems
Dien	7*	?	Mental defic. + P. hosp.	Schizo.	Excess masturbation Pedophilia
Dein & Jeppesen	7	?	IP	Mental deficiency Institute	Excessive masturbation
Laschet (1973)	120	?		Mainly P.D.	50% sexual offenders Hypersexuality
Mothes (1973)	352	?	IP/OP	Mainly P.D. of subnormality	50% sex offenders
Saba et al. (1976)	42*	?	IP	Mental hospital	Pathologic hypersexuality and/or homo-sexuality

*includes female patients.

Drug dose	Time given	Assessment method	Results
100–250 mg	6–18 months	Rating scale	Encouraging for schizo with sexual delusions
100 mg	6 weeks	Rating scale Plethysmography self reports	Decrease in fantasies and self reports
100 mg	Up to 12 months	E.P.I. and other tests Self reports	All who stayed in trial decrease sex drive
50–150 mg	1–6 months	Rating scale Blood Hormone levels	Suppression of sexual responsiveness and general tranquilizing effect
100 mg	2–7 months	Plasma testosterine Clinical	Mixed results
50–200 mg	Several months	Clinical appraisal	sexual activity reduced in intensity, but not direction
50–300 mg	Up to 4 years	Clinical appraisal	5/7 satisfactory results
	4 months	?	No different from placebo
100–200 mg/day	6–57 months	?	Generally good results with specific exceptions
100–200 mg/day	1–4 years	Rating scales Clinical appraisal	70% success rate varying with group
200 mg	?	?	Hypersexuality progressively disappears. Orientation no change

protein deficit have not been confirmed. Care should be taken where there is evidence of thrombophlebitis or thromboembolic changes and unstable diabetes.

Clinical Results

The results of available clinical studies on cyproterone acetate are summarized in Table 1.

In only three of the studies were any attempts made to adequately control parameters. The vast bulk of the clinical data come from studies by Mothes and Laschet (some of the same patients appear to have appeared in both these clinical trials). These trials were carried out in the early days of cyproterone acetate usage and Laschet (1973) comments, "At the outset of these experiments the clinical properties of cyproterone acetate and, therefore, its indication in this type of treatment were unknown. Our attitudes towards its use were somewhat negative. Consequently, although we knew which subjects received treatment, methodology can be termed blind trials." In none of the Laschet papers that are available in English are details given of the assessment of change, although it would seem in her series that while the mentally handicapped and those appearing because of sexual behavioral disorders improved, those with brain damage or schizophrenia showed little change.

Mothes reports on the results of administration of cyproterone acetate to 352 patients varying in age from under twenty to over ninety; ratings were made on previously constructed questionnaires by clinical testers. One interesting parameter they used as a measure of the success of cyproterone acetate treatment was that of social integration. Prior to treatment social integration was rated as disturbed for 63% of the cases. The figures after one year were 45% and after two years 37%. Treatment was rated as successful in 85% of the exhibitionists (51), 70% of those showing pedophiliac interest or homosexuality (28), and in 65%-70% of those presenting with heterosexual, hypersexuality, excessive masturbation, and rapists (82). The success of therapy was greatest among those living at home followed by those interred as punishment than those kept in homes. Worst results of therapy were found in those detained in psychiatric clinics. Apart from the study by Aphelt (1974) there is little to suggest that cyproterone acetate has any influence on sexual delusions when seen as part of schizophrenic syndrome and results with the subnormal possibly vary with the level of subnormality being good in those who are only mildly subnormal but less good in the severely subnormal. Although Laschet's study suggests that those with brain damage do less well, two of the six patients who did well in Baron's (1977) study had histories of organic brain damage. The group, in all studies, who seemed to do best is perhaps not surprisingly the group of patients who desire treatment for sexual deviations which directly and indirectly entail mental stress and/or severe social difficulties, who have good motivation, reasonable personalities, and some positive factors on which other constructive therapies can be based in conjunction with temporary suppression of sexual libido. Shaw (1978) for example has described the use of a Probation run group for the management of sexual problems in conjunction with the use of cyproterone acetate and Bancroft (1979) commented on the potential use of this or such drugs as an adjunct to our other therapies. However, one is left also with his conclusion that "the proper chemical base of these drugs has yet to be clarified but at the present time they should be used with caution and only in those cases where there is obvious clinical need to reduce sexual arousability per se."

In more general terms, it is this author's belief that such treatments can have a part to play, not just with sexual offenders but also in others whose sexuality gives rise to problems for them.

REFERENCES

Appelt, M. and Floru, L. (1974). Erfahungen uber die Beeinflussung der Sexualitat clurch Cyproterinacetat. *Int. Pharompsychiatry* 9:2.

Bancroft, J.II.J. (1979). Trcatment of deviant sexual behavior in R. Gains and B. Hudson (eds.), *Current Themes in Psychiatry* 2. London, Macmillan.

Bancroft, J., Tennent, G., Loucas, K. and Cass, J. (1974). The control of deviant sexual behavior by drugs. *Br. J. Psychiatry* 125:310-315.

Barlow, P.H. (1976). Assessment of sexual behavior in A.R. Gaminero, K.S. Cahoun and H.E. Adams (eds.), *Handbook of Behavioural Assessment.* New York, Wiley.

Baron, D.P. (1977). A clinical trial of cyproterone, acetate for sexual deviancy. *N.Z. Med. J.* 85:366-369.

Bartholomew, A.A. (1968). A long acting phenothiazine as a possible agent to control deviant sexual behavior. *Am. J. Psychiatry* 124:917-923.

Beumont, P.J.V., Harris, G.W., Carr, J., Friesen, H.G., Kolakowska, T., Mackinnon, P.C.B., Mandelbrote, B. and Wiles, D. (1972). Some endocrine effects of phenothiazines: a preliminary report. *J. Psychosom. Res.* 16: 297-304.

Bierer, J. (1950). Stilboestrol in outpatient treatment of sexual offenders. *Br. Med. J.* 1:935-936.

Bobon, J., Collard, J. and Pritchard, A. (1966). Paper presented at Fourth World Conference of Psychiatry. Madrid.

Brown, R.S. and Courtis, R.W. (1977). The castration alternative. *Can. J. Criminol. Corrections* 79:157-169.

B.M.J. (1969). Brain surgery for sexual disorders. *Br. Med. J.* 4:250-251.

Cooper, A.J., Ismail, A.A., Phanjoo, A.L. and Love, D.L. Antiandrogen (Cyproterone Acetate) therapy in Deviant Hypersexuality. *Br. J. Psychiatry* 120: 59-63.

Charney, C.W., Suarez, R. and Sadoughi, N. (1970). Castration in the male. *Med. Aspect Hum. Sexuality* 4:80-83.

Crawford, D.A. (1979). Modification of deviant sexual behavior: the need for a comprehensive approach. *Br. J. Psychiatry* 52:151-156.

Davies, T.S. (1974). Cyproterone acetate for male hypersexuality. *J. Int. Med. Res.* 2:159-163.

Dein, E. (1975). Clinical problems in cyproterone acetate therapy. *J. Int. Med. Res.* 3 Suppl. (4):13-15.

Dein, E. Jeffessen (1973). Antiandrogen in mentally subnormal. *Acta Psychiatrica Scand.* (Suppl.) (1):243-266.

Dunn, C.W. (1940). Stilboestral induced gynecomastia in the male. *J.A.M.A.* 115:2263-2264.

Eibl, E. (1978). Treatment and after care of 300 sex offenders especially with regard to penile plethysmography. In: Proceedings of the German Conference on treatment possibilities for Sex Offenders in Eppingen, 1977. Stutgart.

Edwards, D.A. (1970). Effects of cyproterone acetate on aggressive behavior and the seminal vesicles of male mice. *J. Endocrinol.* 46:477-481.

Fang, S. and Liqo, S. (1969). Antagonistic action of antiandrogens on the formation of a specific dehydrotestosterine-receptor protein complex in rat ventral prostate. *Med. Pharmocol.* 5:420-431.

Ferranti, F. (1976). Medico-Legal Considerations pertaining to Antiandrogens. In L. Martini and M. Motto *Androgens and Antiandrogens*. Raven Press, New York.

Field, L.H. and Williams, M. (1970). The hormonal treatment of sex offenders. *Med. Sci. Law* 10:27-34.

Field, L.H. (1973). Benperidol in the treatment of sexual offenders. *Med. Sci. Law* 13:195-196.

Field, L.H. (1975). The treatment of prisoners: Medico-legal problems. *J. Int. Med. Res.* Suppl. (3):27-29.

Foote, R.M. (1944). Hormone treatment of sex offenders. *J. Nerv. Ment. Dis.* 99:928-929.

Freund, K., Chan, S. and Coulthard, R. (1972). Phallometric diagnosis with non-admitters. *Behav. Res. Ther.* 17:451-457.

Freyhan, F.A. (1961). Loss of ejaculation during Melleril treatment. *Am. J. Psychiatry*. 118:171-172.

Golla, F.L. and Hodge, R.S. (1949). Hormone treatment of the sex offenders. *Lancet* 1:1006-1007.

Hastings, D.W. (1963). *Impotence and Frigity*. Churchill: London.

Heim, N. and Hursch, C.J. (1979). Castration of sex offenders: treatment or punishment? A review and critique of recent European literature. *Arch. Sex Behav.* 8:281-304.

Hinton, J.W., O'Neill, M.T. and Webster, S. (1980). Psychophysiological assessment of sex offenders in a security hospital. *Arch. Sex Behav.* 3:205-216.

Hoffat, H. (1980). The clinical use of antiandrogens in psychiatry. *Gynakologe* 13:33-43.

Itil, T.M. (1976). Rebirth of Hormones in Psychiatry. *Psychiat. J. Univ. Ottawa* 1 (No. 3):105-112.

Johnson, D.C. and Naqubi, B.H. (1969). Effects of cyproterone acetate on L.H. in immature rats. *Endocrinology* 84:421-425.

Kolb, K.H. and Roepke, H. (1968). The pharmacokinetics of cyproterone acetate, a comparative investigation in man and in the baboon. *Int. Zeitschrift fur klinische Pharmakologie, Therapie und Toxikologie* 1,3:187-190.

Laschet, U. (1973). Antiandrogen in the treatment of sex offenders: Mode of action and therapeutic outcome, J. Zublin and J. Money (eds.) In: *Contemporary Sexual Behavior: Critical Issues in the 1970's.* The Johns Hopkins Univ. Press, 311-319.

Laschet, U. and Laschet, L. (1975). Antiandrogens in the treatment of sexual deviations of men. *J. Steroid Biochem.* 6:821-826.

Litkey, I.J. and Feniczy, P. (1967). An approach to the control of homosexual practices. *Int. J. Neuropsychiat.* 3:20-23.

Mandelbrote, B.M. and Wiles, D. (1972). Some endocrine effects of phenothiazines: a preliminary report. *J. Psychosom. Res.* 16:297-304.

Martini, L. and Motta, M. (eds.) (1977). Androgens and Antiandrogens. Raven Press: New York.

Matthews, R. (1975). Comparative study of cyproterone acetate and benperidol. *J. Int. Med. Res.* 3 (Suppl. (4):22-26.

Mothes, C., Lenhert, J., Samimi, F. and Ufer, J. (1973). Clinical trial of cyproterone acetate in sexual deviations — collected assessment. *Schering Medical News* 2:26-41.

Murray, M.A.F., Bancroft, J.H.J., Anderson, D.C., Tennent, T.G. and Carr, P.J. (1975). Endocrine changes in male sexual deviants after treatment with antiandrogens, estrogens or tranquilizers. *J. Endocrinol.* 67:179-188.

Neumann, F. and von Berswordt-Wallraber, R. (1966). Effect of cyproterone acetate on testicular structure, spermatogenerics and accessory sexual glands of the testosterone treated by hypophysectomized rat. *J. Endocrinol.* 35:363.

Neumann, F., von Berswordt-Wallraber, R., Elger, R., Steinbeck, W., Hahn, J.D. and Kramer, M. (1970). Aspects of androgen-dependent events as studied by antiandrogens. *Rec. Prog. Hormone Res.* 26:337-405.

Ott, F. and Hoffet, H. (1968). Beeinflussung von Libido, Potenz und Hodenfunktion durch Antiandrogen. *Schweiz Med. Wschr.* 98:1812-1815.

Petry, R., Mauss, J., Rausch-Strooman, J.G. and Vermeulen, A. (1972). Reversible inhibition of Spermatogenesis in Men. *Horm. Metab. Res.* 4:386-388.

Radznowicz, Turner. (1957). *Sexual Offences.* Macmillan.

Saba, P., Galeone, F., Salvadorinif, F. and Rainer, E. (1976). Investigation on the role of Androgens on sexual behavior in patients with neuropsychiatric disorders. *Int. Symposium in Androgens & Antiandrogens.* Milan.

Sanderson, R.A. (1960). Clinical trial with Melleril in the treatment of schizophrenia. *J. Ment. Sci.* 106:732-741.

Shaw, R. (1978). The persistent sexual offender — control and rehabilitation. *Probation J.* 25:9-13.

Singh, H. (1961). A case of inhibition of ejaculation as a side effect of Melleril. *Am. J. Psychiatry* 117:1041-1042.

Soothill, K.L., Jack, A. and Gibbens, T.C.N. (1976). Rape: A 22-year cohort study. *Med. Sci. Law* 16:61-69.

Sterkmans, P and Geertz, F. (1966). Is Benperidol (R4504) the specific drug for the treatment of excessive and disturbed sexual behavior. *Acta Neuro. Psych. (Belgica)* 66:1030-1040.

Symers, St. C. (1968). Carcinoma of the breast in transexuals after surgical and hormonal interference with primary sex characteristics. *Br. Med. J.* 2: 83-85.

Tennent, G., Fenton, G.W., Fenwick, P.B.C. and Loucas, K. (1974). Male admissions to Broadmoor Hospital. *Br. J. Psychiatry* 125:44-50.

Tennent G., Bancroft, J. and Cass, J. (1974). The control of deviant behavior:
    A double blind controlled study of Benperidol, Chlorpromazine and
    Placebo. *Arch. Sex Behav.* 3:261–271.
Whitaker, L.H. (1959). Estrogen and Psychosexual Disorders. *Med. J. Aust.*
    2:547–549.
Whitehead, T. (1981). Multidisciplinary Approaches to Aggression Research 32.

31

Antiandrogenic Treatment of the Paraphilias

Paul A. Walker, Walter J. Meyer, Lee E. Emory, and Alan L. Rubin

INTRODUCTION

The senior author has been involved in a series of clinical research studies, since 1969, on the use of medroxyprogesterone acetate (Depo-Provera®, Upjohn) in the treatment of sex-offenders. These studies, at Johns Hopkins Hospital, The University of Texas, and now in San Francisco have varied in the extent to which psychotherapies and behavioral assessment techniques, have also been used. Standards of assessment, diagnosis, prescription, and therapy administration have evolved and been modified in the light of experience and ethical concerns. Our experience leads us to believe that antiandrogenic medication, in carefully selected cases, is a valuable adjunct in the treatment of paraphiliac sex offenders.

HISTORY OF ANTIANDROGEN USAGE

Freund (1980) credits Foote (1944) with the first use of an antiandrogenic medication to reduce "sex drive." Foote, and others subsequently used estrogens which may cause unwanted side effects such as gynecomastia. Laschet and Laschet (1975) have written extensively on their experience in Europe using Cyproterone Acetate (Androcur) as an anti-libido medication. Money (1968) described the first case of deviant sexual arousal treated with medroxyprogesterone acetate (MPA). Various reports have followed describing the treatment program at Johns Hopkins Hospital (Money, 1970 and 1972; Money, Wiedeking, Walker and Gain, 1976; Money, Wiedeking, Walker, Migeon, Meyer, and Borgaonkar, 1975; Wiedeking, Money and Walker, 1979; Rivarola, Camacho and Migeon, 1968; Money and Bennett, 1981; Berlin and Meinecke, 1981; Blumer and Migeon, 1975, and Spodak, Falck, and Rappeport, 1978). Walker, 1977, 1978, and 1980; Walker and Meyer, 1981; Meyer, Walker, Wiedeking, et al. 1977; and Meyer, Furlanetto and Walker, 1980; and Meyer, Furlanetto, and Walker, 1982 have reported on the treatment program at The University of Texas. Other authors too have presented data on the effects of MPA on sex offending behavior (Gagné, 1981; Barry and Giccone, 1975; Pinta, 1978; Langevin, Paitich, Hucker, et al., 1979).

However, no large-sample double-blind placebo studies have been conducted, for reasons discussed below. Therefore, the clinical use of this medication for the control of deviant sexual behavior remains investigative.

ANTIANDROGENIC TREATMENT OF AGGRESSIVITY AND DEVIANT SEXUALITY

Blumer and Migeon (1975) in one of the earlier reports on MPA were optimistic regarding its clinical use in controlling aggressive or anti-social behavior. Their patients suffered from both sexual and non-sexual conditions including: temporal lobe epilepsy with "rage reactions" and 47,XYY chromosome males with aggressive impulse control deficits. However, later follow-up studies (Wiedeking, Money and Walker, 1979) questioned the therapeutic success in treating the latter group. Furthermore, Walker and Meyer (1981) reported that MPA treated sex offenders in their sample did not include "violent" sex offenders of the type who deny the sexual aspects of their crime (usually rape) nor those who use gratuitous force and violence.

The accumulated evidence indicates that non-sexual violent offenders, or sexual offenders who use gratuitious violence or who commit "sexual" crimes in which the principal apparent motives are pathological experiences of "power" or "anger" (Groth and Burgess, 1977; Groth, Burgess and Holmstrom, 1977) are not amenable to MPA therapy.

Pedophilia and exhibitionism have been the main paraphilias treated with MPA. However, Gagné (1981) reported its use in 3 rapists and Walker (1980) reported on 4 rapists. Other paraphilias which have been treated with MPA include erotic self mutilation, incest, rape murder, voyeurism, pedophilia with lust murder ideation, transvestism, excessively compulsive and physically injurious impulsive masturbation, frottage, zoophilia and erotic strangulation, and a case of factitious suicidal reaction to compulsive transvestism/masturbation

(Walker, 1980). Gagné (1981) treated 1 case of "indecent assault" and 1 case of "confused sexual orientation." All these varieties of paraphilia seem to respond similarly to MPA.

SEX OFFENDERS: PATIENT SELF SELECTION

Walker (1980) reported on the issue of patient self selection for MPA treatment. Ethical considerations of informed consent, the logistics of clinical out-patient case management, the complex reasons why some sex offenders get caught (perhaps as few as 2%) and others do not, and why some arrested sex offenders are referred for therapy evaluation and others are not, and why some agree to therapy and others do not, and why some non-arrested sex offenders volunteer for therapy and others do not, all combine to produce a highly filtered self-selected sample treated with MPA.

Walker (1980) has reported on 80 "sex offenders" referred to him at The Gender Clinic of The University of Texas Medical Branch, Galveston, over a 4-year period, for evaluation. All subjects either admitted their illegal sexual behavior or had so much evidence against them that the clinician's opinion was that they were "guilty as charged." Cases in which no admission was made, and reasonable doubt about guilt existed were excluded (see Table 1).

Of 80 men evaluated and regarded as guilty by Walker, only 25 (31.3%) became part of his MPA-treated sample. His research results on the use of MPA cannot therefore be applied to all sex offenders.

Walker and Meyer (1981) differentiated four types of sex offenders: *Type 1 (Denial)* deny their crime totally, or they deny the criminal nature of their crime (i.e. they claim that the rape was consensual, or the pedophilia was initiated by the pre-pubertal child). Such men are obviously not amenable to voluntary participation in MPA therapy, or indeed any out-patient therapy. *Type 2 (Disinhibited)*-confess to their crime but blame their behavior totally on non-sexual and non-personal forces such as alcohol, drugs, or job stress. Neither MPA nor sex therapy is usually feasible with this group. *Type 3 (Violent)*-claim or appear to be motivated primarily by some non-sexual gain (e.g. anger, or power). They do not usually receive MPA therapy. *Type 4 (Paraphiliac)*-these males are characterized by a pattern of sexual arousal in which the fantasy or the actuality of a specific deviation accompanies nearly every erection and ejaculation. For example, the fantasy of rape, or voyeurism, is necessary for erection and ejaculation, whether the erection is associated with acting out the behavior in reality, or for masturbatory fantasies, nocturnal emissions, or with a consenting adult partner. For the true paraphiliac, the deviation is released or re-enacted every time there is an ejaculation. This pattern usually dates back to puberty, and has been rehearsed in fantasy with orgasmic reinforcement many thousands of times.

Table 1. Sample and Treatment Description
Sex Offender Program 1976–1980
(The Gender Clinic, University of Texas Medical Branch, Galveston)

N evaluated	80
N who denied illegal behavior and refused any and all therapies	16 (20.0%)
N who admitted some illegal behavior but who refused any and all therapies	13 (16.3%)
N who admitted some sexual problem, MPA not recommended, minimal psychotherapy received	10 (12.5%)
N who admitted to paraphiliac sexual pattern, MPA recommended and refused, minimal psychotherapy received	15 (18.8%)
N who admitted to paraphiliac sexual pattern, volunteered for MPA therapy, and then discovered to be presenting a factitious complaint i.e., falsely claiming a sexual deviation (1 received MPA)	2 (2.5%)
N who admitted to paraphiliac sexual pattern and who received MPA	25 (31.3%)

(Itemized N = 81 as 1 factitious presenter received MPA; one injection only.)

A few paraphiliacs deny this pattern, claiming deviant fantasies only occasionally. Such men, however, report that they have no other sexual fantasies at all: they masturbate and engage in non-deviant sexual activity without visual fantasies. They report instead, when questioned in detail, that they are aware only of tactile stimulation. It is difficult to be certain whether or not these men are in fact devoid of visual fantasies, or whether they are denying or repressing such fantasies. However, these partial-type 4 paraphiliacs usually do report, at least occasional deviant visual fantasies. Because of their prominence, the fantasies accompanying sexual arousal are a primary clinical feature for diagnosis and monitoring progress. The present authors believe that only the full or partial Type 4 paraphiliacs are amenable to MPA therapy. In fact, it is this group, primarily, which has been treated at most centers.

BEHAVIORAL SUB-GROUPS OF THE TYPE 4 PARAPHILIAC

Only some type 4 paraphiliacs express appropriate remorse and feelings of guilt for their behavior. Moreover, only some have insight into the negative consequences their behavior causes them and their victims and only some are motivated to stop their behavior. Of those who are not motivated to change, some were never motivated, others have lost their motivation because of repeated failure of therapy. All of these factors, while not yet systematically studied, affect voluntary acceptance of MPA therapy, and, probably, affect the likelihood of both completion and success of treatment (i.e. therapeutic dropout as discussed below).

Some paraphiliacs reveal what Walker and Meyer (1981) termed "emitted" versus "elicited" deviation: they become conscious of a yearning for "acting out" their deviation (whether ego-syntonic or ego-dystonic) and then spend sometimes hours looking for an opportunity for commission. These men *emit* deviant arousal. Others report being totally unaware of a deviant "need" until they find themselves in a situation which *elicits* or facilitates or triggers the impulse: they suddenly find themselves in the presence of a woman, or child, or bedroom window which they have not actively sought out. The success of the psychotherapies which accompany MPA therapy is probably affected by this variable of elicited versus emitted deviation, but has not yet been systematically studied.

BEHAVIORAL ASSESSMENT OF MULTIPLE DEVIATIONS

Careful clinical histories usually uncover only one paraphiliac pattern in any one offender: e.g., rapists of adult women rarely report fantasies of pedophilia or exhibitionism. Penile plethysmography (Freund, Chan and Coulthard, 1979; Abel and Blanchard, 1976), with standardized visual and/or auditory stimuli, is a useful technique for obtaining objective assessment of sexual arousal patterns to various deviant stimuli. By measuring the percent or absolute volume of erection to such stimuli, one can objectively diagnose arousability. It is also possible to monitor the effectiveness of therapy in reducing arousal to deviant stimuli and of increasing arousal to "acceptable" stimuli.

Penile plethysmography can also confirm, in some cases, what is denied in the clinical interview, i.e., arousability to more than one type of deviant stimulus. Often the patient is unaware of sexual arousal by more than one type of stimulus, and he may honestly report acting-out in response to only one stimulus.

Walker has concluded that clinical work with the paraphiliac must be accompanied by penile plethysmography. Therapeutic attempts to control and eliminate one form of deviation may leave a latent deviation unaffected. The latent deviation may then emerge and be substituted for the deviation eliminated by therapy (Brownell, Hayes and Barlow, 1977). For example, four of the patients treated at the author's Texas clinic who had received psychotherapy for a presenting paraphilia subsequently went on to different and more dangerous paraphilias. One exhibitionist became a rapist after covert sensitization was used to rid him of exhibitionistic fantasies. A voyeur, treated elsewhere, after dynamic-insight-oriented therapy, became an exhibitionist: after this was treated with electric shock aversion therapy, he engaged in pedophilic activity. Prison interrupted his career as a pedophiliac and gave him 5 years to rehearse a new masturbatory fantasy. The potential witnesses to his fantasized pedophilia (his victim children) were slain and dismembered to prevent their giving evidence against him in the future. When released from prison the voyeur-exhibitionist-pedophile was, in his erotic fantasy life, and potentially in reality, a pedophiliac lust murderer. The act of murdering his victims had become eroticized in prison, i.e., the fantasies produced erections. Such potential for multiple deviations must be diagnosed in advance of any form of therapy lest the therapy produce or release a new and more dangerous form of behavior. Penile plethysmography is the best means of diagnosing the potential for multiple deviations.

MPA THERAPY

Rationale and Goals

MPA administered intramuscularly diminishes testicular testosterone production. Sexual arousability in males, believed by many to be mediated or at least facilitated by testosterone, might then be expected to diminish. However, it has not yet been clearly shown (Walker and Meyer, 1981) whether the effect of MPA on sexual arousal is due to its effect on testosterone, or to a direct central nervous system effect (i.e. behavior change correlates most strongly with MPA levels, not with testosterone levels). Intravenous progesterone can be an anesthetic (Merryman, Boiman, Barnes, and Rothchild, 1954), but the biological mechanism by which MPA is effective in the control of deviant sexual arousal is unknown. The claim that MPA, which is a synthetic progesterone, is effective in treating paraphilia, in no way supports a belief that biological factors cause deviant sexual behavior as psychogenic disorders can be treated biologically.

MPA, in the initial Hopkins' studies, produced a near total suppression of emitted sexual arousal in treated patients. In these studies, little or no psychotherapy, other than infrequent crisis-intervention counselling, was given to patients receiving MPA. Placebo effects are possible, and have not been examined systematically. However, over the years, the present author has observed several men alternate, in a double-blind manner, between high and low MPA dosages. Their level of sexual arousability was correlated with the dosages. Such observations, while they suggest that placebo effects are minimal, are not a substitute for a controlled multiple dosage level study.

Blumer and Migeon (1975) reported that sexual arousability diminished within 2 weeks of MPA therapy onset. Gagné (1981) reported favorable response in 40 of his 48 patients within 10 days to 3 weeks. Walker (1980) has observed positive responses within 7-10 days of the first injection of MPA. In some patients the effect was immediate.

The goals of MPA therapy are multiple. The primary behavioral effect (i.e. cessation of unwanted sexual acting-out) is extremely rapid; especially so when compared with the efficacy of psychotherapy alone. Many clinical advantages ensue:

1. Patients become optimistic and hopeful that indeed control of their paraphilia is possible. Many were previously extremely pessimistic and hopeless: they did not think anything could help.

2. Victims are not being harmed while therapy proceeds.

3. As a result of 2., behaviors such as rape and pedophilia are treatable on an outpatient basis, which is less costly than inpatient treatment or incarceration.

4. Issues concerning a clinician's duty to violate confidentiality (child abuse reporting laws, Tarasoff, etc.) become less problematic since the illegal behavior stops early.

5. Concurrent psychotherapies may proceed without the patient having to deal with the discouraging problem of weekly or even daily recidivism causing him to ignore the small gains of weekly psychotherapy.

6. Clinicians are encouraged by the rapid and apparent success of treatment compared to more traditional therapies where effects are less certain.

Usual Treatment Protocol

Walker and Meyer (1981) describe a program in which patients begin therapy with weekly IM injections of 400-500 mg. Gagné (1981) used initial doses of 400-600 mg IM weekly. Such doses rapidly bring circulating testosterone values down to prepubertal male levels. Gagné (1981) used a rather complicated dosage schedule in which the objective was to maintain plasma testosterone at a level lower than 250 ng/100 ml using a minimal dose of MPA. Walker and Meyer (1981) maintain the initial 400-500 mg MPA dose for 6 months. They then lower the dose by 50-100 mg every 2-3 months to zero, or until the patient asks to stop treatment or until unwanted deviant behavior reappears. In the latter case, assuming patient permission, the dosage is maintained at the minimally effective dose for adequate behavior control. Gagné (1981) and Berlin (personal communication) initiate treatment on an inpatient basis for 2-4 weeks. They claim various positive clinical effects. The present author has only rarely initiated treatment on an in-patient basis and then for a few unusually dangerous patients. Where possible, such initial in-patient treatment is probably beneficial in establishing long-term patient/therapist trust and collaboration. Drop-out rates (Walker and Meyer, 1981; Walker, 1980) appear to be higher without that initial in-patient experience.

Walker (1980) reported that 4 of 16 patients were expected to continue indefinitely at high MPA doses as any attempt to lower the dosage resulted, in each case, in a return of unwanted behavior, in spite of concurrent psychotherapies. Thus, therapy protocols, initially different from study to study, are modified within each study on a patient-by-patient basis. Cross study comparisons are thus impossible. A further confusion is due to the fact that the Hopkins and Texas programs used IM MPA while the Canadian studies most often used oral MPA.

RESULTS OF MPA THERAPY

Drop-Outs. Many patients drop out of treatment: 5 of 25 of Walker's (1980) patients, 5 of 48 of Gagné's (1980), 11 of 20 Hopkins' patients (Berlin, 1981), 9 out of 20 (Money and Bennett, 1981), 6 of 23 (Money, Wiedeking, Walker, et al., 1975). Langevin et al. (1979) lost 5 out of 5! Most drop-outs, in every study, leave because they prematurely pronounce themselves cured and no longer in need of therapy. They rarely express dissatisfaction with treatment itself. The psychological make-up of those who drop out is open to speculation. Volunteers usually drop out less often than court or police referred cases.

Footnote: The various reports out of Johns Hopkins, i.e., Blumer and Migeon, 1975; the various reports by Money et al., 1968 to 1981; Spodak, Falck and Rappeport, 1978; and Berlin and Meinecke, 1981; are based on overlapping samples and therefore cannot be combined. Thus the most recent (1981) Hopkins reports by Berlin and Meinecke and Money and Bennett are usually cited in the present paper as representing the Hopkins experience. Similarly, later papers by Walker, and Walker and Meyer, duplicate and expand upon earlier ones.

Behavioral Success on Therapy

Drop-outs excluded, MPA appears highly effective. Walker (1980) reported only 1 patient out of 21 acting out while on therapy. His acting out rate was .25% of the pre-therapy rate, i.e. 2 incidents in 4 years of therapy compared to 3-5 incidents per week pre-therapy. The relapses were related to alcohol abuse. Berlin and Meinecke (1981) and Money and Bennett (1981) reported that only 3 of 20 treated men relapsed while on MPA. Gagné (1981) reported observing only favorable changes and did not report relapses on therapy. However, he noted that 7 men (out of 48 treated) had no favorable response. These 7 all had what he termed "antisocial personalities," (perhaps similar to Walker and

Meyer's Type 3 Violent). Gagné (1981) and Money and Bennet (1981) also report alcohol as a contributing factor to relapse in treated patients.

The above data suggest that MPA is extremely effective in producing near total control of unwanted deviant sexual behavior under the following conditions: 1) The patient volunteers for treatment; 2) lack of concomitant anti-social personality pathology; 3) lack of severe substance abuse; and 4) MPA dosages high enough to suppress testosterone to pre-pubertal male levels; and 5) the availability of a consenting pair-bonded partner (Money and Bennett, 1981). Although no controlled comparative studies have been conducted, it is apparent that MPA is considerably more effective than psychotherapy alone, and even more effective than surgical castration (Heim and Hirsch, 1979).

Sexual Function on Therapy

Various papers claim that patients are "impotent" on therapy or they "can not" or "do not" erect and ejaculate while receiving MPA. This is totally untrue. While patients do not usually have spontaneous erections or ejaculations during treatment, they have no trouble doing so when someone (a researcher, or a consenting sex partner) asks them to do so. Only 1 of 25 patients treated by Walker, Meyer, and Emory could not masturbate to orgasm when asked to do so. All other patients reported only minimal diminution of consensual marital or love-relationship sexual activity. Their penises functioned adequately but the consenting partner or the researcher had to initiate the process. This is not impotence, it is erotic apathy. One exhibitionist currently being treated by Walker and Rubin has stopped exhibiting himself (his pre-therapy rate was 3-8 times per week), and his solitary masturbation (his pre-therapy rate, apart from exhibitionism episodes, was 3-5 times a week), but his consensual intercourse frequency has only diminished from 3-4 times a day to 1-2 times a day; occurring without difficulty upon his partner's initiation.

The above is of great clinical importance. Many men reject the offer of MPA therapy when mistakenly told it will totally deprive them of a sex life. On the other hand, some patients may be led to believe that they are totally "safe" on therapy because of the misconception of alleged "impotence." They can act out, and must be warned of this possibility. The fortuitous and accidental combination of alcohol, situational stress and anxiety, a private place, and the appearance of an unwilling, yet apparently "seductive" victim may, even though the patient is receiving MPA, elicit the paraphilic behavior. Wincze et al. (1982) treated 3 inpatient pedophiles with an A-B, MPA-placebo, protocol. While they report reduction in nocturnal penile tumescence, erection in response to highly erotic visual stimuli is not completely extinguished. However, they do not discount a possible placebo effect. There are verbal reports that paraphilic fantasies diminish while subjects are on placebo.

Physiological Functioning and Side Effects

Walker and Meyer (1981) in their review of published and unpublished data listed the following physiological effects of MPA: 1) no change in blood pressure; 2) no change in blood biochemistry; 3) weight gain while frequently reported, occurred in less than 50% of their own subjects; 4) sperm counts dramatically decreased on therapy and returned to normal within 6–12 months post-therapy (4 of 25 Texas patients, while on MPA, impregnated their wives); 5) all patients, while on MPA, had normal basal insulin levels but also a hyper-insulinaemic response to a glucose load; 6) some attention is warranted regarding possible irregular gallbladder function and possible diverticulitis while on long term MPA therapy; 7) fatigue and/or lethargy was not frequent; 8) the testicular atrophy which occurs is reversible on stopping the drug; 9) increased levels of Somatomedin-C (Meyer, Furlanetto and Walker, 1982); 10) one case of worsening of migraine headaches, and 11) one case of diabetes mellitus; 12) no breast changes have been observed. The worsening of headaches is a known side effect of all progestational agents and diabetes and abnormal glucose tolerance tests have been repeatedly reported in women taking MPA for contraception.

Other investigators have added their observations to the list of MPA side effects; Gagné (1981) mentions fatigue, weight gain, hot and cold flashes, phlebitis, headaches, insomnia, and nausea. Berlin and Meinecke (1981) add nightmares, dyspnea, hyperglycemia, and leg cramps to the list; Baker and Lomis (1980) mention loss of body hair and increased basal body temperature.

Anytime a drug is used for a new purpose, *any* possible side effects should be noted. However, the systematic studies of Walker and Meyer (1981) and Meyer and Walker (in preparation) indicate that the side effects mentioned by other investigators are extremely rare. Yet it is premature and inaccurate to state, as Gagné (1981) has done, that there are no irreversible side effects. Careful long term physiological testing is warranted, especially in cases of high-dosage long-term MPA therapy.

Post-Therapy Sexual Behavior

Long-term, post-MPA therapy behavior change has not been adequately studied. Most reports have been published during the course of the research. Therefore, of the total treatment sample reported upon in any one paper, most patients are still in therapy. Most of those no longer in therapy are considered drop-outs. Some patients who complete therapy volunteer for a resumption of therapy months or years after the first therapy regime. They volunteer when they feel they are in danger of relapse; Walker, Meyer and Emory, have 2 patients, each of whom they have treated 3 times. Others never leave therapy as relapse appears inevitable when the dosage is even slightly lowered, much less stopped.

Berlin and Meinecke (1981) and Money and Bennet (1981) each reported on 20 patients. Nine were considered drop-outs, 8 of whom relapsed. Seven are still in treatment with no relapses. Four were released from treatment, 2 relapsed within one year after treatment and only one is relapse-free after one year. Walker and Meyer (Walker, 1980) reported on 25 men treated with MPA. One had no sexual paraphilia (he presented a factitious complaint); 4 were just beginning MPA therapy when the project data were analyzed; 2 disappeared while on MPA, having skipped bail; 4 are still receiving MPA with only 1 relapse (discussed above); 1 was stopped for medical reasons (severe headaches); 5 dropped out AMA and 8 completed therapy. Of the 8 who finished therapy, one was in jail on therapy and thus is not in a position to re-offend, 3 were not available for follow-up and thus contribute no data; 3 are relapse free after 12–26 months; 1 is in jail having relapsed 6 months after MPA (concurrent with the development of a severe, and hidden, problem of marijuana abuse).

The Hopkins experience (Berlin and Meinecke, 1981; and Money and Bennett, 1981), from 1969–81 produced only 1 patient who is 1 year or more post-treatment and relapse free. The Texas program (Walker, 1980) started with 80 offenders, 25 of whom were treated. Of these, four were released from treatment, and 3 are still relapse free for over 1 year. Gagné (1981) treated 48 men between 1974–1980 and no detailed description of post-therapy long term follow-up was presented. Follow-up periods of only 6 months or 1 year are totally inadequate (Soothill and Gibbens, 1978).

The present authors must conclude that no long-term benefit of MPA therapy alone has been shown after MPA is stopped. However, it must be emphasized that patients and society are relatively safe during MPA therapy.

Concomitant Psychotherapy

Almost all published papers claim that concomitant psychotherapy or "counselling" was given during MPA therapy. These psychotherapies are rarely described. It is likely that psychotherapy was in fact minimal in all studies reported.

Walker (1980) advocates multiple, intensive therapies concomitant with MPA treatment. They include: rational-emotive therapy, sex therapy, sex education, family therapy, couple therapy, and bibliotherapy. In particular he favors the cognitive behavioral therapies such as orgasmic reconditioning and covert sensitization (Cautela and Wisocki, 1971), relapse rehearsal (Marlatt, 1979), and verbal satiation (Laws and Osborn, 1983). The data on psychotherapy together with MPA treatment have not been collected but it is probable they will reveal a long-term success rate at least as high as psychotherapy alone.

Thus MPA is the initial treatment of choice for severe paraphiliacs, but it should be accompanied by other psychotherapies.

ETHICAL CONSIDERATIONS

There are many ethical problems in treating paraphiliacs; especially with MPA. Clinicians must consider the needs of the patient, of the patient's potential victims, and of society. The goals of research vs therapy can become confused and the issue of informed consent, common to nearly everyone in the helping professions, is especially salient in the case of the sex offender.

Outpatient paraphiliacs, who voluntarily present themselves for therapy, must be advised of the limitations to doctor-patient confidentiality, consequent upon child abuse reporting laws, the Tarasoff case etc. These laws, when explained to the patients who had assumed the existence of absolute confidentiality, often cause them to leave or to edit what they say to the clinician. This may limit the data received during the diagnostic assessment and may severely limit the possible benefits of psychotherapy, which requires trust. To refuse paraphiliacs therapy, or to give them placebo therapy, allows the possibility that they may be at continued risk of further acting-out. Furthermore, they run the risk of arrest, and the expense and stigma of a court defense. There is also the danger that delaying treatment may increase the toll of victims. The clinician has an ethical responsibility to potential victims, not just to the presenting patient, and refusing treatment violates this responsibility.

On theoretical grounds, there is a risk of serious side effects to long-term MPA use. Although side effects reported up to the time of writing are not grave, a risk-benefit question remains. While risk studies continue in our research, and that of others, further work is needed in weighing benefit against harm. Therefore, rigidly controlled double blind placebo studies are indicated in samples of in-patient offenders (Wincze et al., 1982) or on outpatient offenders (other than rapists or pedophiles) whose behavior is relatively benign and non-harmful to society.

Because it has been documented (see earlier) that paraphiliacs may have a potential for multiple deviations, and because treatment of one parahilia may release another paraphilia, there is an ethical obligation to test for multiple deviations. All deviations that are found should be specifically treated, lest treatment of the presenting paraphilia alone increase the patient's dangerousness. It then follows that such an effect will increase the chances that future victims may face a worse kind of paraphiliac assault than they would have faced had the paraphiliac never been treated in the first place.

Because existing data are insufficient to justify a promise of long-term effects of MPA, MPA must ethically be used only when accompanied by psychotherapies documented as relevant and effective for the treatment of paraphilia (i.e., behavioral and cognitive behavioral therapies). Providing MPA alone only delays the next assault until the drug is no longer taken.

Because some paraphiliacs receiving MPA drop-out and almost always relapse, patients must be warned that the desire to end therapy is, on statistical grounds, itself a sign of imminent relapse. From the strictly legal viewpoint, patients must be allowed to end therapy if it is voluntary. But some degree of therapist resistance to a patient's desire to stop MPA is warranted. How far the therapist can resist, without entering into duress, is highly problematic.

Medical risks, as they are now known and/or suspected, must be explained to prospective patients if their consent is to be informed. Telling them that there are no irreversible nor long-term negative effects, before such claims have been documented, is unethical. The legal risks to themselves, and the psychological risks to their future victims are well documented.

Halleck (1981) raised the question of the potential misuse of MPA, and other drugs, as a tool for social oppression or of politically motivated behavior control. However, anything, including aspirin and thermometers, can be misused. Anytime a patient's goals match society's goals, it is not always possible to distinguish which of these goals are of prime concern. Halleck hints that we should not use techniques that can be misused.

Sex offenders (all rapists and some assaultive pedophiles) cause great harm to themselves, by risking jail, as well as to others. The harm to others caused by exhibitionists and voyeurs is minimal or absent (Gittelson, Encott, and Mehta, 1978). Alternative therapies to MPA should be considered and tried first with all but rapists and some pedophiles; for the latter, MPA is probably the treatment of first choice. However, MPA should not be denied to the volunteer exhibitionist or voyeur should he so elect after having the risks, and alternative therapies, explained. The victim of an exhibitionist and/or voyeur can in some instances assume attempted rape and be traumatized.

Gagné's (1981) use of MPA in a patient described as being "confused about preferred sexual orientation" (presumably similar to ego-dystonic homosexuality) is problematic. So was Walker's (1980) treatment of a compulsive masturbator. That patient was causing severe tissue damage to his penis, and was imminently suicidal because of the guilt regarding his behavior. MPA was used. Ego-dystonic homosexuality, judging from the furor (e.g., Walker, 1980) being raised by many against the Masters and Johnson (1979) "conversion" program, and similar programs, in the absence of documented and immediate harm to self or others, most probably does not warrant the risks of MPA treatment.

MPA therapy is most often ethically scrutinized and attacked in the context of a prisoner's, or parolee's, or probationer's, or criminally accused person's request for therapy. Some (Halleck, 1981) question whether such people can freely choose a therapy with unknown long-term effects (*as if* other pharmacologic or non-pharmacologic therapies have *all* of their long-term effects known!). When a court puts a man in a position of choosing between prison and a therapy acceptable to the court as probably highly effective, we may answer the prisoner's request for MPA affirmatively only to be accused sometimes of serving as an agent of the state. If we refuse his request (on the grounds of preserving his free will) because we have decided as a profession that people under legal duress cannot, de facto, make a free choice, are we really serving his needs, as he expresses them? The current critics, like Halleck, and some university and hospital institutional review boards, require that in the name of ethical concern over our patient's free will we should condemn these men to have prison as their only choice. That is not choice. The issue is complex and should not be avoided by simply and cavalierly ruling that prisoners must be able to choose. By their very status they can't choose, so must we take the choice of MPA away from them so that they can "freely" choose between the alternatives of prison and prison?

Paraphiliacs, left alone, rarely choose to change. They like what they are doing and they are having fun. Since many, or most, of them are insensitive to the harm they may be causing others, they only ask for therapy because of actual or feared legal duress. Society has already decided to intrude the threat of prison into the paraphiliac's decision making process. The paraphiliac must be given the choice of receiving therapy as an alternative to prison, if there is to be any sense of choice. The choice not to take MPA or any other therapy should not be punished by extended prison time. However, the paraphiliac might be rewarded for choosing MPA or other therapies by a reduction or elimination of otherwise certain prison time. If indeed therapy is his choice, how is that not in his best interest?

ACKNOWLEDGMENT

This study was supported in part by grants from The Upjohn Co. and The Hogg Foundation for Mental Health and by the Clinical Research Center at the University of Texas Medical Branch, and by Grant RR-73 from General Clinical Research Center Program, the Division of Research Resources, National Institute of Health. Serium MPA levels determined courtesy of The Upjohn Company.

REFERENCES

Abel, G.G. and Blanchard, E.B. (1976). The measurement and generation of sexual arousal. In: Hersen, M., Eisler, R.M. and Miller, P.M., (eds.), *Progress in Behavior Modification, V2*. New York: Academic Press.

Baker, L.L. and Lomis, M.J. (1980). Medroxyprogesterone acetate in the treatment of sex offenders: A review of the literature. Offprint from the St. Thomas Psychiatric Hospital, St. Thomas, Ontario.

Barry, D.J. and Ciccone, J.R. (1975). Use of Depo-Provera in the treatment of aggressive sexual offenders: Preliminary report of three cases. *Bull. Am. Acad. Psychiatry and the Law* 3:179–184.

Berlin, F.S. and Meinecke, C.F. (1981). Treatment of sex offenders with antiandrogenic medication: Conceptualization, review of treatment modalities, and preliminary findings. *Am. J. of Psychiatry* 138:5, 601–607.

Blumer, D. and Migeon, C. (1975). Hormone and hormonal agents in the treatment of aggression. *J. Nerv. and Ment. Dis.* 160:2, 127–137.

Brownell, K., Hayes, S. and Barlow, D. (1977). Patterns of appropriate and deviant sexual arousal: The behavioral treatment of multiple sexual deviations. *J. Consult. and Clin. Psychology* 45:1144–1155.

Cautela, J. and Wisocki, P. (1971). Covert sensitization for the treatment of sexual deviation. *Psychological Record* 21:37–48.

Foote, R.M. (1944). Diethylstilbestrol in the management of psychopathological states in males. *J. Nerv. and Ment. Dis.* 99:928–935.

Freund, K., Chan, S. and Coulthard, R. (1979). Phallometric diagnosis with "nonadmitters." *Behav. Res. and Ther.* 17:451–457.

Freund, K. (1980). Therapeutic sex drive reduction. *Acta Psychiatrica Scand. Supple.* 62:1–38.

Gagné, P. (1981). Treatment of sex offenders with medroxyprogesterone acetate. *Am. J. Psychiatry* 138:5, 644–646.

Gittleson, N.L., Eacott, S.E. and Mehta, B.M. (1978). Victims of indecent exposure. *Br. J. Psychiatry* 132:61–66.

Groth, A.N. and Burgess, A. (1977). Sexual dysfunction during rape. *N. Eng. J. Med.* 297:764–766.

Groth, A.N., Burgess, A. and Holmstrom, L. (1977). Rape: Power, anger, and sexuality. *Am. J. Psychiatry* 134:1239–1243.

Halleck, S.L. (1981). Editorial: The ethics of antiandrogen therapy. *Am. J. Psychiatry* 138:5, 642–643.

Heim, N. and Hursch, C.J. (1979). Castration for sex offenders: Treatment or punishment? A review and critique of recent European literature. *Arch. Sex. Behav.* 8:3, 281–304.

Laschet, U. and Laschet, L. (1975). Antiandrogens in the treatment of sexual deviations of men. *J. Ster. Biochem.* 6:821–826.

Langevin, R., Paitich, D., Hucker, S., et al. (1979). The effect of assertiveness training, Provera and sex of therapist in the treatment of genital exhibitionism. *J. Behav. Ther. and Exper. Psychiatry* 10:275–282.

Laws, D.R. and Osborn, C.A. (1983). Setting up shop: How to build and operate a laboratory for the assessment and treatment of sexual deviance. In: Greer, J.G. and Stuart, I., eds., *The Sexual Aggressor: Current Perspectives on Treatment.* New York: Van Nostrand and Reinhold Co., pp. 293–335.

Marlatt, G.A. (1979). Alcohol use and problem drinking: A cognitive-behavioral analysis. In: Kendall, P.C., and Hollon, S.D. (eds.), *Cognitive-Behavioral Interventions: Theory, Research, Procedures.* N.Y.: Academic Press, pp. 319–356.

Masters, W.H. and Johnson, V.E. (1979). Homosexuality in Perspective. Boston: Little, Brown and Company.

Merryman, W., Boiman, R., Barnes, L. and Rothchild, I. (1954). Progesterone "anesthesia" in human subjects. *J. Clin. Endocrin. and Metab.* 14:1567–1569.

Meyer, W.J., Walker, P.A., Wiedeking, C., et al. (1977). Pituitary function in adult males receiving medroxyprogesterone acetate. *Fertility Sterility* 28: 1072–1076.

Meyer, W.J., Furlanetto, R.W. and Walker, P.A. (1980). Medroxyprogesterone acetate (Depo-Provera) increases plasma radioassayable Somatomedin-C concentration. *Pediatric Research* 14:344.

Meyer, W.J., Furlanetto, R.W., and Walker, P.A. (1982). The effect of sex steroids on radioimmunoassayable plasma somatomedin-C concentrations. *J. Clin. Endorcrin. Metab.* 55:1184–1187.

Money, J. (1968). Discussion on hormonal inhibition of libido in male sex offenders. In, Michael, R. ed., *Endocrinology and Human Behavior.* London: Oxford University Press, p. 169.

Money, J. (1970). Use of an androgen depleting hormone in the treatment of male sex offenders. *J. Sex Res.* 6:165–172.

Money, J. (1972). The therapeutic use of androgen-depleting hormone. *Int. Psychiatry Clin.* 8:4, 165–174.

Money, J., Wiedeking, C., Walker, P.A., et al. (1975). 47, XYY and 46, XY males with antisocial and/or sex offending behavior: Antiandrogen therapy plus counseling. *Psychoneuroendocrinology* 1:165–178.

Money, J., Wiedeking, C., Walker, P.A. and Gain, D. (1976). Combined anti-androgenic and counseling program for treatment of 46, XY and 47, XYY sex offenders. In: Sachar, E., ed., *Hormones, Behavior and Psychopathology.* New York: Raven Press, pp. 105–120.

Money, J. and Bennett, R.G. (1981). Postadolescent paraphilic sex offenders: Antiandrogenic and counseling therapy follow-up. *Int. J. of Ment. Health* 10:122–133.

Pinta, E.R. (1978). Treatment of obsessive homosexual pedophilic fantasies with medroxy-progesterone acetate. *Biol. Psychiatry* 13:369–373.

Rivarola, M.A., Camancho, A.M. and Migeon, C.J. (1968). Effect of treatment with medroxyprogesterone acetate (Provera) on testicular function. *J. Clin. Endocrinol.* 28:679–684.

Soothill, K.L. and Gibbens, T.C.N. (1978). Recidivism of sexual offenders: A re-appraisal. *Br. J. Criminol.* 18:267–276.

Spodak, M.K., Falck, Z.A. and Rappeport, J.R. (1978). The hormonal treatment of paraphiliacs with Depo-Provera. *Criminal Justice Behavior* 5: 304–314.

Walker, P.A. (1977). Medroxyprogesterone acetate as an antiandrogen for the rehabilitation of sex offenders. In: Gemme, R. and Wheeler, C. (eds.), *Progress in Sexology.* New York: Plenum Press, pp. 205–207.

Walker, P.A. (1978). The role of antiandrogens in the treatment of sex offenders. In: Qualls, C.B., Wincze, J.P., and Barlow, D.H. (eds.), *The Prevention of Sexual Disorders: Issues and Approaches.* New York: Plenum Press, pp. 117–136.

Walker, P.A. (1980). Antiandrogen treatment of Paraphiliac sex offenders: Eleven years experience. Paper presented at The International Academy of Sex Research, Tucson, Arizona.

Walker, P.A. and Meyer, W.J. (1981). Medroxyprogesterone acetate treatment for paraphiliac sex offenders. In: Hays, J.R., Roberts, T.K., and Solway, K.S., (eds.), *Violence and the Violent Individual.* New York: S.P. Medical and Scientific Books, pp. 353–373.

Wiedeking, C., Money, J. and Walker, P.A. (1979). Follow-up of 11 XYY males with impulsive and/or sex-offending behavior. *Psychological Medicine* 9: 287–292.

Wincze, J.P., Bansal, S., Qualls, C.B. and Binkoff, J. (1982). A controlled investigation of the effects of medroxyprogesterone acetate on the physiological and subjective sexual arousal of male sex offenders. Paper presented at the International Academy of Sex Research meeting, Copenhagen.

32

Limitation and Alternatives to the Use of Drugs in Violent Patients

John Gunn

The practice of forensic psychiatry would be very difficult without the availability of modern medicines. However, medication is a very small part of the total management which can be offered to violent patients.

THE NATURE OF VIOLENCE

Violence is by no means necessarily symptomatic of psychological disturbance. It is a natural, normal part of all mammalian life. It probably serves a number of important biological and social functions. Paradoxically one of its main functions may well be to ensure that peace and order prevail for most of the time. However, whatever its functions there is no argument that violence occurs in a variety of circumstances and is only occasionally associated with psychiatric abnormality. Boys fighting in the street, soldiers going to war, boxers in the ring, robbers holding up a bank, street muggers may all be perfectly healthy individuals. Certainly violence may create a great deal of distress, especially for the victim, and certainly violence may be a symptom of distress in some individuals. When we are considering distress caused by violence or distress that leads to violence, for example, fighting that occurs all too frequently in homes when intense emotions get out of control, it is a matter of debate how far psychiatry, as opposed to other forms of assistance, should be brought in to alleviate the distress.

445

Two important factors need to be balanced in each case; the desire of any identified participant in a violent episode to receive psychiatric help, and the degree of psychological abnormality, perhaps psychiatric illness, which is present within the participant. This second factor is not simply a scientific or clinical issue, it contains within it an important ethical element because the pressure and temptation to intervene psychiatrically, especially with drugs, is quite considerable when violence has occurred and is likely to recur. Recently an English working party (Council for Science and Society, 1981) looked at exactly this problem and came to a firm conclusion that violence should not be dealt with by doctors, drugs, and other forms of medical treatment in a compulsory fashion unless the individual subject to the compulsion can be clearly shown to have a psychiatric disorder. Obviously this conclusion begs a lot of questions about the nature of psychiatric disorder and other matters involving the philosophy of responsibility, but it is an important principle from which to begin any argument. It is a principle which may lead a doctor to have to say to prison governors faced with rioting, violent disobedience, and the like "I'm sorry but I can't help you with any of these individuals unless they are either clearly mentally sick or they themselves wish me to tranquilize them."

As far as the patient who is violent is concerned, the principles are also fairly simply to enunciate although again may give rise to practical problems. The treatment of the violence in such cases is usually the treatment of the disorder from which the violent patient is suffering. Therefore a violent schizophrenic will be treated with all the measures which are available for schizophrenia, including psychotropic medication. A patient who, say, kills during a serious depression should be treated with all the measures available to relieve his melancholia, including ECT, antidepressants, lithium, and the like. However, in each case the type of drug, the dose of drug, will depend upon ordinary clinical factors as much as it will depend upon the severity of the violence.

Perhaps the most debatable issues arise in relation to the patients who suffer from so-called personality disorders. These may include patients who have recurrent rage attacks, patients who say they are easily provoked to violence, patients who are brought by others who say that this man or woman has a history of repeated violence. Much of the debate about the use of drugs in violence, particularly the compulsory use of drugs to control violent behavior is actually about this important group of people. It is probably preferable to ascertain in such individuals whether or not they are willing to take prescribed medicines. Exceptions may, of course, have to be made in dire emergencies where a patient, who is clearly disturbed and distressed within the context of a personality disorder, is likely to harm himself or other people unless immediate medication is given. Apart from that it is probably best not to treat patients with personality disorders against their wishes.

Of course such a clinical approach may condemn an individual to other, less palatable, methods of control. It may mean that he has to be discharged from hospital. It may mean that physical restraints applied by, say, prison officers or policemen, will have to be used. However it is arguable that a patient who is not ill and is able to understand all this when it is put to him is sufficiently responsible, even although he or she may have a personality disorder, to say "no, I don't want your drugs − I'll take my chance the other way." Of course it can also be argued that the threat of non-medical methods of control is sufficient to make some people in this position say "OK I'll have the drugs − it's the less of two evils facing me," and thus he or she is accepting treatment under duress.

It should not be forgotten though that most patients are under some form of duress, whether it is social or biological, and that must in reality be accepted. The important matters are distinguishing between those patients who are competent to make decisions about their treatment for themselves, and those patients who are not, and then allowing the patients who are competent the opportunity to refuse treatment in the knowledge of what may happen instead. The determination of competence is a huge subject which is not appropriate to tackle here, but which is an issue whenever a violent patient is treated psychiatrically whether that is by medication or by some other means.

BEHAVIORAL STRATEGIES

Withdrawal and Reduction of Drugs

In a violence clinic it is frequently necessary to withdraw a drug already prescribed by someone else, or reduce the dosage of a drug, or withdraw a drug taken by the patient without or against advice.

The drug of greatest importance in the study of human aggression is alcohol. There are numerous studies to indicate the association between the intake of alcohol and human violence (see Gunn, 1977 for further information), and many patients presenting for treatment at a violence clinic give clear histories of either persistent heavy drinking, or assaults related to episodic drinking. Why should this be so? Alcohol is a progressive sedative and the so-called higher functions concerned with social graces and inhibitions are among the first functions to be interfered with. It may be therefore that if we meet a frustration or an aggression provoking problem when we have taken a dose of alcohol we are more liable to resort to violence than when we are sober. Vogel-Sprott (1967) has for example found that under conflict subjects who have taken alcohol tend not to be bothered by the inhibitory effect of future punishment but they are just as stimulated by the prospects of reward.

Another important group of drugs which are associated with violence are the stimulants, especially amphetamines (Tinklenberg and Stillman, 1970). The mechanism in this case seems to be through the production of a paranoid psychosis (Allen et al., 1975). The drug intoxicated individual's aggression is a defensive response to frightening delusions.

Ellinwood (1971) examined the histories of 13 people who had committed suicide while intoxicated with amphetamines. In all cases the homicide was clearly related to an amphetamine induced delusional process and/or a state of emotional lability. The author described three fairly distinct phases leading to the violent act. First, a chronic abuse of amphetamines, then an acute change in the individual's state or emotional arousal, and finally a trigger factor which released an ouburst of violence. However, Ellinwood also noted that there were many other variables involved in each case. For example environmental conditions were thought to play a part in most of the killings.

While nothing seems to threaten the pre-eminence of alcohol as the sedative of choice for most of us, the second position in the league table is now held by the ubiquitous benzodiazepine. When they were first marketed, these drugs were sold to us as having particularly powerful tranquilizing properties, and pictures were shown of lions and monkeys tamed with chlordiazepoxide. As always, these advertising gimmicks have given way to a more measured appraisal and it is clear that these drugs have disadvantages even though they are useful as anticonvulsants, hypnotics, and minor tranquilizers. In recent years a number of cases have been reported in which severe aggression or violence appeared in an individual for the first time soon after they started to take one of the benzodiazepines; the so-called paradoxical rage reaction (Lion et al., 1975). In this context it may be of interest that some benzodiazepines are able to induce aggressiveness in mice and rats and Noble and her colleagues (1976) have shown that rheusus monkeys damaged by social isolation are made less shy and more socially aggressive by diazepam. Nevertheless these drugs, especially oxazepam, are useful sedatives in the violence clinic.

The main problem with this group of drugs is the way they are prescribed. People with severe social problems, marital problems, loneliness, and the like, are given these substances and nothing else, when their real needs, practical assistance, counselling, and so on, are ignored. The drug cannot solve the social and psychological problems and before long the patient has the problems plus benzodiazepine dependency, a disorder which is being increasingly recognized as of considerable significance in many patients (Petursson and Lader, 1982).

Finally under this heading of reducing drugs some personal clinical speculations. It's my impression that some psychotic patients prescribed depot psychotropics become less irritable and aggressive when the dose is reduced or the drug removed. I am also very impressed that flupenthixol is a particularly aggravating drug and, I now never use it in patients who have any history of aggression.

Counselling, Support and Environmental Manipulation

A common problem to present itself to the psychiatrist is fighting within the context of interpersonal emotional distress, particularly marital distress. Counselling and support are by no means areas where psychiatry has a monopoly, some would argue that it only has a marginal role. However, as before, it needs to be emphasized that marginal or not, simply prescribing a drug to sedate or calm is not sufficient to deal with the tangle of emotional problems which many people find themselves in. Even if it can be shown at some future date that, for example, the exhibition of a drug such as lithium is useful in lowering the threshold at which people are provoked into violent outbursts, such a pharmacological approach is a small part of the whole. If the violence is symptomatic of a failure of psychological mechanisms to cope in other ways, then simply lowering the threshold at which the violence breaks out may actually reinforce the psychological difficulties rather than alleviate them. Individual support, joint counselling, advice about separation, removal of children to safety all come under this umbrella.

Counselling and support are not, self evident simple remedies which all psychiatrists provide anyway. If carried out properly they are taxing, time-consuming, skilled enterprises. Psychiatrists often choose prescriptions rather than supportive psychotherapy because prescriptions are cheaper and easier. Proper controlled trials of supportive psychotherapy remain to be done and indeed they may be so complex as to be impossible, but for the moment I will argue that clinical experience strongly suggests that the time spent on supportive psychotherapy is not wasted provided the support is expertly handled. The skills involved include being able to accept unpleasant demanding individuals without necessarily accepting their unpleasant behavior; patience in the face of provocative behavior; availability, even outside formal clinic times; and commitment to a long period of treatment, perhaps lasting years.

It is also a fairly well-worn cliche that anybody running a violence clinic must be prepared to offer crisis intervention. For this to be more than an empty phrase there has to be close attention to the details of the patient's life. For full effectiveness, a team of workers is required with someone prepared to carry out domiciliary visits at short notice, someone to spend time dealing with employers, social security officers, and other key figures in the patient's life. It may be particularly important to admit a patient to hospital in an emergency.

These so-called simple and basic techniques lead me to consider the more formal psychotherapies. Matching type of psychotherapy to patient is, however, I believe of critical importance. The uninitiated can quickly run into dangerous transference problems or uncover psychoses. Careful assessment from a skilled psychotherapist is always, therefore, an important first step before embarking on a course of intensive verbal treatment. The options to be considered include traditional interpretative psychotherapy, client centered counselling, reality therapy, group psychotherapy, and directive psychotherapy. The usual emphasis in psychotherapy is on non-directive techniques, allowing the patient to air his thoughts and receive interpretations but giving him no direct advice. Many violent patients, however, are unsophisticated and impulsive and find such an approach irritating. Some of these respond well to a mildly authoritarian approach which includes direct answers to direct questions and an occasional "I think you should do the following . . ."

Others who do not respond well to an individual analytic approach gain support and insight from a group of similar people. Certainly such techniques are used with great success at Grendon prison and at Henderson hospital in England, both of which treat quite a number of violent men. There is some evidence from my own prison studies that group techniques are more effective than individual ones amongst recidivist prisoners (Gunn et al., 1978). However it has to be borne in mind that patients with personality problems are often particularly deficient in relating to groups of people. To plunge someone who is anxious of groups into the nerve wracking experience of a formal psychotherapy group may drive him from the clinic completely. Individual sessions and quasi-social groups may be important preliminaries.

Non-interpretive psychotherapies may also be useful for behavior disordered patients. *Reality therapy* (Glasser, 1975) is simply a treatment which lays a good deal of emphasis on confronting patients with their own responsibility for their behavior. The therapist refuses to accept "excuses" such as "illness" or "bad parental handling" and punishes "bad behavior" while rewarding good. Throughout however the patient is accepted as valued and lovable. *Client centered counselling* refers to the system developed by Rogers (1961), a system which he first developed when working with delinquent adolescents. He identifies the main elements of a helping relationship as (1) genuineness and transparency, in which the helper behaves naturally and does not disguise his real feelings, (2) warm acceptance of and respect for the client as a separate individual and (3) a sensitive ability to see the client's world and self-image as he sees them. Many violent patients have low self esteem and can only begin to control themselves if they feel valued. The therapeutic relationship may be the first in which they have ever experienced this. The therapist's warmth and regard, however, is for the individual rather than for his behavior.

The final psychological treatment I want to mention is *behavior therapy*, particularly in relation to sexual violence. Even in cases appropriate for anti-androgen drugs it does seem that behavioral therapy is required as well if anything other than simple temporary suppression is to be achieved. However there are few studies showing encouraging results for sexual difficulties and deviations which lead to violence. The techniques used include desensitization to anxiety provoking stimuli, simple advice about avoiding provocative situations, aversion to sadistic fantasies, reinforcement of normal fantasies, thought stopping, and discussion of detailed diaries. We have also tried these techniques, on a few patients, who are violent in a non-erotic manner even on a patient who committed arson. Here we have included techniques such as flooding with provocation stimuli and other forms of provocation within the clinic so that reactions can be studied and discussed. It would be nice to give a long list of convincing success stories, but the best that can be said is that some patients change a little by the use of these methods and some learn to control themselves better.

All the techniques mentioned so far can be applied in the outpatient clinic. However the more severe forms of violent behavior may lead to institutionalization of one sort or another. Offenders may be sent to prison as punishment for their violence; patients may be admitted to hospital for treatment. Prisoners are always, and hospital patients sometimes, detained against their own wishes. This compulsory detention may in itself precipitate or increase violent tendencies in some residents; resentment, frustration, anger, and power struggles all may precipitate fighting.

In this discussion it is possible to only touch briefly on the problems of violence in prisons. Nevertheless prisons cannot be ignored entirely, they do suffer a lot of violence, violence directed to the self, and violence directed to others, both inmates and staff. For example Sylvester and others (1977) found that the suicide rate in American prisons was twice as high as in the general population and Topp (1979) has suggested that it may be three times the rate in English prisons. Self-mutilation is also a major problem within most prison systems. In the Grendon prison study mentioned earlier, we observed that Grendon, which is a therapeutic community within the prison system and has frequent group meetings together with a good deal of group psychotherapy and a deliberate attempt to reduce staff prisoner barriers, is much more able to cope with the disruptive and violent prisoner than other places usually are (Gunn et al., 1978). In fact, in spite of the high referral rate of prisoners who are presenting violent problems in other prisons, fighting is almost unknown within Grendon. Perhaps the best known and most spectacular example of controlling violent prisoners by environmental management of this sort is the Barlinnie special unit in Glasgow, Scotland. Several men convicted of murder, who had been punished by every means known to the Scottish prison authorities, were in a state of total impasse having lost all their privileges, all ordinary prisoner rights, and were spending most of their time in solitary confinement and yet were increasingly hostile, unmanageable, and dangerous, attacking officers frequently. They were transferred to a small unit which had few restrictions, except its perimeter, a high staff ratio, and a regime based on a therapeutic community. Almost immediately the new regime had a civilizing effect, violence dropped to zero, and one of the most notable gangland murderers in Scotland became a sculptor and a writer (Boyle, 1977). As policy, psychotropic drugs are not used in either Grendon prison or the Barlinnie special unit.

Although hospitals and prisons are different in many ways, and the types of psychologically disturbed individuals which get admitted to each will be markedly different, some of the principles derived from the management of violence in prisons can be profitably transferred to the hospitals, especially hospitals which have a high ratio of compulsory patients. Therapeutic communities, good staff ratios, and intensive counselling for the especially distressed are all straightforward requirements in any program aimed at reducing violence in hospitals.

In Britain, 90% of all hospital patients are informal and can leave when they wish. This fact in itself makes a big contribution to the low level of violence which British psychiatric hospitals experience.

The predominant forms of violence in mental hospitals are the smashing of property and suicidal behavior. Nevertheless, in one London mental hospital in recent years two nurses have been murdered by patients. A Swedish study of 36 hospitals between 1955 and 1964 suggests that staff shortages increase the risks of aggressive behavior and warns against the mixing of young aggressive patients with the old and feeble. More recently in England, Fottrell (1980) made a study of violent behavior among patients in three mental hospitals, including the hospital which sustained the two murders mentioned above. In spite of the murders, the overall impression was that while incidents of petty violence are common, serious violence was rare. It was also of some interest that the district general hospital unit which caters mainly for acute cases had a violent incident rate nearly twice that of the mental hospital.

Folkard (1959) studied a fairly typical British mental hospital in the late 1950s and found that the younger female patients were responsible for most of the serious aggression. During a typical ten-week period in a female ward averaging 50 patients there were 298 aggressive incidents compared with 53 such incidents in a similar male ward. Aggression included everything from throwing property about to smashing objects such as windows and assaulting other people. An interesting experiment was carried out in that the door of a disturbed female ward was unlocked and this was followed by a reduction in the number of aggressive incidents. In his summary of his work, Folkard concluded that the lessening of restraints had a favorable effect on most patients, but not all. Some patients, especially those labelled "psychopathic," had to be secluded for lengthy periods. Nurses were faced with ambiguities in their role. He advocated ward team discussions, clear therapeutic goals, and a reasonably high tolerance of difficulties.

Effective management of a violent incident on a ward depends upon a number of factors. Architecture arrangements should be designed to minimize the possibility of a patient isolating another person so that the attacked individual cannot raise the alarm. It should always be possible for several staff to be on the scene of a violent incident within a minute or two of the alarm being given. Immediate attention should be given to freeing any victim and preventing any physical assault on another person; any weapons should be removed as rapidly as possible. Information about the aggressor is urgently required at the moment of crisis, for example, diagnosis, medication, medication sensitivities, provoking factors, and so on.

Fear and hurt underlie most angry outbursts; sometimes the patient is feeling humiliated and trying to regain self-esteem by attacking. Staff who know the patient and who are particularly non-provocative should aim to talk to the patient and reassure him that his distress has been properly noted and that nobody is deliberately going to hurt him. It is, therefore, especially important to avoid challenging or daring the patient. "You wouldn't dare hit me" is provocative; on the other hand predictions which are sympathetic and soothing may be helpful, e.g., "I understand how bad you feel and why you want to hit me" tells the patient that his message has been received, understood, and the violence is unnecessary. Often, however, physical restraint will be necessary and that may include compulsory sedation. Another option which should always be available in addition to or perhaps as an alternative to this medication, however, is seclusion. Of course the type of room in which a patient is secluded, the length of time they can be kept there, and the amount of surveillance required are all matters of ward policy.

Turning to ward policies it is important to note that a psychiatric ward or outpatient department which does not have a policy about violence is very vulnerable. Staff should have clear instructions about how to act in a violent emergency. Alarm systems should be available at strategic points, and some instruction should have been given in how to talk to an aggressive patient and in the safe and acceptable techniques of physical restraint. It should also be absolutely clear who will give the instructions during an incident. Democratic procedures must be suspended until calm is achieved. Clear policies about potential weapons are essential. Violent incidents are almost never lethal unless a weapon such as a gun or a knife is available. Which patients are allowed to use sharp implements in occupational therapy, how such sharp instruments are to be stored and who is responsible for them must be discussed. There should be a strict policy about control of personal possessions by patients which may be potential weapons such as knives and scissors.

Following any violent incident, however trivial, there should always be multidisciplinary clinical discussion. The purpose of this discussion is to analyze the reasons for the incident, perhaps make changes in the patient's management, perhaps propose changes in the ward policy, all in an attempt to prevent a recurrence and to defuse the anxiety engendered. The discussion should not include any recriminations or become part of any enquiry or disciplinary procedures.

At a clinical discussion staff should be able to express their feelings including guilt, fear, and anger. If a particular member of staff has erred or been at the center of several incidents this should be discussed frankly but with assistance being offered, either in the group or individually. It is vital that no scapegoats are made, and that it is well understood by all staff, senior and junior that some violence in a psychiatric unit is inevitable.

REFERENCES

Allen, R.P., Safer, D. and Covi, C. (1975). Effects of psychostimulants on aggression. *J. Nerv. and Ment. Dis.* 160:138–145.

Boyle, J. (1977). *A Sense of Freedom.* Pan Books: London.

Council for Science and Society (1981). *Treating the Troublesome.* CSS: London.

Ellinwood, E. (1971). Assault and homicide associated with amphetamine abuse. *Am. J. Psychiatry* 127:1170–1175.

Folkard, M.S. (1959). *A Sociological Contribution to the Understanding of Aggression and its Treatment.* Netherne Monograph No. 1, Coulsdon.

Fottrell, E. (1980). A study of violent behavior among patients in psychiatric hospitals. *Br. J. Psychiatry* 136:216–221.

Glasser, W. (1975). *Reality Therapy.* Harper: New York.

Gunn, J. (1977). Criminal behavior and mental disorder. *Br. J. Psychiatry* 130: 317–329.

Gunn, J., Robertson, G., Dell, S. and Way, C. (1978). *Psychiatric Aspects of Imprisonment.* Academic Press: London.

Lion, J.R., Azcarate, C.L. and Koepke, H.H. (1975). Paradoxical rage reactions during psychotropic medication. *Dis. Nerv. Syst.* 36:557–558.

Noble, A.D., McKinney, W.T., Mohr, C. and Moran, E. (1976). Diazepam treatment of socially isolated monkeys. *Am. J. Psychiatry* 133:1165–1170.

Petursson, H. and Lader, M.H. (1982). *Withdrawal from Tranquillisers* OUP: London (Maudsley Monograph).

Rogers, C.R. (1961). *On Becoming a Person.* Houghton Mifflin: Boston.

Sylvester, S.F., Reed, J.H. and Nelson, D.O. (1977). *Prison Homicide.* Spectrum: New York.

Tinklenberg, J.R. and Stillman, R.C. (1970). Drug use and violence. In: *Violence and the Struggle for Existence* (ed.) D.N. Daniels, M.F. Gilula and F.M. Ochberg, pp. 327–365. Little Brown and Co.: Boston.

Topp, D.O. (1979). Suicide in prison. *Br. J. Psychiatry* 134:24–27.

Vogel-Sprott (1967). Alcohol effects on human behavior under reward and punishment. *Psychopharmacologia* 11:337–344.

Index

tremor
(intention) with tricyclic use in the
aged, 21
with lithium treatment, 4, 5, 98,
110, 115
tricyclic antidepressant (see TCA)
trifluoperazine, 160, 162, 304, 342,
344, 348, 360, 362, 363, 386
trihexyphenidyl, 348
trimipramine (TCA), 85
trimopan (SCH 12679), 397, 402, 406
tryptamine, 79
tryptophan, combined with MAO
inhibitor, 3, 85
tyramine, 78, 79, 83, 86, 87, 299
hypertensive crisis, 78, 87
tyrosine hydroxylase, 263, 265

unipolar depression, 4, 13, 95, 96,
111
lithium therapy for, 13, 95, 96
urinary concentrating defect in long
term lithium treatment, 5

vegetative symptoms of depression
in children, 35
in geriatric population, 19, 20, 27
vegetative syndrome, 20, 28, 119, 331
ventricular arrhythmia in elderly, 23
ventricular function, 1
viral etiology of schizophrenia, 278,
279, 280, 281, 282, 283

violence
acute episode, 399, 400
and alcohol, 447
and stimulants, 448
clinic, 447, 449
in mental hospitals, 452, 453
in prisons, 451
the nature of, 445, 446
violent behavior, 390, 391, 396, 397,
399, 400, 401, 402, 405, 406,
446, 447, 451
assessment, 396
etiology, 400
long term lithium treatment, 345,
405, 406
pharmacotherapy of, 390, 396,
399, 400, 401, 402, 405, 406
psychotherapy, 406, 449, 450, 451
use of drugs for, 446
violent prisoners, environmental
management of, 450, 451, 452
voluntariness, in treatment of violent
behavior, 391, 446, 447
voyeurism, 392, 428, 429, 432, 439

Wilson's disease, dyskinesia related to,
186

zimeldine, 120, 129, 132
zoophilia, 392, 428